Lecture Notes in Medical Informatics

Edited by D. A. B. Lindberg and P. L. Reichertz

17

Biomedical Images and Computers

Selected Papers Presented at the United States-France Seminar on Biomedical Image Processing, St. Pierre de Chartreuse, France, May 27–31, 1980

Edited by J. Sklansky and J.-C. Bisconte

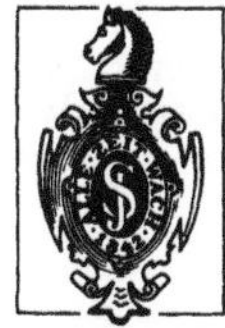

Springer-Verlag
Berlin Heidelberg GmbH

Editors

Jack Sklansky
University of California, School of Engineering
Irvine, California 92717, USA

Jean-Claude Bisconte
Laboratoire de Neurobiologie Quantitative, U.E.R. Biomédicale
74, rue Marcel Cachin, 93012 Bobigny Cedex

DOI 10.1007/978-3-642-93218-2

Library of Congress Cataloging in Publication Data
United States-France Seminar on Biomedical Image Processing (1980: Saint Pierre de Chartreuse, France) Computer-aided formation and analysis of biomedical images. (Lecture notes in medical informatics; 17) Bibliography: p. Includes index. 1. Imaging systems in medicine--Data processing--Congresses. I. Bisconte, J. C. (Jean-Claude) II. Sklansky, Jack. III. Title. IV. Series. [DNLM: 1. Image enhancement--Methods--Congresses. 2. Radiographic image enhancement--Methods--Congresses. 3. Computers--Congresses. 4. Microscopy--Instrumentation--Congresses. 5. Technology, Radiologic--Instrumentation--Congresses. WI LE 334N v. 17 / WN 160 U56 1980c] R857.O6U56 1980 616.07'5
82-10521

Originally published by Springer-Verlag Berlin Heidelberg New York in 1982
MyCopy version of the original edition 1982

2145/3140-543210
www.springer.com/mycopy

PREFACE

The technology of automatic pattern recognition and digital image processing, after over two decades of basic research, is now appearing in important applications in biology and medicine as well as industrial, military and aerospace systems. In response to a suggestion from Mr. Norman Caplan, the Program Director for Automation, Bioengineering and Sensing at the United States National Science Foundation, the authors of this book organized the first United States-France Seminar on Biomedical Image Processing. The seminar met at the Hotel Beau Site, St. Pierre de Chartreuse, France on May 27-31, 1980. This book contains most of the papers presented at this seminar, as well as two papers (by Bisconte *et al.* and by Ploem *et al.*) discussed at the seminar but not appearing on the program.

We view the subject matter of this seminar as a confluence among three broad scientific and engineering disciplines: 1) biology and medicine, 2) imaging and optics, and 3) computer science and computer engineering.

The seminar had three objectives: 1) to discuss the state of the art of biomedical image processing with emphasis on four themes: microscopic image analysis, radiological image analysis, tomography, and image processing technology; 2) to place values on directions for future research so as to give guidance to agencies supporting such research; and 3) to explore and encourage various areas of cooperative research between French and United States scientists within the field of Biomedical Image Processing.

The attendees at this seminar consisted of fifteen scientists from the United States, thirty-two from France, one from Germany, one from the Netherlands, and one from Italy. These participants are listed in the Appendix. The participants were selected from United States and French universities, industries and government agencies to represent a cross section of biomedical image processing: theory and practice; physics, engineering, and computer science; hardware and software; research, design and operation.

During the conference several areas of potentially useful collaborations between French and American scientists were identified. These areas included the sharing of special purpose expensive equipment; the exchange of data, algorithms, and computer programs; the establishment of United States-France workshops on specialized subjects such as aspiration needle biopsy, proton emission tomography, and computer graphics for the three-dimensional display of anatomical, cellular and molecular structures. Preliminary steps along these directions have been taken, as well as the organizing of a second United States-France Seminar on Biomedical Image Processing.

This book, following the organization of the Seminar, is divided into four Themes: Microscopic Image Analysis, Radiological Image Analysis, Tomography, and Image Processing Technology.

The discussion of Microscopic Image Analysis includes the automated analysis of chromosomes, blood cells, bone marrow cells, and human tissue. The detection and imaging techniques include color photometry, visual optics, acoustics, electron optics, and three-dimensional reconstruction.

The discussion of Radiological Image Analysis includes the imaging of coronary arteries, cerebral blood vessels, the heart, the lung, lung tumors, the kidney, and the liver. The imaging techniques include x-ray film, fluoroscopy, and ultrasound.

The discussion of Tomography is mainly concerned with new tomographic imaging techniques, including high-speed computed x-ray tomography, region-of-interest tomography, coded aperture tomography, positron emission tomography, ultrasound tomography, and the display of the digital three dimensional structures obtained by computed tomography.

The discussion of Image Processing Technology includes the latest developments in high-speed image-processing computer architecture and automated microscopy, and a recently developed mathematical theory supporting a parallel image-processing architecture.

The editors of this book are grateful to the authors of the papers for making the Seminar and this book possible. They are grateful for the organizational advice and financial support of the National Science Foundation (in particular, Dr. Henryk Uznanski and Mr. Norman Caplan), the Centre National de la Recherche Scientifique and the Délégation Générale à la Recherche Scientifique et Technique, and for the financial support of the Compagnie Générale de Radiologie. The editors are much indebted to Victoria von Hagen for her diplomacy and energy in assisting the organizing of the seminar and the editing of this volume, and to Mr. Masamitsu Hashimoto for his assistance in the technical review.

We are grateful to the Seminar's organizing committee for their contributions to the Seminar's success. The members of this committee were: B. Boesso, G. Brugal, P. Chibon, F. Delourme, J. F. Feldman, P. Garderet, R. Gariod, F. Veillon, and V. von Hagen.

Jack Sklansky
United States

Jean-Claude Bisconte
France

Seminar Co-Chairmen

TABLE OF CONTENTS

Theme 1: Microscopic Image Analysis

Theme 2: Radiological Image Analysis

THE APPLICATION OF COMPUTERIZED HIGH RESOLUTION SCANNING TECHNIQUES TO THE IDENTIFICATION OF HUMAN CELLS AND TISSUES

By

Leopold G. Koss, M.D.

Professor and Chairman, Department of Pathology,
Montefiore Hospital and Medical Center, Albert
Einstein College of Medicine, Bronx, New York 10467
U.S.A.

Supported in part by Grant No. 5-R26-CA-15803
of the National Cancer Institute through the National
Bladder Cancer Project, Worcester, Massachusetts 01604

ABSTRACT

The purpose of this paper is to summarize the basic information on cell morphology useful in the microscopic diagnosis of human disease with special emphasis on morphologic identification of cancer cells. The rationale for computerized analysis of digitized cell images and the principal targets of this approach, namely, cytology of the uterine cervix, urine and sputum have been discussed. The technical and legal problems of sample preparation and the problems of sample interpretation have been outlined. A summary of present and future research trends concludes this paper.

1. INTRODUCTION

The introduction of the microscope to the study of tissue and cell samples of human origin during the latter part of the 18th and mainly during the 19th century has led to the current concepts of human disease. It has been firmly established that disease processes are the result of an altered state of cells or their components and products, and consequently of tissues which are best defined as aggregates of cells sharing common purpose. Many of the common disease processes cause changes in microscopic configuration of tissues and cells which may be quantitative or qualitative. The quantitative changes may be the result either of an increase or a decrease in the number of cells composing a tissue or an organ. The qualitative changes pertain to the microscopic or submicroscopic modifications in the structure or in the function of cells (1).

In 1866 Paul Broca, the great French surgeon and cancerologist, said this about the microscopic study (2): "Les recherches microscopiques sont minutieuses et fatiguantes; elles exigent une patience à toute épreuve une persévérance prolongée, et les premiers observateurs auraient été bientôt découragés s'ils n'eussent été soutenus dans cette étude ingrate et difficile par l'appât puissant d'une brillante théorie." (The microscopic research is very precise and demanding; it calls for endless patience and perseverance. The early observers would have been rapidly discouraged in this thankless and difficult task were it not for the powerful appeal of a brilliant theory). Broca was referring to Virchow's concept of cell pathology with which he incidentally disagreed, much to the detriment of future developments in French pathology.

Nonetheless, the basic truth of Broca's words is still valid today and many of the common diagnostic procedures based on microscopic study are difficult, tedious, repetitious and time-consuming. Furthermore, the interpretation of the findings often depends on the experience, skill, and talent of the observer.

It is evident, therefore, that new approaches to the study of cells that may induce diagnostic objectivity in the identification of disease and relieve the tedium of microscopy would be of great benefit to the society. Image analytical techniques offer considerable promise in this regard.

It is beyond the scope of this summary to indicate the enormous variety of microscopic images that may be encountered in the study of human disease. Furthermore, these images may vary significantly from organ to organ and even from tissue to tissue, thus preventing the establishment of general and simple classification rules that could have universal applicability. Therefore, image analysis techniques must seek specific and selective targets that would provide optimal cost:benefit ratio.

It is, of course, conceivable that the analysis of objective computer-based information could yield new data on the biologic nature of the disease studied and, in the case of cancer, data on sequence of cellular events, and even data of prognostic nature. The creation of appropriate computer algorithms coupled with simple and practical technical approaches, may prove to be a highly beneficial commodity that could be made available to the entire human race at a moderate cost, thus raising the level of microscopic diagnosis throughout the world without the need for extensive and time-consuming training of personnel. While this may be an utopic concept at this time, I am personally convinced that given adequate resources the target is achievable within the available technology.

2. CELL MORPHOLOGY

The obvious primary target of image processing are cells rather than tissues. The task is facilitated by the relatively small size of the cell and the relative ease with which it can be reduced to a digital form. With the exception of mature red blood cells and some epithelial cells which are composed of a cytoplasmic matrix alone, all other human cells display the 2 essential components: the nucleus and the cytoplasm. The nucleus is the site of the reproductive apparatus of the cells and contains deoxyribonucleic acid (DNA), whereas the cytoplasm is the site of metabolic events which are expressed morphologically and may provide the observer with information regarding cell function and destiny (1).

2.1. Resting cells

In the resting cell, the nucleus generally has a spherical configuration. The nuclear DNA and associated proteins, or the so-called nuclear chromatin, are hydrated, hence not visible except for granules of the so called heterochromatin which remain in condensed state throughout the resting phase. In duplicating cells, i.e., cells undergoing mitotic division, the amount of DNA will double during the synthetic or S-phase of the cell cycle with resulting nuclear enlargement. During mitosis the DNA condenses in the form of chromosomes. The chromosome complement and morphology is characteristic of each species. The chromosomes can be classified according to their size, configuration, and internal structural differences, expressed as alternating darker and lighter bands which can be brought out and classified by special techniques (3).

An important component of the normal nucleus is the nucleolus which is the center of formation of ribonucleic acid (RNA), the messenger substance that provides the communication between the nucleus and the cytoplasm. The number and the size of the nucleoli may vary according to the level of cell activity and other factors.

With a very few exceptions of highly specialized cells such as polymorphonuclear leukocytes, the configuration and the texture of the nuclei are not specific for normal cells and thus their images cannot be utilized for cell classification. On the other hand, the cytoplasm of the normal cells mirrors their origin and activity. Thus, a great variety of cytoplasmic images may occur which serve to classify many normal cell types. The size, texture, content and activity of the cytoplasm can be readily analyzed.

2.2. Reactions of cells to injury

Under abnormal or pathologic circumstances, the cells may undergo morphologic modifications which may be reflected either in the nucleus, or the cytoplasm, or both. In general, the reactions of the cells to injury, regardless of its nature, may take 3 pathways:

1. The cells die.

2. The cells respond by adapting to the changed environment and then return to normal.

3. The cells undergo a permanent modification of structure which is inherited by their progeny.

The injury may signal the need for cell multiplication with increased number of mitotic events, reflected in the nucleus. The need for a modification of cell function may reflect itself in alteration of the cytoplasmic structure, texture, and configuration. These changes may be either temporary or permanent. Cell death may affect either the cytoplasm or the nucleus and cause severe modification in both.

2.3. Cancer cells

Cancer and events leading to cancer may induce significant changes in the morphology of cells. The summary of principal morphologic changes that may be observed in cancer cells is shown in Table I.

TABLE I

MORPHOLOGIC CELL FEATURES THAT MAY BE MODIFIED IN CANCER

1. CELL SIZE AND CONFIGURATION
2. NUCLEAR SIZE AND CONFIGURATION
3. CHROMATIN TEXTURE
4. NUCLEOLAR SIZE, CONFIGURATION, AND NUMBER
5. RELATIONSHIPS OF CELLS TO EACH OTHER
6. CONFIGURATION OF CELL SURFACES
7. MITOTIC ACTIVITY

The most significant morphologic features of cancer cells reside in a modification of the nuclear structure and texture. An irregularly increased amount of nuclear DNA and its altered packaging are particularly characteristic and are reflected in increased binding of certain stains to nuclear chromatin. This results in darker staining or hyperchromatic and coarsely granular nuclei. The size and shape of the nucleus may change, and there is often an increase in the number and size of the nucleoli. The cytoplasmic changes are much less characteristic. The degree of morphologic deviation from the normal cell of origin may vary significantly depending on factors generally known as "tumor differentiation." (1).

Table II lists the measurable morphologic or cytochemical parameters of cells that may prove of particular value in objective evaluation of cell structure and function. It must be stressed that the difficulties in cancer cell identification are not due to some extravagant properties of cancer cells but to their essential similarity to benign cells. At best, these features represent a set of changing and dynamic values that vary from organ to organ, from tissue to tissue, from individual to individual, and from tumor to tumor.

TABLE II

MEASURABLE PARAMETERS OF CELLS SUITABLE FOR IMAGE PROCESSING OR FLOW CYTOMETRY*
CELL SIZE, SHAPE, MASS, VOLUME
NUCLEIC ACID CONTENT AND CONFIGURATION
DNA, RNA, NUCLEAR TEXTURE (CHROMATIN CONFIGURATION)
NUCLEOLAR SIZE, NUMBER, AND FUNCTION
IMMUNOLOGIC PROPERTIES
CELL SURFACE AND INTERIOR
CERTAIN CYTOCHEMICAL PROPERTIES
ENZYMES
STAINING REACTIONS OF VARIOUS CELL COMPONENTS

*Modified from Bahr *et al.*: Automated Cytology in Koss, L.G.: *Diagnostic Cytology and Its Histopathologic Bases*, 3rd ed., Philadelphia, Lippincott, 1979.

3. TARGETS FOR IMAGE ANALYSIS

The benefits of cytology automation are most evident in 2 areas:

A. Procedures that are frequently performed, labor-intensive, tedious and, therefore, costly. Targets belonging to this category are:

1. Analysis of smears of peripheral blood.
2. Cervical smears (Papanicolaou smears) for the detection of precancerous states of the uterine cervix.
3. Smears of urinary sediment for detection and diagnosis of cancer of the bladder and lower urinary tract.
4. Other cytologic preparations, for example: smears of sputum, fluids such as pleural effusion or ascites.
5. Karyotyping (analysis of chromosomes).

C. Procedures that offer diagnostic and prognostic options not otherwise available by microscopic examination of the samples. Targets belonging to the second category have not been fully and clearly identified as yet. Some of the potential targets are:

1. Identification of sub-populations of lymphocytes (B, T, Null).
2. Evaluation of smears of cancers for prognostic purposes (for example: prostate or breast cancer).
3. Evaluation of response of tumors to therapeutic agents (radiotherapy, cytotoxic agents).

4. COMMON CYTOLOGIC PROCEDURES AS TARGETS FOR CELL ANALYSIS

4.1. Fundamental differences in the targets of automated analysis

Although all of the procedures identified above have in common a large population of cells that have to be analyzed, there are some basic and fundamental differences among them: For example, the evaluation of peripheral blood smears calls for the identification of cell images in a representative portion of the sample. The number of cell types in the sample is limited and does not vary from individual to individual. Therefore, a limited number of algorithms is required for cell identification. For this reason, the art and science of computerized analysis of peripheral blood smears is advanced and several commercial instruments are on the market. This target will be discussed by others, hence I will not return to it.

On the other hand, the analysis of cervical smears or of sputum for purposes of cancer detection or diagnosis calls for identification of rare events, i.e., the infrequent cancer cells dispersed in a large and complex population of benign cells of several origins. The examination of the urinary sediment or body fluids (effusions) represents specific targets of intermediate difficulty: the identification of fairly frequent event (cancer cells) in a relatively small population of benign cells of moderate complexity (Table III).

TABLE III
FUNDAMENTAL DIFFERENCES IN TARGETING OF AUTOMATED PROCEDURES IN HUMAN CYTOLOGY

TARGET	PURPOSE	PROCEDURE
PERIPHERAL BLOOD SMEARS	IDENTIFICATION OF COMMON ABNORMALITIES OF LEUKOCYTES AND ERYTHROCYTES	EVALUATION OF A REPRESENTATIVE SAMPLE WITH LIMITED NUMBER OF CELL TYPES
CERVICAL SMEARS OR SPUTUM	DETECTION OR DIAGNOSIS OF CANCER AND PRECANCEROUS STATES	SEARCH FOR A RARE EVENT (CANCER CELLS) IN A VERY COMPLEX POPULATION OF BENIGN CELLS
URINARY SEDIMENT	DIAGNOSIS OF SPECIFIC TYPES OF CANCER WITH KNOWN GRAVE PROGNOSIS	SEARCH FOR SPECIFIC CELL TYPES IN A POPULATION OF BENIGN CELLS OF LIMITED COMPLEXITY
OTHER CANCERS (SAMPLES OF CANCER CELLS)	INFORMATION OF POSSIBLE DIAGNOSTIC OR PROGNOSTIC SIGNIFICANCE	STUDY OF CHARACTERISTICS OF THE POPULATION OF CANCER CELLS (FOR EXAMPLE, PLOIDY)

4.2. Technical requirements

In order to transform cell images into a form amenable to analysis by computer, certain basic principles apply to all biologic targets. The material must be presented in a manner that is not confusing to the computer. If, for example, the computer is capable of identifying a cancer cell based on nuclear size, which is twice as large as the nuclear size observed in the corresponding benign cells, the superposition of 2 benign cell nuclei may also result in a false alarm (4). This problem which is virtually non-existent with peripheral blood cells which form no attachments to each other, is particularly important in evaluation of cell samples originating from epithelial lining tissues such as the uterine cervix, the bladder, or the bronchus.

A number of methods of cell separation have been described, most commonly based on mechanical shearing or syringing of the sample (5). It has been shown by our group that vigorous cell separation by enzymatic or chemical means usually results in cell destruction (6). Weak enzymatic action of pepsine combined with mechanical shearing has been successfully applied by some observers (7,8). In order to achieve a constant concentration of cells per unit of sample, an ingenious apparatus has been devised by Bahr *et al.* in which the opacity of the cell suspension is controlled by a laser beam (9).

Another important problem is visual cell identification which is particularly important during the initial process of establishing appropriate algorithms for various cell categories. Because cells are usually identified in stained preparations, it is of advantage to use stained cells for such purposes. Staining of cells introduces a number of artifacts and requires rigid control over the quality of the stains and the timing of the staining procedure (10). Thus, it is of advantage to have this aspect of the procedure automated as well. Some investigators utilize special stains not commonly used in the diagnostic procedures. Such stains may enhance one cell feature, for example, the DNA content of the nucleus, better than routine stains and thus facilitate the automation process based on this one feature. While this approach may serve certain purposes, it does not facilitate cell identification and classification.

The speed with which a sample is processed may be of critical importance. Very slow systems may be accurate but not practical. Very rapid automated processing by high resolution systems, even using television equipment, may cause a very high signal to noise ratio with resulting distortion of messages. Flow systems, which offer a very high rate of information are currently limited to the study of very few parameters such as cell size or DNA content (11,12). However, it is my judgment that, for the time-being at least, the primary target of the technology is to achieve high quality of imaging and interpretation rather than high speed.

5. THE LEGAL REQUIREMENTS OF AUTOMATION

Automation of human cell samples other than blood should theoretically match or improve diagnostic achievements of the experienced human observer. It must be stressed that while a sample may be obtained primarily for one purpose, for example, the detection of cancer of the uterine cervix, the sample may reflect a number of disease states other than cancer, i.e., the presence of various infectious agents, or of cell changes caused by such agents. Furthermore, the patient may also harbor other cancers, for example, carcinoma of the endometrium. The cells from endometrial cancer differ in size, nuclear and cytoplasmic configuration and DNA content from cells of carcinoma of the cervix. The critical point of this aspect of automation is the legal responsibility of the investigator towards the patient.

In the United States any automated diagnostic apparatus must be licensed by the Food and Drug Administration of the Federal Government before actual human use. It is evident that this agency will demand proof that such a device or machine will perform according to the diagnostic criteria established by the human eye. Should this not be the case, the agency will require that the examinee or the patient be so informed in clear language.

6. APPLICATION OF BIOMEDICAL IMAGE PROCESSING TO EPITHELIAL CELLS

6.1. The cervical smear

The cytologic detection of precancerous changes and occult cancer of the uterine cervix (Papanicolaou smear) has been one of the most successful applications of contemporary biology to the solution of a major public health problem. Evidence at hand clearly indicates that cancer of the uterine cervix, which previously was the most frequent form of genital cancer, can be controlled by cytology (1). In Western countries where screening of women has become an accepted public health procedure, the rate of cancer of the cervix has dropped in a statistically significant fashion.

While the technical approaches to the practical solution of the problem may vary and have been summarized elsewhere (13), the strategy of automation remains essentially the same and involves several steps which are summarized in Table IV.

TABLE IV
STRATEGY OF AUTOMATION OF HUMAN CELL SAMPLES BY HIGH RESOLUTION SCANNING

1. PREPARATION OF SAMPLE SUITABLE FOR AUTOMATED PROCESSING
2. ANALYTICAL ASSESSMENT OF CELLS
    a. Acquisition of cell images
    b. Isolation of cell images (cleaning)
    c. Scene segmentation:identification of cell components (nucleus and cytoplasm)
    d. Extraction of cell features and determination of their value
    e. Classification of known cells (teaching set) and unknown cells (object set)
3. DIAGNOSTIC ASSESSMENT OF SAMPLE

The diagnostic assessment of the sample may be based on simultaneous classification of all cell images into several possible cell types or on hierarchic decision sequence (11,14). It has been our experience that hierarchic classification is more reliable when more than 3 cell types are involved.

Several strategies are also available in reference to sample interpretation (13). One can establish an arbitrary figure for the number of specific signals. For example, if an algorithm is established for the identification of cancer cells, the sample is automatically considered abnormal whenever this signal occurs. This approach carries with it the likelihood of a very high number of misclassifications due to false positive signals.

Alternately, a predetermined threshold may be established in which each sample with a specified number of such signals (for example, 5 or more) will be considered as abnormal. This approach, while limiting the number of false positive samples, risks the possibility that a sample with a very small number of true cancer cells will be misclassified as normal. The third approach consists of careful, high resolution assessment of every positive signal for further analysis by computer or the human eye. Obviously, this last procedure, while highly reliable, is time-consuming and will slow down the analytical process. Finally, it is possible to evaluate the entire sample by establishing "indices of atypia" in which the entire sample will be evaluated and classified as an arbitrary value (15).

Calculations have been performed to indicate the optimal number of cells that have to be examined in a cervical sample for optimal diagnosis of cervix cancer precursors. This is approximately 50,000 cells, provided that the coefficient of variation among samples is not greater than 50% (16). This brings into focus yet another aspect of cytology automation, namely, optimization of clinical sampling. It is evident that the entire automation procedure will fail if the sample submitted for automation is not representative of the disease. In the case of the uterine cervix, this basic failure of the screening procedure has been variously estimated at 4 to 40% of the premalignant lesions (1). Thus, the success of the automation process depends not only on the excellence of the technical approach but also on the biologic aspects of the target tissue which unfortunately is variable and the least likely to be controlled by objective scientific factors. Inspite of these caveats, several teams in the United States, Europe, and Japan have developed sophisticated approaches to the solution of these many problems (17). While the technical approaches vary, the purpose is the same, and the very large number of publications on this subject suggest that one or more solutions may become available in the foreseeable future.

6.2. The urinary sediment

Cancer of the urinary bladder is one of several human cancers associated with industrial pollution. For this reason, this group of diseases is the subject of intensive inquiry in the United States. Cancer of the bladder presents a very different dilemma from that of the uterine cervix. Approximately 90% of bladder tumors are initially of papillary configuration and are composed of cells that differ very little from normal. This type of disease is usually discovered because of clinical symptoms. Within the recent years, it has been determined that the prognosis of most bladder tumors depends to a large extent not on the appearance and classification of papillary disease but on the presence of epithelial abnormalities known as non-papillary (flat) carcinoma in situ. On the one hand, such lesions are difficult to identify clinically and, on the other hand, they shed in the urine clearly identifiable cancer cells, hence represent an important target of cytology automation (18).

The technical problems in the automation process of cells in the urinary sediment are quite different from those described for the uterine cervix (19). There is usually a high ratio of cancer cells to benign cells. The urine, however, is not a hospitable medium for cells and, therefore, causes varying degrees of degeneration of benign and malignant urothelial cells. Such degenerated cells represent significant problems in cell identification.

The work performed to date clearly suggests that algorithms for the identification of the various subpopulations of urothelial cells can be determined. Furthermore, hierarchical classification recently performed strongly suggests that an automated system may be based on elimination from analysis of cells that are difficult to classify (20). Thus, the final determination may be based on cell images of diagnostic value. In a preliminary study of patients' profiles the feasibility of this approach was determined (21).

To date, the work on cells in the urinary sediment was based on the slow high resolution scanning techniques. The introduction of high speed scanning technology may result in a practical system within a few years.

6.2. Other targets of automation

High resolution scanning has been applied to the identification of cancer cells in sputum for the diagnosis of lung cancer (22) to the study of cells in effusions (23). It has also been shown that discrimination of T-lymphocytes from B-lymphocytes can be accomplished by computer although these 2 cell types cannot be differentiated by microscopic study in the absence of special procedures (24,25).

7. DISCUSSION

The brief summary of the state of the art in the application of high resolution image analytical techniques to human cells is, of necessity, limited and incomplete. Important contributions by many investigators have been omitted because personal choices had to be made in the selection of information fitting the limited space. The interested reader is referred to several excellent recent summaries either previously published or in print (1,11,13,17).

It is evident that techniques are in place to analyze human cells by computer and that the information derived from such studies has the potential for benefitting mankind in several areas (Table V).

TABLE V

POTENTIAL BENEFITS OF HIGH RESOLUTION SCANNING OF CELLS

1. REDUCTION OF LABOR AND COST
2. OBJECTIVIZATION OF DIAGNOSTIC CRITERIA
3. IMPROVEMENT IN INTERPRETATION OF BIOLOGIC DATA (PROGNOSIS, RESPONSE TO TREATMENT)
4. AVAILABILITY OF HIGH LEVEL MEDICAL TECHNOLOGY TO UNDERDEVELOPED COUNTRIES

This optimistic assessment must be balanced by a great many difficulties still ahead, listed briefly in Table VI. There is little doubt that suitable computer hardware and software and optical systems can be provided at a moderate cost. Problems of biologic nature pertaining to uniformity of sampling, sample collection and processing, and diagnostic control are more difficult to solve because they are not subject to the progress of machine technology. Some of these problems may be bypassed by studying multiple samples from the same patient. In fact, this may prove to be the best and ultimately the least expensive approach to cytology automation, once fully automated systems are in place.

TABLE VI

FACTORS GOVERNING THE SUCCESS OF THE HIGH RESOLUTION SCANNING OF HUMAN CELLS FOR DIAGNOSTIC PURPOSES IN INCREASING ORDER OF DIFFICULTY

1. HARDWARE AND SOFTWARE
2. SAMPLE PREPARATION
3. BIOLOGIC PITFALLS
4. CLINICAL SAMPLING VARIABILITY

Can a universal automatic system of microscopy fully replacing the human observer, ever be built? Probably not in the near future mainly because of the complexities of the human sample which will require many additional years of work to create a data base for the identification of the key modalities of cell morphology. On the other hand, systems with specific, limited, well-defined targets probably can be built and operated within a few years. It is clearly incumbent upon the investigators to inform the licensing authorities and the public of such limitations. Otherwise, citizens who ultimately pay for this research one way or another may be misled as to what can and what cannot be achieved.

REFERENCES

1. L.G. Koss, Diagnostic Cytology and Its Histopathologic Bases, 3rd ed. Lippincott, Philadelphia, 1979.
2. P. Broca, Traîté des Tumeurs, P. Asselin, Paris, 1866.
3. M.L. Mendelsohn (Ed.), "Automation of Cytogenetics." Asilomar Workshop, Pacific Grove, California, 1976; sponsored by Div. Biomed Environ. Res., U.S. Energy Res. and Develop. Admin.
4. J.J. Sychra, P.H. Bartels, M. Bibbo, J. Taylor, and G.L. Wied, Computer recognition of binucleation with overlapping in epithelial cells, Acta Cytol., 22: 1978, pp. 22-28.
5. J.S. Mead, P.K. Horan, and L.L. Wheeless, Syringing as a method of cell dispersal. I. Effect on intermediate and superficial squamous cells, Acta Cytol., 22: 1978, pp. 86-90.
6. R.C. Wolley, F. Herz, H.M. Dembitzer, K. Schreiber, and L.G. Koss, The monodisperse cervical smear. Quantitative analysis of cell dispersion and loss with enzymatic and chemical agents. Analyt. Quant. Cytol. 1: 1979, pp.43-49.
7. J. Zante, J. Schumann, B. Barlogie, W. Goehde, Th. Buchner, "New preparing and staining procedures for specific and rapid analysis of DNA distributions." In Pulse Cytophotometry, II. Goehde, W. et al. (eds.) European Press Medikon, Ghent, 1976, pp. 97-1060.
8. B. Tribukait, H. Gustafson, and P. Esposti, Ploidy and proliferation in human bladder tumors as measured by flow-cytofluorometric DNA-analysis and its relations to histopathology and cytology, Cancer, 43: 1979, pp. 1742-1751.
9. G.F. Bahr, M. Bibbo, M. Oehme, J.H. Puls, F.R. Reale, and G.L. Wied, An automated device for the production of cell preparations suitable for automatic assessment, Acta Cytol., 22: 1978, pp. 243-249.
10. P.H. Bartels, G.F. Bahr, M. Bibbo, D.L. Richards, M.G. Sonek, and G.L. Wied, Analysis of variance of the Papanicolaou staining reaction. Acta Cytol., 18: 1974, 522-531.
11. G.F. Bahr, P.H. Bartels, G.L. Wied, and L.G. Koss, "Automated Cytology" in L.G. Koss: Diagnostic Cytology and Its Histopathologic Bases, 3rd ed., Lippincott, Philadelphia, 1979.
12. W. Goehde, J. Schumann, T. Buchner, F. Otto, and B. Barlogie, "Pulse cytophotometry: Application in tumor cell biology and clinical oncology." In Flow Cytometry and Sorting (Melamed, M.R., Mullaney, P.F., Mendelsohn, M.L., eds.) John Wiley & Sons, New York, 1979, pp. 599-620.
13. P.H. Bartels, L.G. Koss, and G.L. Wied, "Cytology automation by computerized high resolution scanning." Advances in Clinical Cytology, Butterworths, London and Boston, 1980 (in print).
14. J. Taylor, P.H. Bartels, M. Bibbo, G.L. Wied, Automated hierarchic decision structures for multiple category cell classification by TICAS. Acta Cytol. 22: 1978, pp. 261-267.
15. P.H. Bartels, L.G. Koss, J.J. Sychra, and G.L. Wied, Indices of cell atypia in urinary tract cytology, Acta Cytol., 22: 1978, pp. 387-391.
16. P.H. Bartels, "Statistical sampling requirements," in The Automation of Uterine Cancer Cytology (Wied, G.L., Bahr, G.F., and Bartels, P.H., eds.) Tutorials of Cytology, Chicago, 1976, pp. 268-288.
17. N.J. Pressman and G.L. Wied, eds., "The Automation of cancer cytology and cell image analysis" Chicago, Tutorials of Cytology, 1979.
18. L.G. Koss, Mapping of the urinary bladder: its impact on the concepts of bladder cancer, Human Pathol. 10: 1979, pp. 533-548.
19. L.G. Koss, P.H. Bartels, Urinary cytology. Device capabilities and requirements, Analyt. Quant. Cytol. 2: 1980, pp. 59-65.

20. L.G. Koss, A. Sherman, P.H. Bartels, J.J. Sychra, and G.L. Wied, Hierarchic classification of multiple types of urothelial cells by computer (in preparation).
21. L.G. Koss, P.H. Bartels, J.J. Sychra, and G.L. Wied, Diagnostic cytologic sample profiles in patients with bladder cancer using TICAS system. Acta Cytol, 22: 1978, pp. 392-397.
22. J.K. Frost, H.W. Tyrer, N.J. Pressman, C.D. Albright, M.H. Vansickel, G.W. Gill, Automatic cell identification and enrichment in lung cancer: I. Light scatter and fluorescence parameters, J. Histochem. Cytochem., 27:1979, pp. 545-551.
23. E. Jahoda, P.H. Bartels, M. Bibbo, G.F. Bahr, J.H. Holzner, and G.L. Wied, Computer discrimination of cells in serous effusions. I. Pleural fluids. II. Peritoneal fluid. Acta Cytol. 17: 1973, 94-105 and 533-537.
24. P.H. Bartels, G.B. Olson, J.M. Layton, R.E. Anderson, and G.L. Wied, Computer discrimination of T and B lymphocytes. Acta Cytol. 19: 1975, pp. 53-57.
25. P.H. Bartels, Y-P. Chen, B.G.M. Durie, G.B. Olson, L. Vaught, S.E. Salmon, Discrimination between human T and B lymphocytes by computer analysis of digitized data from scanning microphotometry. II. Discrimination and automated classification. Acta Cytol. 22: 1978, pp. 530-537.

AUTOMATED ANALYSIS OF PAPANICOLAOU STAINED CERVICAL SPECIMENS USING A TELEVISION-BASED ANALYSIS SYSTEM (LEYTAS)

by

Johan S. PLOEM and Anneke M.J. VAN DRIEL-KULKER
Department of Histochemistry and Cytochemistry,
University Medical Center, Sylvius Laboratories,
P.O. Box 772, LEIDEN, THE NETHERLANDS.

ABSTRACT

An image analysis program for automated screening of entire Papanicolaou stained slides, using a television based analysis system (LEYTAS), is described. A series of 45 specimens has been screened to test this program, that consists principally of nuclear contour finding, size and thresholding operations on the nucleus and artefact rejection procedures, using image transformations. The significance of the total number of alarms and the number of detected nuclei per 10.000 epithelial cells as discriminatory factors is discussed with regard to future improvements and developments.

1. INTRODUCTION

Automated prescreening of cervical specimens for malignant and premalignant lesions has been investigated during the past few years by several groups, using both flow systems (BARRETT et al., 1979 ; CAMBIER et al., 1979 and STÖHR et al., 1979) and slide based systems (ABMAYR et al., 1979 ; AL et al., 1979 ; READ et al., 1979 ; TANAKA et al., 1979 ; TUCKER, 1979 ; ZAHNISER et al., 1979). After defining and optimizing the cell classification parameters, only a few groups working with slide based instruments have now published results obtained by the analysis of entire slides, stained according either to Papanicolaou (TANAKA et al., 1979) or with a quantitative cytochemical method (TUCKER, 1979 ; ZAHNISER et al., 1979). The Leyden Television Analysis System (LEYTAS), as it is used in our laboratory for the screening for precancerous and cancerous lesions of the cervix, has principally been applied to the analysis of entire slides, stained according a quantitative staining procedure (acriflavine-Feulgen SITS) (AL et al., 1979 ; DRIEL-KULKER et al., 1980; TANKE et al., 1979).

The use of the conventional Papanicolaou stained cervical smear has found world-wide acceptance for the visual cytomorphological diagnosis of exfoliated cervical cells. Automated analysis however, requires additional preparation techniques in order to reduce the number of overlapping cells, standardize and reduce the thickness of the cell layer on the glass slide and slightly modify the Papanicolaou staining to increase the contrast between the nucleus and the cytoplasm. Therefore, laboratories working in the field of automation of cytology, have devised procedures to obtain the required monolayer specimens using either centrifugation techniques (BAHR et al., 1978 ; DRIEL-KULKER et al., In press ; LEIF et al., 1975 ; LEIF et al., 1977 ; OTTO et al., 1979), spinning methods (WOLLEY et al., 1979) or other droplet/smear methods (EASON et al., 1979 ; HUSAIN et al., 1978 ; ROSENTHAL et al., 1979). Several papers report on the suitability of such preparations for cytomorphological evaluation (BARRETT et al., 1978 ; HÖFFKEN et al., 1979). In conjunction with our LEYTAS work we have chosen centrifugal cytology in order to obtain a relatively high number of well flattened cells deposited onto a small defined area of the glass slide DRIEL-KULKER et al., In press).

The conventional staining procedure according to Papanicolaou however, even when used on especially prepared monolayer specimens, has still been shown to cause problems for several image analysis systems (AL et al., 1979 ; DRIEL-KULKER et al.; 1980; TUCKER, 1979 ; ZAHNISER et al., 1979). This was mainly due to the spectral overlap of the stained nucleus and the cytoplasm, as well as to the non-quantitative character of the staining result. This prompted the development of quantitative staining methods such as gallocyanine (EASON et al., 1979), thionine-congo red (ZAHNISER et al., 1979) and acriflavine-Feulgen-SITS (TANKE et al., 1979). These staining procedures have in common that they provide quantitative information about important macromolecules like DNA and protein in the cell. In addition image analysis methods can often provide valuable data, due to the effective separation of nucleus and cytoplasm which results from several of these cytochemical staining methods (TANKE et al., 1979 ; ZAHNISER et al., 1979).

On the other hand, during the interactive learning phase of automated cytology, it is desirable to use as much a priori cytological knowledge as possible, which is often not available yet for specimens stained with quantitative cytochemical methods. As the cytological knowledge of cervical cells has primarily been obtained by cytomorphological evaluation of Papanicolaou stained cells, we investigated the possibility of using LEYTAS for the automated analysis of entire Papanicolaou stained slides.

This project has been carried out in collaboration with F. Meyer from the Centre of Mathematical Morphology in Fontainebleau, France, who developed a set of image transformations for the analysis of Papanicolaou stained specimens (MEYER et al., 1980). This method first selects interesting objects and subsequently rejects most of the artefacts using shape analysis. The detection of abnormal cells is mainly based on nuclear features. Investigation is in progress on the addition of cytoplasmic parameters.

2. PREPARATION OF CERVICAL MATERIAL

Cells are sampled with an acryl cotton tipped applicator, thereafter the applicator is immersed in a buffered salt solution (Polyonic: 0.09 M sodium chloride; 0.03 M sodium acetate; 0.03 M sodium gluconate; 6 mM potassium chloride; 1.5 mM magnesium chloride. pH = 7.4), containing 25% ethanol. The cell samples are sent to our laboratory by mail, where they are further processed. After centrifugation and replacement of the supernatant by Carbowax fixative (2% poly ethylene glycol in 50% ethanol), the cell concentration is estimated by measuring the 90° scatter of laser light (DRIEL-KULKER et al., In press). The cell suspension is then syringed automatically using 21 gauge needles to break up cell clumps. For slide preparation use is made of a recently developed centrifugation bucket, which centrifuges the prefixed cells onto the slide at 1250 G (DRIEL-KULKER et al., In press). After disassembling the bucket, the slides are airdried and left at room temperature. Directly before staining the cells are further fixed in a mixture of methanol / 40% formaldehyde / acetic acid = 85 / 10 / 5 v/v (Boehm-Sprenger fixative). Staining is performed in a staining machine (Shandon, England). A Papanicolaou staining procedure is used which is adapted in order to obtain optimal contrast between the intensity of the nucleus and the cytoplasm using light at 570 nm (GALBRAITH et al., 1979).

3. SYSTEM DESCRIPTION

HARDWARE

The Leyden Television Analysis System (LEYTAS) consists of a microscope, a Plumbicon TV camera, the Texture Analysis System (TAS, Leitz, West-Germany) a 4 bit grey value memory and a PDP 11-03 computer (VROLIJK et al., 1980)(fig. 1).

The microscope is composed of a Leitz Orthoplan stand with a Leitz 5 μm stepping stage permitting maximum speed of 800 steps per second. The microscope is equipped with a projective rotor to change magnification. Autofocus is carried out by stepping-motor control of the fine focus knob following video analysis of the field. All microscope functions are operated by the computer. For screening purposes a 40x objective is used resulting in a microscopic field available for picture processing of 250x250 μm with a spatial resolution of 1 μm. A detailed description of this automated microscope is given by PLOEM et al.(1979).

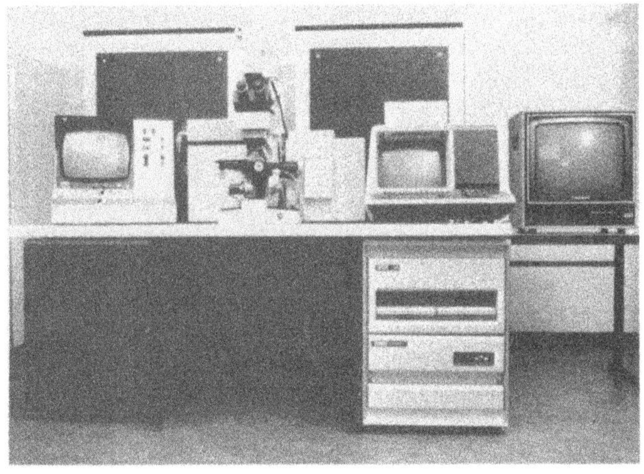

Figure 1 - The Leyden Television Analysis System (LEYTAS) consists of an automated microscope (centre), a Texture Analysis System (TAS, left), a PDP 11-03 computer (below) and a TV monitor for display of grey value memory images (right).

Figure 2 - Displays of the computer terminal at several steps of the analysis.

```
A

WELCOME TO TAS-2
PREPARATION ID:HIJ    OPERATOR ID:02          DATE: 02-JUL-80
1-NUMBER OF FIELDS/LINE:     40     5-FILE NUMBER(FIRST): 1
2-NUMBER OF LINES:           40     6-EVALUATION SET:     2
3-MAXIMUM NUMBER OF ALARMS:  99     7-CRITERIUM SET A:    5
4-FOCUS FREQUENCY:            5     8-CRITERIUM SET B:    0
FIELDNUMBER:                        NUMBER OF EPITHELIAL:
NUMBER OF ALARMS:                   NUMBER OF LEUKOCYTES:
CELL:     OVER:     GROU:     DIRT:     PLAS:
ENTER < CR > TO ACTIVATE SCREENING
```

```
B

WELCOME TO TAS-2
PREPARATION ID:       OPERATOR ID:            DATE:
1-NUMBER OF FIELDS/LINE:            5-FILE NUMBER(FIRST):
2-NUMBER OF LINES:                  6-EVALUATION SET:
3-MAXIMUM NUMBER OF ALARMS:         7-CRITERIUM SET A:
4-FOCUS FREQUENCY:                  8-CRITERIUM SET B:
FIELDNUMBER:                        NUMBER OF EPITHELIAL:
NUMBER OF ALARMS:                   NUMBER OF LEUKOCYTES:
CELL:     OVER:     GROU:     DIRT:     PLAS:
PLEASE ENTER PREPARATION ID: _
```

```
C

MEMORY DISPLAY
PREPARATION ID:HIJ    OPERATOR ID:02          DATE: 02-JUL-80
1-NUMBER OF FIELDS/LINE:     40     5-FILE NUMBER(FIRST): 1
2-NUMBER OF LINES:           40     6-EVALUATION SET:     2
3-MAXIMUM NUMBER OF ALARMS:  99     7-CRITERIUM SET A:    5
4-FOCUS FREQUENCY:            5     8-CRITERIUM SET B:    0
FIELDNUMBER:               1600     NUMBER OF EPITHELIAL: 24518
NUMBER OF ALARMS:            45     NUMBER OF LEUKOCYTES: 10357
CELL:     OVER:     GROU:     DIRT:     PLAS:
RESULTS OF AUTOMATED SCREENING; SYSTEM WAITS FOR INTERACTION!
```

```
D

FINAL RESULTS
PREPARATION ID:HIJ    OPERATOR ID:02          DATE: 02-JUL-80
1-NUMBER OF FIELDS/LINE:     40     5-FILE NUMBER(FIRST): 1
2-NUMBER OF LINES:           40     6-EVALUATION SET:     2
3-MAXIMUM NUMBER OF ALARMS:  99     7-CRITERIUM SET A:    5
4-FOCUS FREQUENCY:            5     8-CRITERIUM SET B:    0
FIELDNUMBER:               1600     NUMBER OF EPITHELIAL: 24518
NUMBER OF ALARMS:            45     NUMBER OF LEUKOCYTES: 10357
CELL: 23   OVER: 4   GROU: 4   DIRT: 14   PLAS:
```

a: Start of the program by the display of a simple protocol. b: The analysis characteristics have been determined by the user. c: End of machine analysis; the results are displayed. d: Using rapid visual inspection of alarms stored in grey value memory and displayed on the TV screen; a subdivision has been obtained in 'cells', 'overlaps', 'groups' and 'dirt'.

The image transformations are carried out using the 16 1-bit planes of the TAS in which binary images can be stored. The 4 bit grey value memory serves for storage of detected objects (alarms). Sixteen stored alarms are visualized in one TV display; all other alarms, up to a maximum of 99, are temporarily stored on disk.

The system also permits 8 bit TV scanning at 0.3 μm spatial resolution. These data are stored on disk to allow further software analysis (SMEULDERS et al., 1980). A second minicomputer will be implemented in the near future, permitting software processing of detected objects simultaneously with the screening procedure.

SOFTWARE

Because LEYTAS should be suited not only to programmers but also to cytopathologists and cytotechnologists, a program was developed, written in FORTRAN, which is highly interactive, resulting in the display of the simple protocols on the computer terminal. After starting this program, the computer terminal displays some questions concerning the preparation identification, the number of fields to be analysed etc. (fig. 2a). When these variables are determined (fig. 2b), screening is activated. During the automated screening, the computer terminal permanently displays the number of fields, the number of epithelial cells and the number of leukocytes that have been analysed, as well as the number of alarms that have been detected. These alarms are simultaneously visualized on a separate TV monitor as they are stored in the grey value buffer memory. After machine analysis is completed (fig. 2c), the first 16 alarms are displayed (fig. 5a) and the user can classify all alarms by inspection of the grey value memory (fig. 5a, b, c). After this interactive portion (fig. 2d), which takes about 1 minute per 16 alarms, since they are simultaneously displayed on 1 TV screen, the results are printed. When an alarm classification is not possible on the basis of the image on the TV screen, or when further software analysis has to be performed, the alarms are relocated in the microscope using the computer controlled stepping stage after automatic change of magnification (fig. 6a-e). Although perhaps not directly evident from the photographic reproduction of the TV screen (fig. 5), comparison of visual classification of the TV screen (grey value memory) and the microscopic image showed good accordance in as far as dividing alarms in single epithelial cells, overlapping nuclei, groups of cells and dirt.

IMAGE ANALYSIS PROGRAM

The image analysis routines used for the detection of abnormal cells and rejection of artefacts are based on image transformations which work in parallel on the entire microscopic field. These transformations belong to the field of mathematical morphology as described by Serra (SERRA). All transformations described in this paper were developed by Meyer from the Center of Mathematical Morphology, Fontainebleau, France (MEYER et al., 1980).

A hierarchical tree structure (see fig. 3) is used for the classification of cells. The conclusion as to whether the microscopic field under investigation shall continue in decision tree is based on the results of the transformations which have been performed.

First the nuclear contours are detected by means of a gradient method (fig. 3, step 2). Zones of the gradient which result in a closed contour (fig. 3, step 3 and fig. 4a, b) are further investigated by several combinations of size and intensity (fig. 3, step 5). Those objects which are thus detected (fig. 3, step 7 and fig. 4c) are tested by several artefact rejection routines, primarily based on the shape of the object as it is defined by the skeletonization of its conditional bissectrix (MEYER, 1979; MEYER et al., 1980). Objects which have past the tree are counted as 'alarms' (fig. 4d). After the location of the alarms in the field is determined, they are automatically stored in a 4 bit buffer memory which is visualized permanently during the entire screening procedure. The x and y coordinates of the alarms are stored in the computer to allow relocation in the microscope after machine analysis.

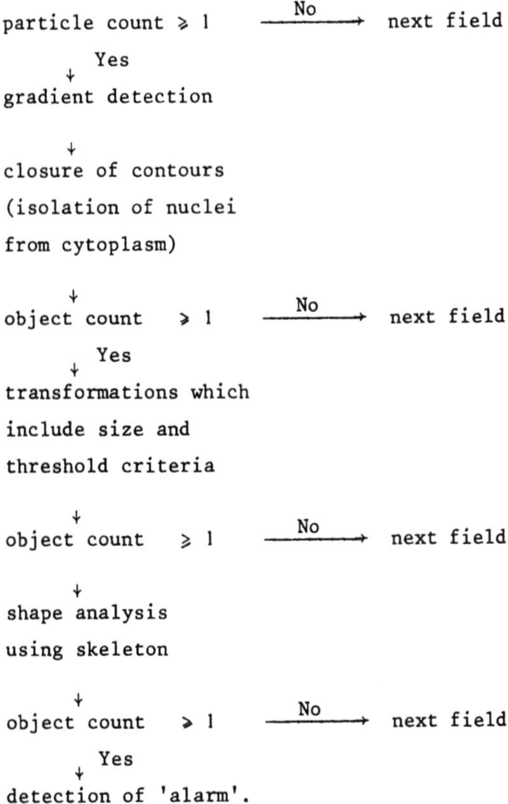

Figure 3 - Hierarchical decision tree through which the image transformations are invoked, performed on entire microscopical fields. Alarms have to survive each set of image transformations.

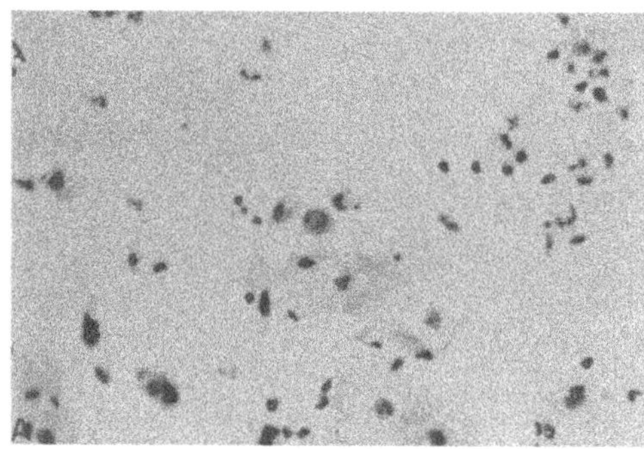

Figure 4 - Results of several image transformations demonstrated on a Papanicolaou stained cervical specimen.

a: The analogue image of a microscopical field displayed on the TAS monitor.

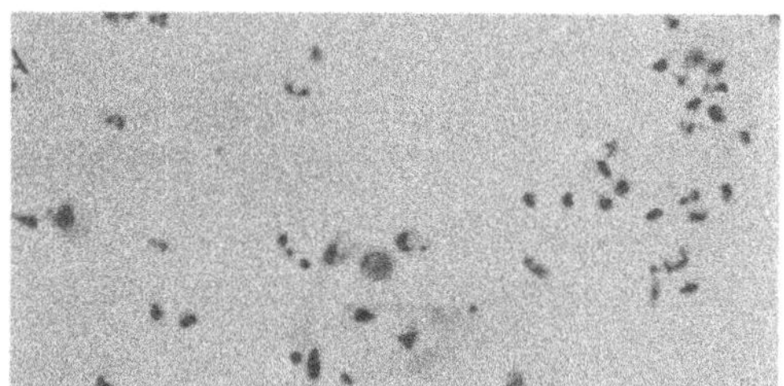

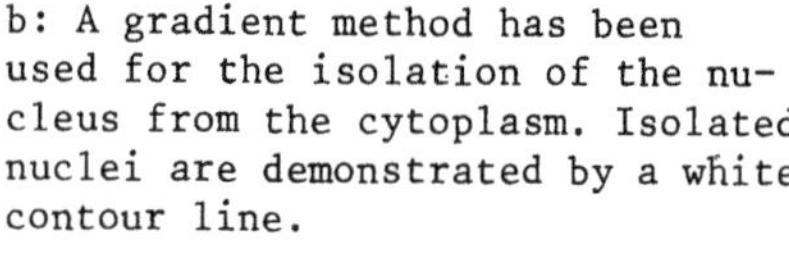

b: A gradient method has been used for the isolation of the nucleus from the cytoplasm. Isolated nuclei are demonstrated by a white contour line.

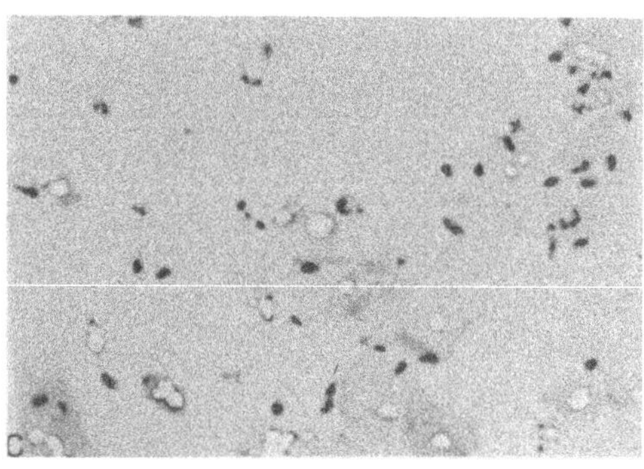

c: The nuclei which have been isolated (white) are further analysed with image transformations, using size and threshold criteria.

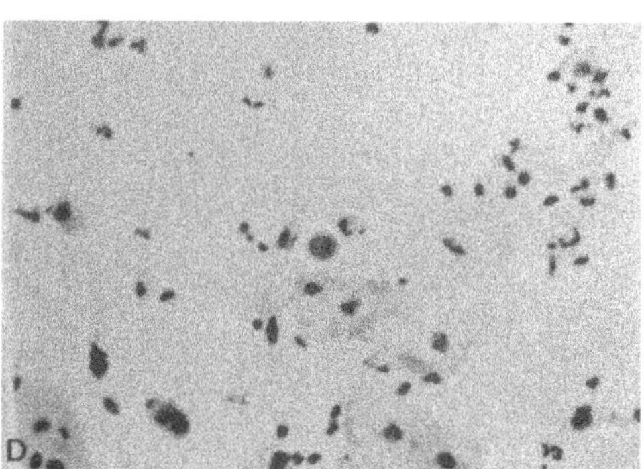

d: Final result of the automated analysis: Only the suspect cell in the center has been detected.

RESULTS

In this preliminary study which has been performed to test the effectiveness of the developed image transformations and the reliability of the automated microscope, a series of 45 Papanicolaou stained cervical specimens was investigated. It consisted of 21 negative specimens, 13 specimens of which the cytological diagnosis was mild dysplasia and 11 positive specimens (severe dysplasia, carcinoma in situ and invasive carcinoma). The cytological diagnoses made on the suspension preparations were all in accordance with the cytological diagnosis of a conventionally made Papanicolaou stained smear and if available with the histological diagnosis.
Further restrictions to admission of specimens to the test were that the preparations had to contain a sufficient number of cells and that fixation and staining were adequate.

For each specimen 1600 fields of 250x250 μm were analysed without human intervention. Focus could be automatically maintained during the entire analysis of the 1600 fields in all 45 specimens due to the robustness of the focus algorithmes and the flatness of cells obtained by centrifugal cytology (DRIEL-KULKER et al., in press).

The results which are obtained by the machine without visual interaction are depicted in table 1 (colums 3, 4, 5 and 6). The subdivision of the alarms in "nuclei" and "artefacts" (table 2) is made by visual inspection of the alarms stored in the grey value memory and displayed on the TV screen. These classifications were checked by automated relocation of the alarms in the microscope. Relocation of the alarms using the computer controlled stepping stage is not sufficiently accurate to locate the alarm exactly in the center of the microscopic field. Comparison with the stored grey value image of the alarm displayed on the TV screen insures that the correct alarm is examined in the Papanicolaou stained microscope image.

An average of 30,000 epithelial cells and 9,000 leukocytes have been analysed per specimen (see table 1). The average number of automatically detected alarms was 36 in the negative specimens, 47 in the specimens diagnosed as mild dysplasia, and 154 in the positive specimens. The number of alarms per 10,000 epithelial cells analysed is given in column 6 of table 1. The mean number of alarms per 10,000 epithelial cells detected in the negative specimens is 15 ± 13 (mean ± S.D.), in the specimens classified as mild dysplasia, this ratio is 27 ± 20, whereas in the positive specimens an average of 36 ± 21 alarms was detected.
Although the average ratio of detected alarms in the positive specimens is higher then the average ratio in negative specimens, there are large variations within each specimen category which are mainly due to the variation in artefacts detected (see table 2).
All the results just described have been obtained by automated analysis without any human visual interaction. It is clear that a diagnosis with the machine alone is not possible at present due to the varying number of alarms caused by artefacts.

At this state of the analysis, the results obtained are shown on the computer terminal (fig. 2c) and the first 16 detected alarms are simultaneously displayed on a separate TV monitor (fig. 5a). The user can request the subsequent display of all alarms stored in the grey value memory and an alarm classification can be given.
In table 2, the alarms are visually subdivided into 'nuclei' (alarms caused by epithelial cell nuclei) and 'artefacts' (all other alarms e.g. caused by groups of leukocytes, bacteria, intensely stained cytoplasm and dirt). The number of non-eliminated artefacts is on the average 31 for all slides under investigation.
The average number of detected nuclei in the negative specimens is 3. In the specimens which were cytologically classified as mild dysplasia, the average number of detected nuclei is 26, whereas in the positive specimens an average of 117 nuclei per specimen were detected after the analysis of 1600 microscopic fields. The mean number of detected nuclei per 10,000 epithelial cells analysed (table 2, column 5) is 1 ± 2 (mean ± S.D.) for negative specimens. In the specimens classified as mild dysplasia, the mean number of detected nuclei is 17 ± 19, whereas in the positive specimens an average of 25 ± 19 nuclei were detected per 10,000 epithelial cells.

specimen number	cytological diagnosis	number of epithelial cells	number of leucocytes	total number of alarms	number of alarms / 10.000 epithelial cells
1	negative	12,395	3,027	23	19
2	negative	7,310	1,327	11	15
3	negative	11,824	1,447	18	15
4	negative	22,547	3,319	14	6
5	negative	101,536	28,564	58	6
6	negative	54,268	21,476	101	19
7	negative	27,822	2,602	10	4
8	negative	80,192	30,087	208	26
9	negative	10,444	2,243	10	10
10	negative	11,120	1,843	15	14
11	negative	12,807	3,815	49	38
12	negative	31,802	13,133	151	48
13	negative	2,337	388	1	4
14	negative	3,752	676	1	3
15	negative	13,521	2,451	6	4
16	negative	7,364	1,113	0	0
17	negative	18,855	5,012	17	9
18	negative	17,598	2,926	16	9
19	negative	12,753	2,018	6	5
20	negative	38,127	6,739	37	10
21	negative	9,247	2,152	10	11
22	mild dysplasia	7,289	1,106	14	19
23	mild dysplasia	62,265	18,864	129	21
24	mild dysplasia	43,295	6,894	36	8
25	mild dysplasia	12,862	1,657	16	12
26	mild dysplasia	44,008	11,335	119	27
27	mild dysplasia	14,332	4,091	46	32
28	mild dysplasia	32,625	5,091	45	14
29	mild dysplasia	4,331	869	18	42
30	mild dysplasia	2,950	458	21	71
31	mild dysplasia	19,852	2,673	3	2
32	mild dysplasia	23,738	5,627	36	15
33	mild dysplasia	12,707	3,682	64	50
34	mild dysplasia	16,512	4,321	70	42
35	severe dysplasia	31,547	5,880	87	28
36	carcinoma in situ	58,618	25,474	168	29
37	carcinoma in situ	122,893	39,278	173	14
38	invasive carcinoma	101,953	37,421	644	63
39	severe dysplasia	13,910	2,525	27	19
40	severe dysplasia	7,893	1,606	45	57
41	invasive carcinoma	41,458	10,437	130	31
42	invasive carcinoma	13,646	3,362	78	57
43	invasive carcinoma	37,756	9,670	99	26
44	severe dysplasia	135,520	39,591	61	5
45	severe dysplasia	27,835	9,452	178	64

Table 1

Results of the automated analysis of 45 cervical specimens by LEYTAS. All results have been obtained by machine analysis only after the investigation of the entire slides of 1600 microscopical fields each.

specimen number	cytological diagnosis	number of alarms caused by dirt	nuclei	number of nuclear alarms / 10.000 epithelial cells
1	negative	20	3	2
2	negative	11	0	0
3	negative	16	2	2
4	negative	9	5	2
5	negative	54	4	0
6	negative	85	16	3
7	negative	6	4	1
8	negative	208	0	0
9	negative	3	7	7
10	negative	13	2	2
11	negative	49	0	0
12	negative	151	0	0
13	negative	0	1	4
14	negative	1	0	0
15	negative	4	2	1
16	negative	0	0	0
17	negative	16	1	1
18	negative	14	2	1
19	negative	4	2	2
20	negative	37	0	0
21	negative	8	2	2
22	mild dysplasia	10	4	5
23	mild dysplasia	60	69	11
24	mild dysplasia	14	22	5
25	mild dysplasia	10	6	5
26	mild dysplasia	52	67	15
27	mild dysplasia	35	11	8
28	mild dysplasia	12	33	10
29	mild dysplasia	2	16	37
30	mild dysplasia	1	20	68
31	mild dysplasia	2	1	1
32	mild dysplasia	20	16	7
33	mild dysplasia	26	38	30
34	mild dysplasia	39	31	19
35	severe dysplasia	31	56	18
36	carcinoma in situ	32	136	23
37	carcinoma in situ	63	110	9
38	invasive carcinoma	46	598	59
39	severe dysplasia	14	13	9
40	severe dysplasia	0	45	57
41	invasive carcinoma	36	94	23
42	invasive carcinoma	22	56	41
43	invasive carcinoma	19	80	21
44	severe dysplasia	20	41	3
45	severe dysplasia	119	59	21

Table 2

Results of the analysis of the same 45 specimens mentioned in table 1. All automatically detected objects (alarms) have been visually subdivided in 'dirt' and 'nuclei' by using the 4 bit image of the alarms as they are stored in the grey value memory and displayed on a TV monitor.

DISCUSSION AND CONCLUSION

For the LEYTAS analysis of cervical specimens, a cell classification strategy is applied in which only a very few false positively classified cells are allowed. With the cell classifiers for Papanicolaou stained specimens that we have available at present, this means that we cannot detect all abnormal cells. This in accordance with the theoretical predictions made by Castleman and White (CASTLEMAN et al., in press) for the efficiency of a cell classifier in automated cervical cytology. The number of detected artefacts must therefore be extremely low in order not to outrange the number of detected abnormal cells.

To evaluate the LEYTAS performance in analysing entire Papanicolaou stained cervical specimens, results can be analysed at three steps of the procedure: directly after the machine analysis has terminated (see table 1); no human interaction has taken place. Due to the large variation in the number of detected alarms within each specimen category, mainly caused by artefacts, no specimen classification can be obtained at this step of the analysis. The number of artefacts, being an average of 31 per specimen, although very low compared to the number of epithelial cells analysed (approx. 30,000) it is still too high to allow a specimen classification without human intervention. For this reason much effort is being made at present to develop additional artefact rejection methods using both TAS algorithmes and software pattern recognition.

By inspection of the grey value memory displayed on a TV screen subsequent visual subdivision of alarms in 'nuclei' and 'artefacts' is possible. This is a rapid procedure since 16 alarms are displayed simultaneously on 1 TV screen (see fig. 5a, b, c). The number of nuclear alarms per 10,000 epithelial cells analysed (table 2, column 5) permits a specimen classification. We have untill now not counted the number of cytomorphologically abnormal cells present in the positive specimens under investigation. However, comparison with a study performed by Barrett et al. (BARRETT et al., 1978), who published a percentage of abnormal cells present ranging from 0.049 to 1.52%, shows that the percentage of detected nuclei in the positive specimens, ranging from 0.03 to 0.59, is slightly lower. If we consider e.g. that 5 detected nuclei per 10,000 epithelial cells is the upper limit in negative specimens and a number higher then 5 may occur only in positive specimens, this would result in 1 false positively classified specimen (nr. 9), whereas 1 positive specimen had been missed (specimen number 44). The specimens which were cytologically classified as mild dysplasia would then be classified as positive and 4 would be negatively classified using this criterium. In the automated analysis of cervical specimens we aimed at the detection of cases with a cytological diagnosis of severe dysplasia, carcinoma in situ or invasive carcinoma. It is of importance, however, that a proportion of the specimens classified as mild dysplasia, is also brought to the attention of the cytologist.

Finally, the nuclear alarms are relocated in the microscope under computer control and a cytomorphological diagnosis of the detected cells can be given. The difficulty of giving a cytomorphological diagnosis based on a single cell must be stressed. We found that it can be especially difficult to distinguish isolated atypical cells as occur in inflammatory specimens, from dysplastic cells. Nevertheless some of the 41 detected nuclei in specimen 44 (see table 2, column 4) were cytomorphologically diagnosed as 'very abnormal'. This specimen had to be classified as a 'false negative' case after the number of detected nuclei per 10,000 epithelial cells was calculated (for this case the ratio was 3). Using visual inspection of automated relocated cells in the microscope, this false negative case could be detected in a relatively easy way. As a result no positive specimen would be missed in this preliminary study in which, however, only a relatively small number of cases was tested.

Although this preliminary study still includes visual spection to arrive at a specimen classification, LEYTAS and the program have been designed in such a way that further software implementations can easily be performed. The possibility to automatically separate detected artefacts from detected epithelial cells at a higher resolution is e.g. at present being studied, as is the possibility to identify

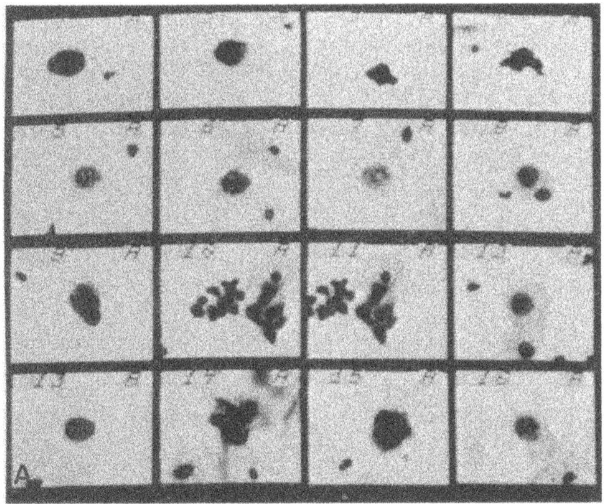

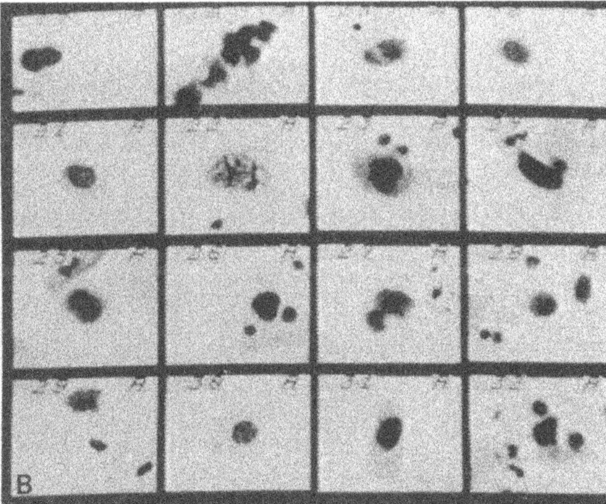

Figure 5a, b, c - After automated screening of an entire slide which was cytologically classified as 'moderate to severe dysplasia', 45 alarms have been detected, stored in the buffer memory and subsequently displayed. Detected non-cellular alarms can thus be visually eliminated.

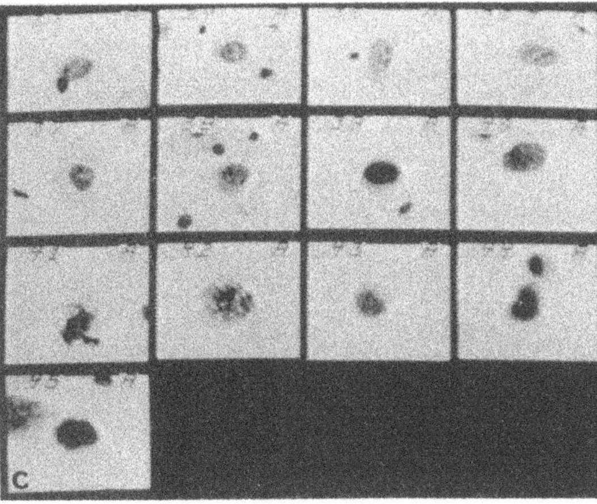

Next page.

Figure 6 - Some of the alarms detected in the specimen mentioned in fig. 5, have been automatically relocated using the computer controlled stepping stage. On the left (fig. 6a, c, e, g) the cellular image is displayed on the TV monitor after automatic change of magnification. On the right (fig. 6b, d, f, h) the Papanicolaou stained microscope image of the same cell is demonstrated.

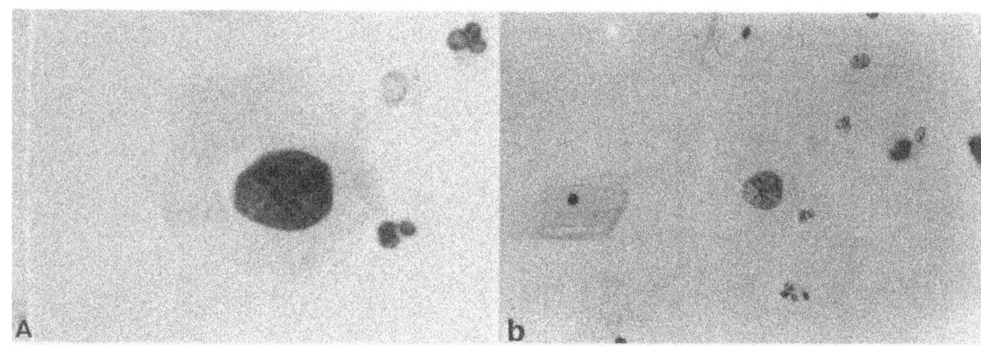

a,b: alarm number 1; abnormal cell.

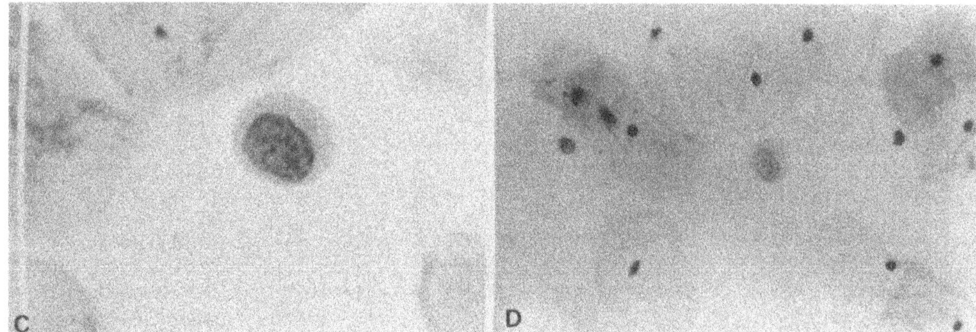

c,d: alarm number 20: abnormal cell.

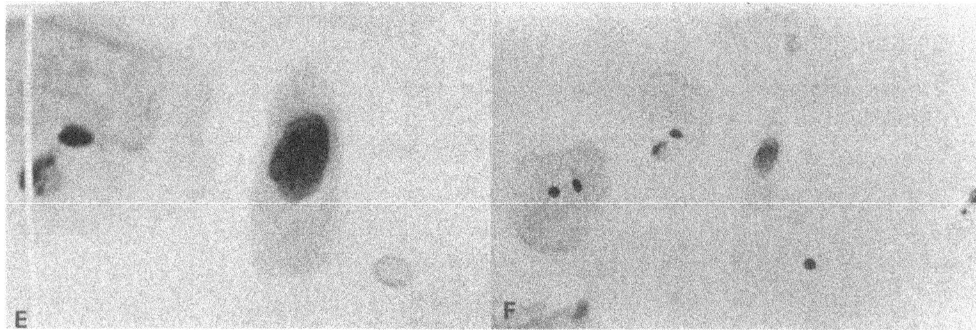

e,f: alarm number 31; abnormal cell.

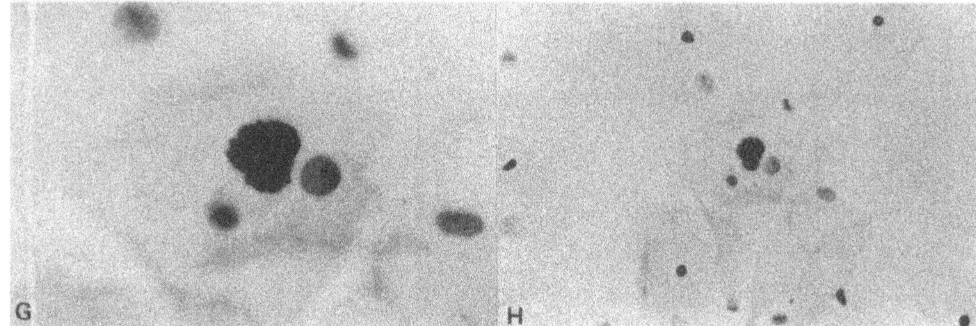

g,h: alarm number 26; an artefact, consisting of a clump of intensely stained dirt lying on top of an epithelial cell, which could not be automatically eliminated by the used image transformations.

different classes of detected epithelial cells. Due to the grey value images displayed on the TV screen and the relocation option such a study can at least technically easily be performed.
The possibility to follow the entire screening procedure visually on a TV monitor and to interprete the detected objects visually during and after the screening constitutes one of the main advantages of LEYTAS. It allows a high interaction of the observer at any stage of the screening program and it also means that LEYTAS can be used for other purposes, such as investigation of aspiration biopsy material. Furthermore we have a direct insight of the kind of detected cells that contribute to the diagnosis.
A disadvantage of LEYTAS in comparison to other systems such as CYBEST (TANAKA et al., 1979) and BIOPEPR (ZAHNISER et al., 1979) is its slowness. The next version of LEYTAS will, however, be much faster.

The used image analysis program was designed in such a way that few artefacts are finally to be detected, meaning that also relatively few abnormal cells are detected. Here the program differs from the programs used in other groups that mostly permit many more artefacts to detect more abnormal cells. We are of the opinion, however, that as long as monolayer specimens contain many artefacts, the main problem consists of rejecting artefacts and not of detecting abnormal cells. We feel therefore, that LEYTAS analysis as used in this study has all possibilities for a complete automated analysis of cellular material.

ACKNOWLEDGEMENT

This study was financially supported by the Bundesministerium für Forschung und Technologie, West Germany.

REFERENCES

ABMAYR, W. ; BURGER, G. and SOOST, H.J., Progress report of the TUDAB project for automated cancer cell detection. J. Histochem. Cytochem., 27 : 604-612 (1979).

AL, I. and PLOEM, J.S., Detection of suspicious cells and rejection of artefacts in cervical cytology using LEYTAS. J. Histochem. Cytochem., 27 ; 629-634 (1979).

BAHR, G.F. ; BIBBO, M. ; OEHME, M. ; PULS, J.H. ; REALE, F.R. and WIED, G.L., An automated device for the production of cell preparations suitable for automatic assessment. Acta Cytol., 22 : 243-249 (1978).

BARRETT, D.L. ; JENSEN, R.H. ; KING, E.B. ; DEAN, P.N. and MAYALL, B., Flow cytometry of human gynecologic specimens using log chromomysin A3 fluorescence and log 90° light scatter. J. Histochem. Cytochem., 27 : 573-578 (1979).

BARRETT, D.L. ; KING, E.B. ; JENSEN, R.H. and MERRILL, J.T., Cytomorphology of gynecologic specimens analyzed and sorted by two-parameter flow cytometry. Acta Cytol., 22 : 7-14 (1978).

CAMBIER, J.L. ; KAY, D.B. and WHEELESS, L.L., A multidimensional slit-scan flow system. J. Histochem. Cytochem., 27 : 321-324 (1979).

CASTLEMAN, K.R. and WHITE, B.S., Optimizing cervical cell classifiers. Analyt. and Quant. Cytol. In Press.

DRIEL-KULKER, A.M.J. van ; MEYER, F. and PLOEM, J.S., Automated analysis of cervical specimens using the TAS. Acta Microscopica, Suppl. 4. Quantitative Image Analysis and Microphotometry. S. Hirzel Verlag Stuttgart (1980).

DRIEL-KULKER, A.M.J. van ; PLOEM-ZAAIJER, J.J. ; ZWAN-VAN DER ZWAN, M. van der and TANKE, H.J., A preparation technique for exfoliated and aspirated cells allowing different staining procedures. Proceedings of Third Intern. Conf. on Automation of Diagnostic Cytology and Cell Image Analysis. Analyt. and Quant. Cytol. In Press

EASON, P.J. and TUCKER, J.H., The preparation of cervical scrape material for automated cytology using gallocyanin chrome-alum stain. J. Histochem. Cytochem., 27 : 25-31 (1979).

GALBRAITH, W. ; MARSHALL, P.N. ; LEE, E.S. and BACUS, J.W., Studies on Papanicolaou staining: I. visible light spectra of stained cervical cells. Analyt. and Quant. Cytol., 1 : 160-168 (1979).

HÖFFKEN, H. ; OTTO, K. and SOOST, H.J., Cytomorphologic results of preparation experiments for monolayer deposition of cervical material. J. Histochem. Cytochem., 27 : 19-24 (1979).

HUSAIN, O.A.N. ; PAGE ROBERTS, B.A. and MILLET, J.A., A sample preparation for automated cervical cancer screening. Acta Cytol., 22 : 15-21 (1978).

LEIF, R.C. ; GALL, S. ; DUNLAP, L.A. ; RAILEY, C. ; ZUCKER, R.M. and LEIF, S.B., Centrifugal cytology in the preparation of fixed stained dispersions of gynecological cells. Acta Cytol., 19, 159-168 (1975).

LEIF, R.C. ; NORDQVIST, S. ; CLAY, S. ; CAYER, M. ; INGRAM, D. ; CAMERON, B.F. ; BOBBIT, D. ; GADDIS, R. ; LEIF, S.B. and CABANAS, A., A procedure for dissociating ayre scrape samples. J. Histochem. Cytochem., 25 : 525-537 (1977).

MEYER, F., Interactive image transformations for an automatic screening of cervical smears. J. Histochem. Cytochem., 27 : 128-135 (1979).

MEYER, F. and DRIEL-KULKER, A.M.J. van, Automatic screening of Papanicolaou stained cervical smears with the TAS. Acta Microscopica. Suppl. 4. Quantitative Image Analysis and Microphotometry. S. Hirzel Verlag, Stuttgart (1980).

OTTO, K. ; HÖFFKEN, H. and SOOST, H.J., Sedimentation velocity separation: A preparation method for cervical samples. J. Histochem. Cytochem., 27 : 14-18 (1979).

PLOEM, J.S. ; VERWOERD, N. ; BONNET, J. and KOPER, G., An automated microscope for quantitative cytology combining television image analysis and stage scanning microphotometry. J. Histochem. Cytochem., 27 : 136-143 (1979).

READ, J.S. ; BOROVEC, R.T. ; BARTELS, P.H. ; BIBBO, M. ; PULS, J.H. ; REALE, V.R. ; TAYLOR, J. and WIED, G.L., A fast image processor for locating cell nuclei in uterine specimens. Proceedings of the Second Internat. Conf. on the Automation of Cancer Cytology and Cell Image Analysis. Eds. N.J. Pressman and G.L. Wied (1979).

ROSENTHAL, D.L. ; STERN, E. ; LATCHIE, C.Mc. ; WU, A. ; LABASSE, L.D. ; WALL, R. and CASTLEMAN, K.R., A simple method of producing a monolayer of cervical cells for digital image processing. Analyt. and Quant. Cytol., 1 : 84 (1979).

SERRA, J., Lectures on image analysis by mathematical morphology. Fontainebleau, France.

SMEULDERS, A.M.J. ; LEYTE-VELDSTRA, L. ; DRIEL-KULKER, A.M.J. van ; PLOEM, J.S. and CORNELISSE, C.J., Towards real time cell recognition of breast and cervical samples of LEYTAS preselected events. Submitted for publication. Analyt. and Quant. Cytol.

STÖHR, M. and GOERTTLER, K., The Heidelberg flow analyzer and sorter (HEIFAS) approach on the prescreening of uterine cancer. J. Histochem. Cytochem., 27 : 564-566 (1979).

TANAKA, N. ; IKEDA, H. ; UENO, T. ; MUKAWA, A. and KAMITSUMA, K., Field test and experimental use of CYBEST model 2 for practical gynecologic mass screening. Analyt. and Quant. Cytol., 1 : 122-126 (1979).

TANKE, H.J. ; INGEN, E.M. van and PLOEM, J.S., Acriflavine-Feulgen stilbene (AFS) staining: a procedure for automated cervical cytology with a television based system (LEYTAS). J. Histochem. Cytochem., 27 : 84-86 (1979).

TUCKER, J.H., An image analysis system for cervical cytology automation using nuclear DNA content. J. Histochem. Cytochem., 27 : 613-620 (1979).

VROLIJK, J. ; PEARSON, P.L. and PLOEM, J.S., LEYTAS, a system for the processing of microscopic images. Analyt. and Quant. Cytol., 2 : 41-48 (1980)

WOLLEY, R.C. ; HERZ, F. ; DEMBITZER, H.M. ; SCHREIBER, K. and KOSS, L.G., The monodisperse cervical smear. Analyt. and Quant. Cytol., 1 : 43-49 (1979).

ZAHNISER, D.J. ; OUD, P.S. ; RAAIJMAKERS, M.C.T. ; VOOYS, B.P. and WALLE, R.T. van de, Biopepr: A system for the automatic prescreening of cervical smears. J. Histochem. Cytochem., 27 : 635-641 (1979).

RECOGNITION AND QUANTIFICATION OF COMPLEX HISTOLOGICAL TISSUES : APPLICATIONS TO NERVOUS TISSUES

by

J.-C. BISCONTE, V. VON HAGEN, R. GARDETTE, C. SAVY
Laboratoire de Neurobiologie Quantitative
UER Expérimentale de Santé, Médecine et Biologie Humaine
74, rue Marcel Cachin
93012 BOBIGNY CEDEX (France)

ABSTRACT

An overview of image analysis applications by video systems is presented. The analysis of histological sections involves specific problems such as segmentation, large amounts of information, transformation from to 2 to 3 D (stereology). The device including a TAS (Leitz) interfaced to a PDP 11-34 computer is used in two applications to the nervous system : the analysis of trigeminal ganglionic sections and the quantification of cerebellar structures. In the first case, only the basic image transformation capabilities of the TAS are used. In the second one, a statistical method of analysis of grey-level histograms had to be developed in order to automatically recognize the various cerebellar zones. The advantages of both methods are discussed. Image analysis will be soon applied more generally to histology. Indeed, tissue sections provide essential architecture information often difficult to apprehend by traditional methods.

1. INTRODUCTION

Current techniques in biomedical image analysis by TV camera are now giving satisfactory results in certain biologic applications particularly those related to the study of blood (Ingram and Preston, 1970). Since these tissues include essentially well-separated cellular elements that also possess morphological and staining characteristics which are particularly appropriate to such analyses, it is easy to see why the first clinical applications were developed in this area. In the last few years cost effective instruments (LARC, Abbot 500, Diff 3, HEMATRAC, etc.) have become standard hospital equipment. They are completely automatic even with respect to the preparation and staining of tissue samples under rigorously standard conditions. Although it is tempting to speculate on what the next stages will be in the vast domain of biomedical image processing trends, we will only develop in this article those applications relating to the study of cells and tissues *in vivo*.

CURRENT TRENDS

As the many different lectures of this seminar have shown, certain areas of biomedical image processing are being more intensively explored than others. The first, automatic karyotyping, has long awaited the development of instrumentation applicable to routine examinations. Although there now exist partial solutions to the problem, the investment required to make instrumentation effective appears to be too costly for the results so far obtained (Castleman and Melynk, 1976 ; Vrolijk et al., 1980). The second area however shows more immediate promise : the detection of cancerous cells of the epithelium, particularly of the cervix (Driel et al., 1980). It is certain that the development of instrumentation and algorithms for exfoliative cell analysis will lead to efficient screening procedures for high-risk populations. However, the inherent problems have not been entirely resolved. Processing time is still unwieldy and artifacts as well as false negatives and false positives are still a matter of concern. To these problems must be added sociological, economic and methodological considerations. But none of these problems are considered to be insoluble and we expect the development of cost effective instrumentation in the near future. Moreover, it is likely that such instrumentation can be adapted to other exfoliative cancers such as the trachia and bladder (Liedtke and Aeikens, 1980).

There is a field that was not discussed at the symposium but which is also an important application of TV image processing : the analysis of bacterial colonies (Kaminska et al., 1978). In this case we can process an automatic determination of the antibiogram as well as automatic studies of toxicities (mutagenic tests). Here the problem is relatively simple and reduces to the study of the size and densities of tens, hundreds and even thousands of colonies dispersed in Petri dishes (Grimm et al., 1979).

Another field presently being explored is the analysis of the cell constituents of bone marrow. In this case the difficulty arises from the marked variability of the hemopoietic material. The images to be digitized consist of cellular elements that are relatively well-separated but which combine 30 or so different cell types. Furthermore, these cell types must be grouped as a function of the cell cycle (Brenner et al., 1977 ; Adelh et al., 1978).

There is no doubt that image analysis will in future deal with material of a much more complex nature such as living cells and histological sections. Present cell culture methods, whether relating to prokaryotes or eukaryotes are developing rapidly. The applications of real time image analysis to cell culture material can lead to the determination of toxicity parameters. But more generally, they can be applied to cell to cell and cell to medium interactions, and even the characteristics of spontaneous motility (i.e. spermatozoïds, Schoevaert and David, 1979) can be studied (Bell et al., 1979). It is obvious that the classical methods of time lapse cinematography are both time consuming and complex and can only relate to a single microscopic field. Such images are difficult to analyse sequentially based on elementary film images.

In our laboratory, we have recently shown that image analysis can be carried out in real time with preparations maintained under constant conditions (Bisconte and Margules, 1979). We even showed that it was possible to extract results from 30 fields sampled every five minutes in sequential form. The object of these studies was to observe the phenomena of cellular aggregation by measuring the number of clumps of the different size categories as a function of time. More recently we showed that the T.A.S. coupled to a PDP-11 allowed the reconstruction of the trajectory of one or several isolated cells located in a microscopic field. The preliminary findings underline the necessity of innovating new systems of optic illumination since living cells obviously cannot be stained. Moreover, an increase in the memory capacity of the cell analyser hardware is essential for such complex studies. Recent advances in cellular hybridization techniques make it possible to develop cloned cultures. Such monoclonal material will be of considerable importance as an exploratory biological and therapeutic tool in the very near future. This again underlines the importance of automatic culture analysis (Monk et al., 1973).

If we now consider histological sections, we are led to study tissues that either cannot be dissociated, such as bone, or should not be, such as nervous tissue, because the tissue architecture itself is meaningful. The use of currently available image analysers therefore poses problems very different from those already mentioned. In general the images are complex and can be divided into at least 4 sub-categories which constitute the whole image :

- cells of variable types (differing in size and stain affinity),
- fibers (neural, connective, muscular) and walls,
- vessels,
- spaces (ventricles).

In each of these cases one wishes to obtain information representative of an organ from a histological section which must have a thickness of about 10 µm. Thus we must deal with a stereological effect. But a section can only provide partial and not necessarily representative information. Thus we are obliged to formulate suppositions with respect to the size and the initial characteristics of the objects. For example, let us consider the texture of the chromatin of a cell sectioned at different levels. The chromatin will have a very different aspect depending on the level of the cut.

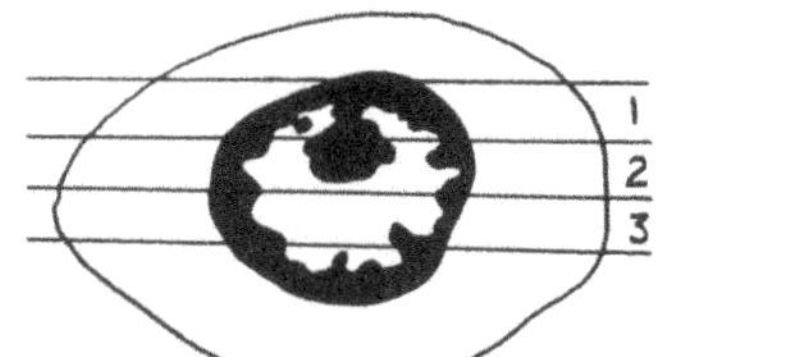

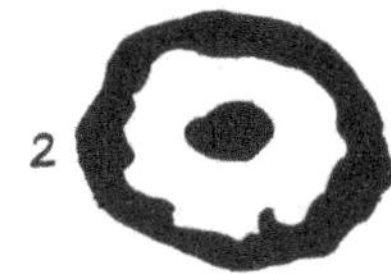

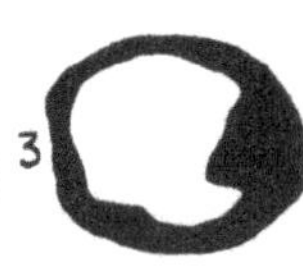

For the architecturally complex organs, analyses based on sampling areas of one section is problematic, although a priori the process is possible for smears. Thus it is necessary to correlate the results of an analysis with the true position of the object within the section. From these observations it should be apparent that image analysis will constitute an indispensable method for complex tissues. This is not the case for the analysis of smears which can, at least in part, be replaced by flow cytometry (Horan and Wheeless, 1977). It is apparent that this technique can be used to analyse complex tissue which has been dissociated but in this case the cellular architecture will have been destroyed.

Future applications of complex tissue analysis are extremely varied, ranging from the analysis of biopsy sections to the examination of post mortem material, without excluding many basic biomedical problems in research. The inherent difficulties of complex tissue image analysis are nevertheless considerable. The most fundamental of these is related to the difficulty in obtaining satisfactory image segmentation by the use of grey level thresholding procedures (nervous system, kidneys, pancreas, epithelia : Meyer, 1977 ; Bradbury, 1978). If the tissue sample is large, the memory capacity of present image analysers is quickly exceeded and auxillary memories must be added, particularly if it is necessary to reconstruct the organ from appropriately sampled sections (Underwood, 1970 ; Teckhans et al., 1980).

We shall present two different approaches to this type of problem in neurobiology. The first one involves the analysis of ganglionic sections. This tissue is relatively easy to analyse since the organs are small and are composed of only two categories of objects : cells and fibers. The approach used is classic and only requires the memory capacity of the T.A.S. The second application, on the other hand, is far more ambitious because it involves the automatic analysis of a central nervous system structure, the cerebellum.

For this study the T.A.S. is only used to digitize the image. The data thus obtained are then analysed by statistical programs run on the PDP-11. It is a basic premise that in a highly organized tissue each microscopic field has a characteristic signature related to a specific distribution of cells, fibers, intercellular spaces etc. This signature is already expressed in a simple densitometric analysis since we know that each class of objects is characterized by a spectrum of specific densities (deeply staining nuclei, moderately grey cytoplasm, pale cell spaces). This method is related to general methods used for the identification of earth resources.

II. AUTOMATED MORPHOMETRIC STUDY OF MOUSE TRIGEMINAL GANGLION AFTER SENSORY RECEPTOR DESTRUCTION (Savy et al., in press)

The model chosen is that of Van der Loos and Woolsey (1979) which consists in a deafferentation by coagulation of the vibrissae follicles of the muzzle of new born mice. The first relay studied in this model is the trigeminal ganglion where the peripheral sensorial neurons whose axons innervate the vibrissae are located. The trigeminal ganglion has two parts : the ophthalmomaxillary rostral part and the caudal which is common to the ophthalmomaxillary branch and the mandibular branch. While classical histological examination of serial sections of the trigeminal ganglion gives a general idea of neural depletion after vibrissae follicle destruction, morphometric methods are needed to make these studies quantitative and more objective. Therefore, the purpose of the present study is to quantify the effects of sensory receptor destruction on elements of the peripheral nervous system.

All the vibrissae follicles of newborn mice were destroyed on one side of the muzzle. The other side and its trigeminal relay were used as the control. Histological serial sections of both trigeminals were prepared and stained with cresyl violet. Every tenth section was retained for analysis, giving a total of about 100 sections per mouse : the total ganglionic section area and the total surface occupied by neuronal cell bodies were measured (Fig. 1). The total ganglionic section area was delineated by light pen initially in order to estimate digitalization error. Neuronal cell body area was measured by grey level detection : cell bodies stain more intensely than other ganglionic elements such as nerve fibers. The measurement of the surface occupied by the neuronal bodies is global and includes the satellite cells which surround the neurons. The measurements obtained by this method permitted the calculation of the respective volumes of the different parts of the ganglion as well as their constituents, such as the ophthalmomaxillary part which is reduced both longitudinally and transversally. The reduction of the total ganglionic section area is significant at all levels with respect to the control side. The latter was evaluated by the difference between the total ganglionic surface and that occupied by the cell bodies.

For the calculation of the volumes, the surface measurements were multiplied by the section thickness (7.5 μm) ; (Davies, 1978 ; Hamburger, 1934 ; Hendry, 1976) and by the number of sections contained in the interval between the sections analysed. The average results for 5 mice sacrified at 2 months show that there is a decrease of 43 % in the total volume of the ganglion on the deafferented side with respect to the control, and a reduction of 61.5 % in its ophthalmomaxillary part and of 24 % in its common part. The total volume occupied by the neuronal cell bodies in the ganglion is diminished by 55 % in the ophthalmomaxillary part of the ganglion while it is unchanged in the common part. Thus, we confirmed that the neurons whose axons innervate the vibrissae are exclusively situated in the ophthalmomaxillary part of the ganglion as suggested by Mazza and Dixon (1972), Zucker and Welker (1969) and Farkas-Bargeton et al., (1980). We also found that the volume occupied by the nerve fibers was reduced by 64.5 % in the ophthalmomaxillary part of the ganglion and by 28 % in the common part. The ophthalmomaxillary part is reduced both longitudinally and transversally. The reduction of the total ganglionic surface is significant at all levels with respect to the control side. The difference in surfaces between the control and experimental side occupied by the neuronal cell bodies is clearly significant only in the central zone of the ophthalmomaxillary part of the ganglion. On the other hand, the surface occupied by the nerve fibers was significantly decreased in a homogeneous fashion through the whole length of the ganglion (fig. 2). We should note that the reduction of measured surfaces and calculated volumes of the neuronal cell bodies and nerve fibers observed for the denervated side can be explained, in part, by a loss in the number of neurons as was verified by counting the latter at different levels of sections in 3 mice. We found the neuronal loss to be on the order of 36.5 %. However, the reduction in the size of certain neurons cannot be excluded.

We can conclude by pointing out that the quantitative histological study of this model allowed us to show that destruction of the peripheral receptor in the immature animal provokes the death of the sensory neurons situated in the corresponding ganglion. Studies in progress use more automated methods and focus on the quantitative morphometry of the proximal and distal portions of the nerve and its relays in the C.N.S.

III. AUTOMATIC QUANTIFICATION OF MOUSE CEREBELLUM (Gardette et al., in press)

The central nervous system of all superior organisms has one of the most complex histological organizations of all tissues. It is composed of a large number of varied regions, each having its own specific function, and the equilibrium of its functions is dependant on the interaction between the different regions. A quantitative variation in a particular nervous zone not only induces alterations in the functioning of that zone, but also in other nervous structures connected to it. Alterations at the histological level are in relation with those at the level of the integration of higher functions. For instance, they can involve an abnormal behaviour of the animal as is the case for most of the neurological mutants of the mouse (Sidman et al., 1965). This is why the precise quantification of the set of structures composing the central nervous system is fundamentally important.

By training and experience, a biologist can recognize a particular nervous zone, while an image analyser still cannot (for a review concerning image analysis applied to the central nervous system, see Miller et al., 1979). Moreover, the advantage in having an automatic quantification instrument is its rapidity and reliability. Thus it is necessary to "teach" the analyser to recognize the exact nature of the microscopic field of a complex nervous structure during quantification.

As initial step, we chose a nervous structure whose architecture was well-known so that we could study the problem of automatic recognition. We have shown that the cerebellum can be described as being composed of a maximum of 9 zones arranged in regular arrays (Gardette, 1980). Some of these zones can be considered as cellularly homogeneous. These are : the outside of the section (index 1), the molecular layer (index 4), the granular cell layer (index 6), the white matter (index 8), and the deep cerebellar nuclei (index 9). The other layers are mixed zones formed by the association of two or three of the aforementioned homogeneous zones. The Purkinje cells situated on the border between the molecular layer and the granular cell layer cannot be separated automatically at present from the other cellular components and have to be included in the granular cell layer.

A densitometric study carried out on each of these zones on a learning sample of 490 microscopic fields has shown that each characteristic zone generated a typical histogram of areas as a function of grey levels (Gardette et al., in press). The learning procedure (Mallet et al., 1980) permits the generation of 9 mean histograms that are stored in the PDP 11-34 interfaced to the TAS. The histogram of each new field (actual field) analysed is compared to the 9 mean histograms as these fields are acquired and is classed automatically (predicted field). This operation was first carried out on the learning sample and then on a test sample of the 204 fields for which the histograms had not been integrated into the mean histograms stored in memory. The results obtained are presented in tables IIIa and IIIb.

After automatic recognition of the microscopic field under study, an automatic quantification can only be carried out on the pure cellular components. Thus, in the case of the pure cerebellar zones the quantification step can be performed directly. But for the mixed zones it is first necessary to separate the different fractions corresponding to pure cellular zones by a procedure of histogram decomposition. An illustration of this method is presented in Figure 3. From an index 5 field it is thus possible to find the respective percentages of the indices 4 and 6 zones including it. We have some reason to think that the classification percentages (respectively 70 % and 72 % for the test samples) can be improved by the use of complementary parameters such as the distribution of the cells in the field.

Automatic quantification is based on the same rules of apprenticeship recognition and comparison of the histograms. A preliminary study carried out on the molecular layer has shown a difference of less than 2 % between manual and automatic quantification (table IV). This leads us to expect that a method will be shortly developed which will be both reliable and cost effective.

IV. DISCUSSION AND CONCLUSION

The two examples given here illustrate two very different strategies for the analysis of histological sections : the first consists in using the normal capacity of the T.A.S., that is to say thresholding by grey level, image transformation, individual analysis, parametrisation and classification. User interaction is indispensable to correct imperfections in segmentation functions. This interaction is acceptable because the surface studied is small. Although the procedure is slow, it does yield precise results. The second is based on a statistical analytic procedure and is on the contrary very rapid since a fraction of a second is needed to obtain the field histogram. Statistical analysis and automatic classification of the 20 dimension histograms so obtained is more time consuming. But this step can be achieved much faster when using a computer as we do with the PDP 11-34. However, even if it is surprising that so much information from simple grey level histograms can be obtained, all ambiguities in histological zone identification cannot be resolved by these methods. The histogram analysis can be greatly improved by apprenticeship and it is clear that important progress in this area can be expected.

A knowledge of even the approximative coordinates of the fields already explored reduces uncertainties after histogram analysis. It is also possible to extract essential complementary information such as the spectral analysis of colour, "texture" (cytoarchitecture) and above all essential information related to the presence of specific radioactive or fluorescent markers. The latter provide dynamic data (tritiated thymidine and deoxyglucose detected by autoradiography) or functional data (detection of specificity of the membrane, or neuromediators, hormones, etc.).

Under these conditions it is probable that the initial inconvenience of working with serial sections can become an enormous advantage. In fact the use of two or several neighbouring sections permits the application of different complementary stains. This approach requires the recombination of data from different sections. For these applications to histology an effort is necessary to achieve total automatization : contouring of the organ, automatic switching of microscope objectives – without altering the coordinates, recombination of data from the analysis of neighbouring sections, etc. One may speculate that the considerable progress already achieved in earth resource survey science can now be used profitably in biomedical research. Similarly it will be necessary to use methods of geometric correction and interpolation which, though relatively classic, are still slow. These methods can be used to correct tissue deformation introduced by the microtome, for example, while interpolation can be used to reconstruct an organ from the serial sections (Nach, 1976 ; Teckhans et al., 1980). If it appears at present that these methods need computers which are too large and complex, this will not necessarily be the case in the near future, if we are to judge from the pace of current advances in computer technology (Strome and Goodenough, 1978).

ACKNOWLEDGEMENTS

This work has been supported by a C.N.R.S. grant and was carried out with the technical help of S. Margules, X. Albe and R. Joubert.

REFERENCES

Adelh, D., Garbay, C., Brugal, G. and Veillon, F. : Etude et réalisation d'une méthode automatique de reconnaissance de types cellulaires dans les tissus hématopoïétiques. Reconnaissance des formes et traitement des images, IRIA ed., 863-871 (1978).

Bell, E., Levinstone, D., Sher, S., March, L., Merill, C., Young, I. and Eden, M. : An interactive computer system for the analysis of cell lineages. J. Histochem. Cytochem. 27, 458-462 (1979).

Bisconte, J.C. and Margules, S. : Real-time continuous quantitative analysis of cultured living cells. Mikroskopie (in press).

Bradbury, S. : Microspical image analysis : problems and approaches. J. Microsc., 115, 137-150 (1978).

Brenner, J.F., Necheles, T.F., Bonacossa, I.A., Fristensky, R., Weintraub, B.A. and Neurath, P.W. : Scene segmentation techniques for the analysis of routine bone marrow smears from acute lymphoblastic Leukemia patients. J. Histochem. Cytochem. 25, 601-613 (1977).

Castleman, K.R. and Melynk, J.H. : An automatic system for chromosome analysis. Final Report JPL, 5040-30 (1976).

Davies, D.C. : Neuronal numbers in the superior cervical ganglion of the neonatal rat. J. Anat., 27, 43-51 (1978).

Driel, A.M.J. van, Meyer, F. and Ploem, J.S. : Automated analysis of cervical specimens using the T.A.S. Microsc. Acta, Suppl. 4, 73-81 (1980).

Farkas-Bargeton, E., Savy, C., Verney, C., Hopkins, Y. and Verley, R. : A quantitative and qualitative study of mice trigeminal ganglion and nerve after destruction of vibrissae follicles since birth. Acta Neuropath., suppl VII (in press).

Gardette, R. : Chronoarchitectonie par radioautographie et quantification par analyse d'images dans le Système Nerveux Central de la souris normale et de la souris mutante Staggerer. Doctorat de 3ème Cycle, Paris (1980).

Gardette, R., Mallet, A. and Bisconte, J.C. : Automatic recognition of nervous structures by image analysis. A pattern recognition method applied to the study of mouse cerebellum. J. Neuroscience Methods (in press).

Grimm, J., Bhend, H., Lüthy, R. and Siegenthaler, W. : On-line measurement of antibiotic concentrations. Microsc. Acta, Suppl. 3, 179-184 (1979).

Hamburger, V. : The effects of wing bud extirpation on the development of the central nervous system in the chick embryo. J. Exp. Zool., 68, 449-494 (1934).

Hendry, I.A. : A method to correct adequately for the changes in neuronal size when estimating neuronal numbers after nerve growth treatment. J. Neurocytol., 5, 337-349 (1976).

Horan, P.K. and Wheeless, L.L. : Quantitative single cell analysis and sorting. Science, 198, 149 (1977).

Ingram, M. and Preston, K. : Automatic analysis of blood cells. Scientific Americain, 223, 72 (1970).

Kaminska, G., Kaminski, M., Blaton, O., Szymkowiah, W. and Ostrowski, K. : One-step method for direct, quick and accurate measurement of three different migration inhibition test modifications using the automatic image analyser Quantimet B. Archiv. Immunol, 26, 401-405 (1978).

Liedtke, C.E. and Aeikens, B. : The segmentation of urinary cells – a first step in the automated processing in urine cytology. Microsc. Acta, Suppl. 4, 230-234 (1980).

Mallet, A., Gardette, R., Nakache, J.P., Steimer, J.L., Boisvieux, J.F. and Bisconte, J.C. : Automatic recognition and quantitative analysis of cerebellum densitometric patterns. Medinfo 1980, Tokyo, (1980).

Mazza, J.P. and Dixon, A.D. : A histological study of chromatolytic cell groups in the trigeminal ganglion of the rat. Archs Oral Biol., 17, 377-387 (1972).

Meyer, F. : Contrast features extraction. Special issues of practical metallography, Vol. 8, Riederer Verlag GmbH, Stuttgart (1977).

Miller, A.K.H., Alston, R.L. and Corsellis, J.A.N. : The practical application of image analysing systems to neuropathology : principles and possible scopes. In Recent advances in Neuropathology. (Smith, W.T. and Cavanagh, J.B., eds), Vol. 1, Churchill, Livingstone, pp 113-128, (1979).

Monk, I.B., Malone, J.F., Smith, D.A. and Orr, J.S. : The use of a television image analysis system to determine the number and size distribution of mammalian cell clones. Brit. J. Radiol., 46, 388 (1973).

Nach, M.L. : Final report on image registration research. Computer Science Corporation (1976).

Savy, C., Margules, S., Farkas-Bargeton, E. and Verley, R. : A morphometric study of mice trigeminal ganglion after unilateral destruction of vibrissae follicles at birth. Brain Research (in press).

Schoevaert-Brossault, D. and David, G. : Reconnaissance et classification automatique des spermatozoïdes humains. 2ème Congrès AFCET-IRIA, 3, 34-41 (1979).

Sidman, R.L., Green, M.C. and Appel, S.H. : Catalogue of the neurological mutants of the mouse. Harvard University Press, Cambridge, Mass. (1965).

Strome, W.M. and Goodenough, D.G. : The use of array processors in image analysis. In Machine-aided image analysis, Gardner ed., Institute of Physics publisher, Bristol (1978).

Teckhans, L., Lübbers, D.W. and Rager, G. : A new method of three-dimensional reconstruction of complicated structures by combining an automatic and interactive computer technique. Microsc. Acta., Suppl. 4 (1980).

Underwood, E.E. : Quantitative stereology, Addison Wesley Publishing Company, Reading-Massachusetts, (1970).

Van der Loos, H. and Woosley, T.A. : Somato-sensory cortex : structural alterations following early injury to sence organs. Science, 395-398 (1979).

Vrolijk, J., Ten Brinke, H., Ploem, J.S., and Pearson, P.L. : Video techniques applied to chromosome analysis. Microsc. Acta, Suppl. 4, 108-115 (1980).

Zucker, E. and Welker, W.H. : Coding of somatic sensory input by vibrissae neurons in the rat's trigeminal ganglion. Brain Research, 12, 138-156 (1969).

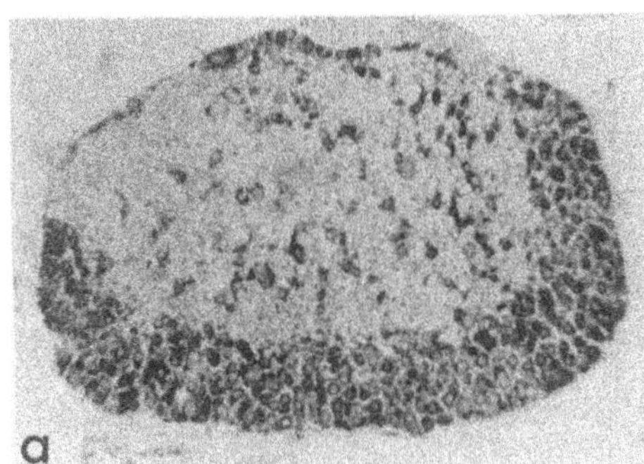

Fig. 1

a. Transverse section of trigeminal ganglion.

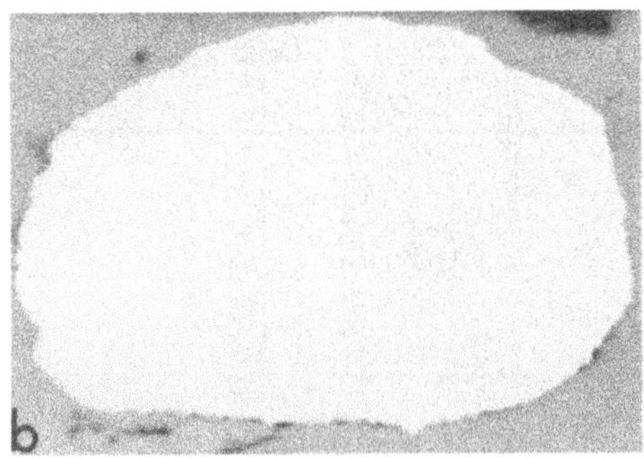

b. Detection of the total ganglionic section area.

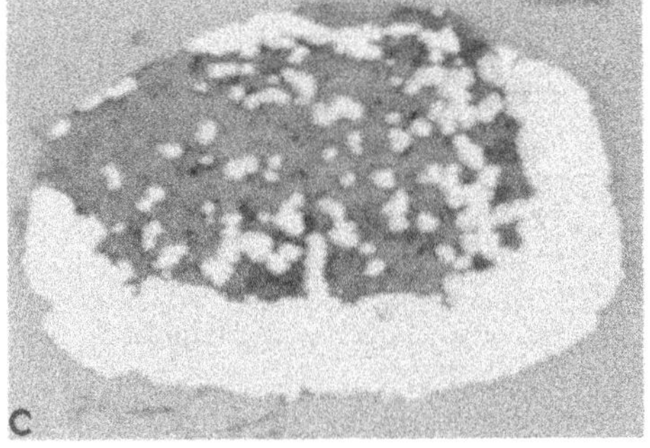

c. Detection of the neuronal cell bodies area.

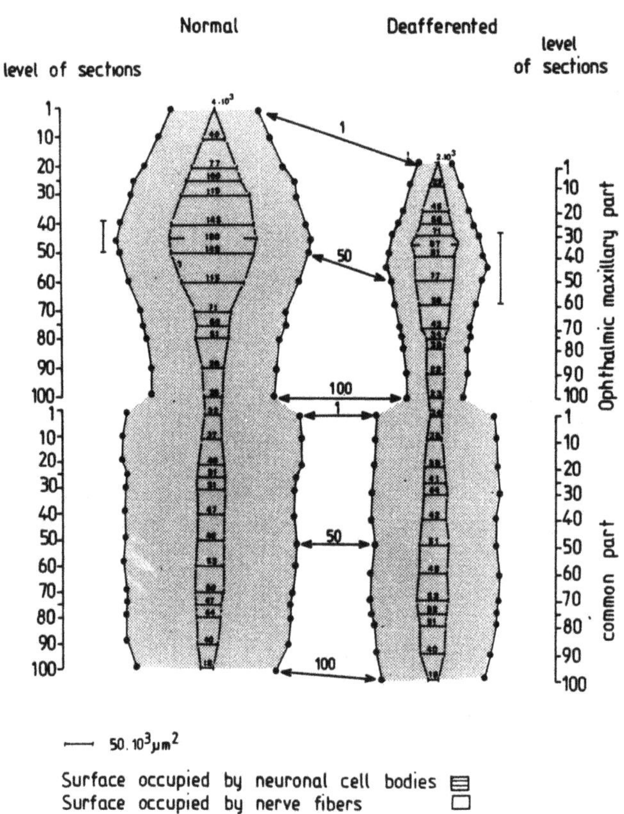

Fig. 2

Decrease of the nerve fibers areas as a function of the ganglionic level

IIIa

PF / AF	1	2	3	4	5	6	7	8	9	% well class.
1	38									100
2		47	1							98
3			29		3				1	88
4		1	1	55	2				3	89
5			3		54	2				92
6					1	58				98
7						1	69			99
8							5	67		93
9								2	47	96
% well pred.	100	98	85	100	90	95	93	97	92	95 / 94

IIIb

PF / AF	1	2	3	4	5	6	7	8	9	% well class.
1	4	1						3		50
2		15	2	1						83
3		1	6	1	1					67
4		1		14	2			2	2	67
5		1	1	1	21	1	2		6	64
6					1	10				91
7		3		1		4	26	2	2	68
8				2			5	22	4	67
9		1		1	1		3	4	23	70
% well pred.	100	65	67	67	81	67	72	67	62	70 / 72

Table III

Results
of automatic classification

a. Learning sample (490 fields)
b. Test sample (204 fields)

P.F. : predicted field index
A.F. : actual field index

NUMBER OF CELLS	
Manual Quantification	**Automatic Quantification**
732	743.8

Table IV

Preliminary results
of automatic quantification

(molecular layer – 30 fields)

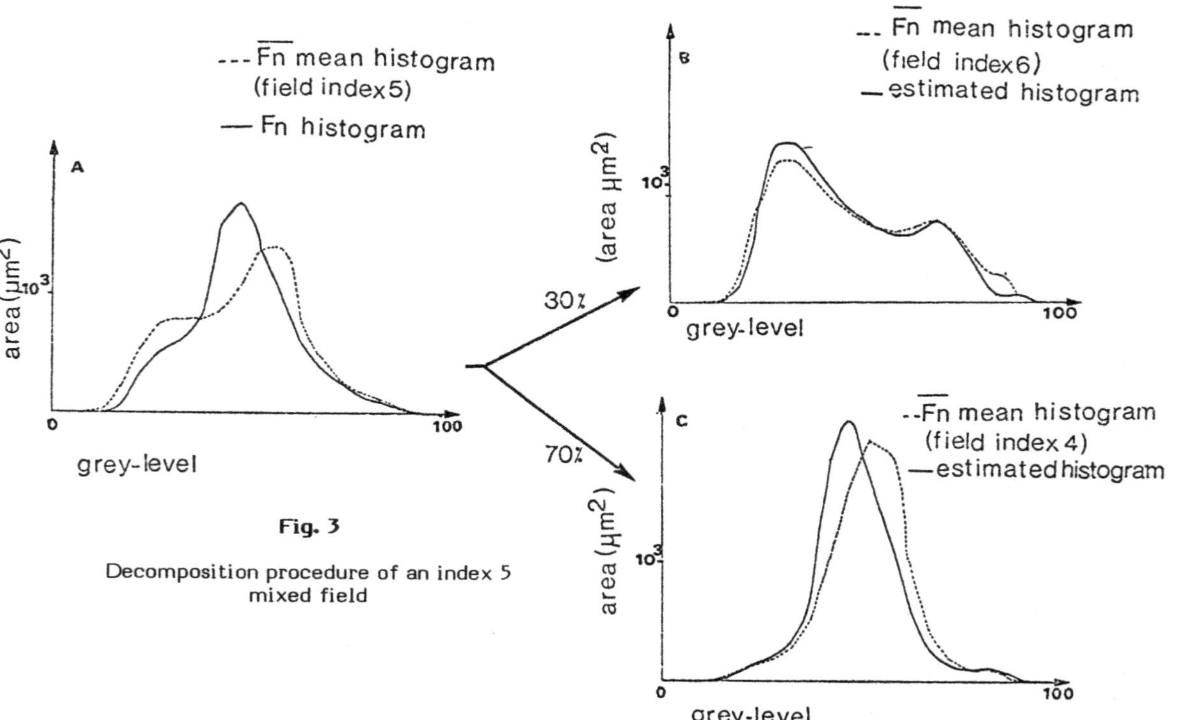

Fig. 3

Decomposition procedure of an index 5 mixed field

BONE MARROW CELL IMAGE ANALYSIS
BY COLOR CYTOPHOTOMETRY

by

Gérard BRUGAL
Equipe de Microscopie Quantitative - C.E.R.M.O.
Université Scientifique et Médicale de Grenoble
B.P. 53 X - 38 041 GRENOBLE Cedex. FRANCE.

ABSTRACT

A cell image analyzing system is described and recent advances in color processing algorithms are reported. Images of human bone marrow cells are acquired using red, green and blue broad band filters and processed according to a model based on the perceptual vision of color. The discriminatory power of hue, luminance and saturation computed on cells is discussed.

1. INTRODUCTION

CELL IMAGE ANTAGONISMS. The visual observation of biological specimens has been improved in the last three decades by quantitative assessment of the images given by a microscope. The theoretical and technological developments evolved from the pioneering works of MERTZ and GRAY (1934) and CASPERSSON (1936) have not resolved two main antagonisms over the current requirements in the field of cell image analysis.

The first antagonism lies in the choice of scanning microphotemetric versus TV (or solid state) camera image acquisition systems. Image analysis by means of microphotometric methods has the advantage of permitting insights into the chemical composition and the local mass distribution of various substances in both the nucleus (DNA, RNA) and the cytoplasm (RNA, structural and enzymatic proteins) of cells. The concept that quantization of cell components may be conclusive as regards to cell type description and recognition has led to the design and the construction of various cytoanalytical machines including a photomultiplier tube as light detector. These machines are namely the CYTOANALYZER (TOLLES, 1955), the CYDAC (NADEL, 1965) and the TICAS (WIED *et al.*, 1968) systems among the best known.

Conversely, either a TV (vidicon, plumbicon) or a solid state (photo diode array scanner) camera is used when the computation of both the shape and the texture cell features are considered to be effective for characterization and recognition of cell types. A great deal of mathematical and technological work has been carried out in the field of digital picture analysis (see ROSENFELD review, 1976) and mathematical morphology (MATHERON, 1969), and has led to the development of many image analyzing systems including a TV camera such as the QUANTIMET (IMANCO METAL RESEARCH) and the TAS (WILD-LEITZ) or a diode array scanner such as the ADC 500 white blood cell analyzer (ABBOTT LABORATORIES).

Simultaneous acquisition of the photometric and pattern information contained in the cell image with both the high densitometric resolution of a photomultiplier tube and the fast scanning speed associated to high spatial resolution of a camera remains a technological challenge.

The second antagonism concerns the goals of cell image processing and results from some eagerness to reach two different objectives : prescreening and powerful cell description. In prescreening, one wishes to process the minimum required information to perform a fast discrimination between a very few classes such as normal and abnormal cells ; on the other hand the objective description and characterization of cells - which promotes analytical cytology to a measuring quantitative science - involves the computation of maximum extractable information related to shape, texture, densitometry and cell color. Owing to the fact that the prescreening as well as the objective cell description cannot be performed independently in nearly all cytological applications of image processing, a methodological challenge arises.

One may place different emphasis on one's own approach to cell image processing, but an up-to-date compilation on the state of the art in biomedical pattern recognition (FU and PAVLIDIS, 1979) illustrates that image processing methods as well as image analyzing systems are respectively mathematical and technological compromises due to the inherent above mentioned antagonisms.

The bone marrow cell description, recognition and classification by means of image processing may show the difficulties which arise within the development of hardware and software compromises in a project to subclassify patients with the classical varieties of acute leukemias.

CHALLENGE IN BONE MARROW CELL IMAGE ANALYSIS

A large number of possible prognosis factors has been investigated to improve the leukemia therapy and includes : clinical features, cytogenetic tests, electron microscopy observations, cytochemical staining and immunofluorescent markers. Potentially, some of the most hopeful prognosis parameters are based upon the rate of occurence and morphology of normal and leukemic cell types (NECHELES et al., 1971 ; PANTAZOPOULOS and SINKS, 1974) which suggests that the occurrence ratio and morphology of leukemic cells are closely related to patient's survival and response to the therapy. Unfortunately, the microscopic observations advanced to support this evidence are "eye-brain" processed and therefore subjective ; they thus do not replicate well from one cytotechnologist to another (MURPHY et al., 1975). Consequently, the first goal of our work has been to carry out the methods of computer analysis to perform quantitative, objective and reliable morphologic description of bone marrow cells (BMC). The second goal, presently in progress, is to correlate these data with the cytotechnologist classification of BMC types. The third goal will be to provide the clinician with an automatic BMC image processing instrument.

It is our belief that one of the possible approaches for successful BMC recognition is to base the analyzing method upon the cytotechnologist experience, i.e. to compute cell descriptors strongly correlated with the perceptual features taken into account by the human observer (area, shape, texture and color of cell nucleus and cytoplasm). This approach is thus in opposition with the microspectrophotometric method proposed by BACUS (1976), BRENNER et al. (1974, 1977) AUS et al.(1977), GREEN (1979) and others. These methods have been classically used to get an insight into biochemical composition of cells in order to provide an evaluation of cell components in quantitative terms not perceptible to the eye. We think, however, that the microspectrophotometric methods may be effective only when applied to stoechiometric stained cells. Unfortunately, current cytochemistry offers only a very limited number of dyes which may be considered really stoechiometric. Moreover, the choice of accurate wavelengths used in multispectral cell image analysis depends on the color of the stained cells which are to be processed so that a combination of 2 to 3 wavelengths suitable for a given cell type may not be adequate for another cell type or for the case of slight staining variations. Our approach, on the other hand, involves a computation of the color displayed by the cells in terms of luminance, hue and saturation (color purity). To this end, we have proposed a model of the major transformations of the external light stimulus in the course of its travel from the eye to the cerebral cortex (GARBAY, 1979).

2. INSTRUMENTATION

The design and the construction of a cytoanalytical instrument started on 1974 in our laboratory. The basic principles of our machine were the same as those of the CYTO-ANALYZER and the CYDAC systems since we were convinced that the photomultiplier tube is the only light detector able to pick-up the densitometric information on cell images with the accuracy we expected to be necessary. Our system, called SAMBA (Système d'Analyse Microphotométrique à Balayage Automatique) (BRUGAL et al., 1979), was initially devoted to both the measurement of nuclear DNA content and the computation of the pattern of chromatin network. A software was elaborated to recognize cells in the various phases of the mitotic cycle (G_1, S, G_2, M) as well as resting cells (G_0) (GIROUD, 1979). In order to enlarge the cytological applications of SAMBA and to render the system suitable for routine work a second generation was designed and will be commercially available before long.

SAMBA 1st GENERATION

As shown in figure 1 and 2, the microphotemetric image analyzing system SAMBA includes:

- a microphotometer fitted with a motorized X, Y stepping stage (2.5 μm/step ; 400 Hz) ;
- a mechanical disk scanner associated with a photomultiplier tube : the resolution power of the scanner depends on the objective used and can reach the 0.25 μm upper limit. The frame format is 43 x 45 pixels, the frame time is either 0,5 s or 1 s and the sampling frequency is about 4 KHz ;
- a driving electronic module which controls the digitization (8 bits corresponding to 256 grey shades), commands the shifting of the scanning stage and manages the relationships between the image acquisition module and the picture processing computer (NORSK DATA NORD 10/S, 64 Kwords 16 bits). The local mini-computer is linked to a HB68 CIIHONEYWELL-BULL computer via the telephonic channel.

The successive elementary fields of 43 x 45 pixels each are processed in real-time and connected line/line and column/column to the possible 8 neighbouring fields. As shown in figure 4, a close superposition is observed between the microscopic image and the corresponding binary picture display covering several elementary fields acquired successively according to the meandering path of the microscope stage. The SAMBA system thus allows an iterative alternation between the scanning of the microscope elementary field and the displacement of the slide so that a continuous image of a cell population can be processed in its integrity regardless of the size and magnification. The algorithms involved in the one-pass computation required for field to field connection and features extraction have been already described (ADELH et al., 1978 ; VEILLON, 1979 ; CHASSERY, 1979).

SAMBA 2nd GENERATION

The new analyzing system now ready to be manufactured, was designed jointly with TITN and SORO laboratories. As shown in figure 3, it is a dual resolution system.

The low resolution path includes a linear photodiode scanner (256 elements) involved in both the cell location and the focusing processes. The same light detector is used in alternation for search mode and focusing mode. The video signal is quantized into 8 bits. The scanned band is 160 μm large and the pixel size is either 2.5 μm (search mode) or 0.6 μm (focusing mode) at the object plane.

The high resolution path involves X, Y vibrating mirrors focused on a photomultiplier tube. The image including 64 x 64 pixels is scanned and processed within 0.4 s. the spatial resolution power is 0.4 μm. This imaging system involves three R, G, B broad bandwith filters allowing picture acquisition and subsequent processing in color. The scanning stage (2.5 μm/step, 156 Hz) is used in search mode to drive and to center the successive cell images within the boundaries of the high resolution field.

The computer hardware comprises a driving and control processor which shares an image memory with the picture analyzing processor. The time necessary for the acquisition and processing of 300 cells by means of standard programs stored on a cassette tape is expected to average 2.30 mn depending on the quality of cell dispersion within the slide.

As early as 1966, PREWITT and MENDELSOHN emphasized the importance of spectral composition of the light transmitted through the constituent parts of cells in the recognition of the particular cell type illuminated. Later on, YOUNG (1969), MILLER et al. (1974) and others have carried this concept further and their extensive studies have led to the manufacture of various white blood cell processing machines by CORNING, GEOMETRICAL DATA, PERKIN-ELMER and ABBOTT Laboratories. These picture analyzing systems involve some color processing technique and include various kinds of light sensors and processors. They are all special-purpose on account of either their hardware or their software. On the other hand, the optimized cell image analyzing instruments capable of processing cell color, shape, geometry and texture information are neither widely known nor distributed although they can be expected to perform several kinds of both routine and experimental cell image analysis. The SAMBA 2nd generation system falls into this category since it includes a programmable cell analysis oriented processor and, above all, because it is provided with a multipurpose color software.

3. COLOR VISION MODEL

HUMAN COLOR PERCEPTION

The perceptual color vision model we used is already described elsewhere (GARBAY, 1979). Only the basic principles will be briefly presented below.
When entering the eyes, the light stimulus is absorbed by the R, G, B retinal pigments and generates three R, G, B nervous signals proportionnal to the logarithm of the external stimulus intensity. When processed by the lateral geniculate body, the signals are converted into one achromatic R, G, B additive signal (A) and two chromatic R, G, B differential signals (C_1, C_2) which are responsible for the appreciation of color in the cerebral cortex (figure 5).

COLOR VISION MODEL

In order to preprocess pictures according to the above scheme of human color vision, the acquisition of cell images by means of SAMBA system is performed using 3 broad bandwith filters characterized by spectral transmission curves similar to the absorbance properties of the retinal pigments (figure 6). As shown in figure 7, the three successive R, G and B images of an object are transformed into one achromatic (A) and two chromatic (C_1 and C_2) images. According to the perceptual mechanisms, the achromatic image supports the luminance information when the chromatic images support the color information in terms of differential visible spectrum information.

COLOR PROCESSING

According to the perceptual model, a given color is represented by a particular point (Q) in a three dimensionned perceptual space (A, C_1, C_2) as shown in figure 8. The notion of perceptual space leads to the parametrisation of colors in terms of luminance, saturation and hue which are compatible with human color vision experience :
- the luminance (L) is related to quantity of light emitted by a colored object and is supported by the A axis of the perceptual space (figure 8) ;
- the hue (H) is the attribute of color denoted by blue, green, yellow, red... and is measured by the angle opened between the C_1 axis and the projection OP of OQ within the C_1, C_2 plane as shown in figure 8 ;
- the saturation (S) is a purity factor of color depending on the amount of white altering the hue ; it is measured by the distance OP between the axis origin (O) and the projection P of Q within the C_1, C_2 plane.

4. BONE MARROW CELL PROCESSING

The bone marrow smears used for our studies were collected from the "Institut de Cancérologie et Immuno-Génétique" of VILLEJUIF. These routine PAPPENHEIM-GIEMSA stained cell preparations exhibit large disparities regarding the intensity of staining and the efficiency of cell dispersion. The PAPPENHEIM-GIEMSA staining procedure is preferred to the WRIGHT because cytoplasmic granulation of leucocytes, and especially neutrophil granulocytes, is more pronounced while the various hues among cell types are well contrasted. It would be, however, necessary to improve standardization of that staining procedure.

IMAGE ACQUISITION

Bone marrow cells belonging to various types were examined on the SAMBA 1st generation acquisition system. Specifically, the data acquisition process consists of scanning the cell images in a 43 x 45 pixels raster with a 0.66 µm spatial resolution power. The photometric signal is quantized into one of 256 grey levels. This scanning process is repeated through the three successive R, G, B broad bandwith filters and cell images are recorded on magnetic disk memory.

SCENE SEGMENTATION

Segmentation is the process by which the computer isolates cells of interest from the surrounding region containing a transparent background and other objects such as erythrocytes, leucocytes, cell debris, stain blobs and various artefacts. Segmentation is one of the most challenging steps in image processing although it is the easiest one for humans.

In manually prepared BMC smears, many cell clusters occur. These clusters can be processed by computer separating methods such as those proposed by AUS et al. (1977) and BRENNER et al. (1977). Since these highly performing methods are time consuming and may alter the integrity of touching or overlapping cells, it is our opinion that one must avoid them for routine purpose. To this end, mechanical dispersion of cells by spinner type techniques must be improved for bone marrow aspirates. It is not known, however, whether spinner - prepared bone marrow smears contain a valuable diagnostic information similar to that of routine preparations.

The BMC image segmentation involves the recognition of 4 classes of objects, namely the background, the erythrocytes the cytoplasm and the nucleus of leucocytes.

The first method we have carried out consists of thresholding the luminance, hue and saturation of image using the corresponding histograms as shown in figure 9. When considering the hue and saturation thresholds in addition to the luminance one, the scene segmentation efficiency is greatly enhanced as demonstrated in figure 10. Unfortunately, the thresholds are dependent upon the particular smear under consideration because of the poor reliability of the PAPPENHEIN-GIEMSA staining used for this work.

Even in standardized staining circumstances some slight variations of cell colors may be expected. It is thus usefull to provide the picture analyzing algorithm with an automatic, self-adaptative scene segmentation procedure. A statistically based segmentation algorithm was thus used and involves the partitioning of the space generated by the vectors V (H, L, S) into 4 clusters corresponding to the above mentioned 4 classes of objects. Using a training set discriminant functions are calculated from a number of vectors computed under the different staining conditions which may be encountered. This learning stage is performed once and only once. The efficiency of these functions was tested using various cell images and the results were quite encouraging since in most cases the cell separation thus obtained is as suitable as that observed using the previous single H, L, S thresholding methods as shown in figure 11.

In some cases, the BMC and specially those belonging to the neutrophil lineage exhibit very pale cytoplasmic regions ; moreover, the nucleus of the basophil white cells is often hidden by as heavy granulation. These peculiarities render the BMC segmentation sometimes so confusing that either the thresholding methods or the statistical one may fail to succeed in a perfect delineation of cytoplasm and nuclear boundaries. Therefore, various complementary separating methods must be carried out. It is our belief that the contextual information may remove potential local uncertainties. Since an object may be considered as a particular spatial organisation of points characterized by the same label, some relations in terms of probabilities must exist which promote or discredit some configurations of spatially associated labels. Consequently, we have calculated - using a training set of images - the probabilities of occurrence of all possible configurations regarding 4 of the neighbouring points surrounding each given point of an image. During the segmentation process involving contextual information, the labelling decision for the current point under interest thus can be balanced by the labels involved in the particular surrounding configuration. When the statistical automatic segmentation method is improved by the contextual probabilities

this case, we attempted to determine the most pertinent features of the normal and abnormal cell types before trying to carry out a final BMC automated classifier. Consequently, in order to test the discriminatory power of the color parameters computed on the BMC, a discriminant analysis was performed.

The 20 cell types taken into account are given in table 1 which displays their lineage relationships. The parameters involved in the composition of a training set are presented in table 2 and were computed on 20 cells per type.

To select the most pertinent parameters, the stepwise linear discriminant analysis program BMD 07M of the University of California was used ; it provides a ranking of the parameters according to their discriminatory power and allows the computation of a confusion matrix. The parameters are listed in table 3 according to the descending discriminatory order calculated by the program. Only the parameters ranked first to tenth among the whole set of parameters are recorded. One may observe in table 3 that nine of the ten first best discriminating parameters are related to color features of the cell, namely the hue (order 1, 4, 7, 8, 9), the nuclear integrated luminance (order 2) and the low cytoplasmic stauration (order 3, 5, 10). Only one geometrical parameter, namely the cytoplasmic area, is ranked (order 6) among the ten most discriminatory parameters. Other geometrical features such as nuclear area (A), nuclear and cytoplasmic perimeter (P) and curvature (P^2/A) have been computed : they are listed among the less discriminatory parameters.

The confusion matrix between the cytotechnologist (rows) and the classifier (columns) is given in table 4. The numbers of correctly classified cells lie on the matrix diagonal while the numbers scattered elsewhere represent the misclassified cells. Since two successive stages within a given cell lineage are not clear-cut the correctly classified cells are found in the underlined extended diagonal. This assumption allows us to calculate that the rate of correct classification is 92 %. Among the incorrectly classified cells, one may observe that :
- 24 % may be attributed to confusion between various maturation stages within a given lineage ;
- 50 % may be attributed to confusion between cells at the same stage of maturation but belonging to different lineages ;
- 26 % may be attributed to confusion between cells at different stages of maturation and belonging to different lineages.

At the present stage of our work, the above distribution of error within the 8 % misclassified cells need not be discussed with regard to either an ideal or absolute cell classifier design for automatic BMC recognition and counting, but rather in terms of parameter performances.

It is essential to notice that only color parameters associated to the classical area, perimeter and curvature geometrical parameters are involved in the discriminant analysis performed. In spite of the lack of any cell shape or texture parameter (excepted the ineffective curvature parameter), the rate of correct classification is 92 %, thus obviously demonstrating the expected efficiency of the color parameters processed according to the perceptual model of human color vision as described above.

The classification results presented above are inferred from a small size training set 400 cells and thus may be so noisy that it cannot support valid evaluation of the classifier adequacy. Nevertheless, for large scale experiments of BMC classification involving shape, texture and color features, the linear discriminant analysis may not be expected *a priori* to be the most optimal classifying tool because the discriminatory power of a given parameter strongly depends on the cell types to be recognized. Therefore, the combination of discriminant analysis with hierarchical classification schemes should probably offer a powerful classifier for cell image processing.

5. CONCLUSIONS

The experiments reported in this paper should be considered as feasibility studies carried out on SAMBA 1st generation, and useful for the design of SAMBA 2nd genera-

processing, possible misinterpreted parts of objects are rejected, as shown in figure 12.

BACUS (1976), BRENNER et al. (1977), AUS et al. (1977) and others before us have emphasized the necessity of taking into account the color information of blood and bone marrow cells to achieve computer segmentation, but the dilemna remains whether the microspectrophotometric (multispectral marrow band analysis) or the perceptual method provides the best approach to color information processing. A valid comparison between these methods is not still available, nevertheless, the assumption that the segmentation is a difficult task for a computer when compared to the "eye-brain" ability to separate objects in a scene, allows us to claim intuitively that perceptual based processing must provide a very powerful segmenting tool.

FEATURE EXTRACTION

It is not the aim of the present paper to emphasize the traditionnal shape and texture parameters so useful in discrimating between cell types. Rather our purpose is limited to demonstrating the potential efficiency of the luminance, hue and saturation color parameters with respect to the cell type description and recognition.

The luminance, hue and saturation values calculated for each point of a cell image allow the computation of the averages, variances and histograms of luminance, hue and saturation over the cell components. Among these parameters, the histogram appears to be the most disciminating. Figure 13 presents the luminance, hue and saturation histograms at some significant stages of the differenciation of BMC belonging to the erythroblast and eosinophil granulocyte lineages.

Erythroblastic lineage (Figure 13 a) : the beginning of the erythroblast maturation, mainly characterized by a discrete enhancement of the nuclear to cytoplasm contrast, demonstrates clearly the descriptive power of luminance and saturation cell parameters. Namely, the maturation of the pronormoblast into a basophil normoblast is characterized by a slight lightening of the cytoplasm which corresponds to a small shift of the blue peak in the hue clock histogram. The differentiation of the basophil normoblast into a polychromatophil normoblast is marked by an alteration of the saturation of the cytoplasmic blue staining which is expressed by an evident bimodal evolution of the saturation histogram ; in addition, the enhancement of the nucleus to cytoplasm contrast is closely related to a similar bimodal transformation of the luminance histogram.

Eosinophil granulocyte lineage (Figure 13 b) : the different stages of the myeloblast transformation into the eosinophil granulocyte may exemplify the importance of the hue parameter in determining the identity of the particular cell under consideration: namely, the myeloblast differentiation into the eosinophil myelocyte is marked by the apparition of an acidophil granulation which strongly attenuates the cytoplasmic blue color : a blue peak disappearence is noted in the corresponding clock histograms of the hue. The eosinophil maturation, which takes place during the transformation of the myelocyte into the eosinophil metamyelocyte is characterized by an overcrowding of the cytoplasm by eosinophil granules. This phenomenon leads to a subsequent appearance of a new red peak in the corresponding clock histograms of the hue.

The above examples, although limited, illustrate the kind of considerations that have motivated our work. As stated previously, these motivations are to preserve the close relationships between the significance of the computed color parameters and the conceptual and experienced cytological knowledge and related visual interpretation.

BONE MARROW CELL CLASSIFICATION

An automated classifier, such as that involved in the white blood cell classification for example, is classically compared to a competent human observer. In some cytological applications, however, equally competent authorities may disagree upon the proper categorization of some cells. Given such a handicap, the evaluation of a classifier performance may become exceedingly difficult. Since the BMC recognition falls into

tion system as was our first goal. Our second goal, which involves a statistically based and standardized comparison between cytotechnologists and the computer automatic cell diagnostic, will benefit greatly from the present analyzing tool ; moreover further analyses will obviously include a set of cell shape and texture parameters respectively related to the bending energy and the co-occurence matrix, in addition to the primary color features. The evaluation of the discriminatory power of the above named cell shape and texture parameters is in progress and the routine classifier for BMC will be included in the SAMBA 2nd generation software.

ACKNOWLEDGEMENT

This work was supported by grants from D.G.R.S.T., I.N.S.E.R.M. and C.N.R.S.

REFERENCES

ADELH, D. ; BRUGAL, G. ; CHASSERY, J. M. ; CHIBON, P. and GARBAY, C., Microscopic image analysis system. Applications to biology : cell cycle, cancerous blood and bone marrow cells. Proc. IV th Int. Joint Conf. on Pattern Recog. Kyoto (Japon) : 864-871 (1978)

AUS, H. M. ; RUTER, A. ; MEULEN, V. T. ; GUNZER, U. and NURNBERGER, R., Bone marrow cell scene segmentation by computer-aided color cytophotometry. J. Histochem. Cytochem., 25 : 662-667 (1977).

BACUS, J. W., A whitening transformation for two-color blood cell images. In Pattern Recognition. Pergamon Press, 8 : 53-60 (1976).

BRENNER, J. F. ; GELSEMA, E. S. ; NECHELES, E. S. ; NECHELES, T. F. ; NEURATH, P. W.; SELLES, W. D. and VASTOLA, E., Automated classification of normal and abnormal leucocytes. J. Histochem. Cytochem., 22 : 697-706 (1974).

BRENNER, J. F. ; NECHELES, T. F. ; BONACOSSA, I. A. ; FRISTENSKY, R., WEINTRAUB, B. A. and NEURATH, P. W., Scene segmentation techniques for the analysis of routine bone marrow smears from acute lymphoblastic leukemia patients. J. Histochem. Cytochem., 25 : 601-613 (1977).

BRUGAL, G. ; GARBAY, C. ; GIROUD, F. and ADELH, D., A double-scanning microphotometer for image analysis : hardware, software and biomedical applications. J. Histochem. Cytochem., 21 : 144-152 (1979)

CASPERSSON, T., Uber den Chemischen Aufbau der Strukturen des Zellkernes. Scand. Arch. Physiol., 73, suppl. 8 : 1-151 (1936).

CHASSERY, J. M., Connectivity and consecutivity in digital pictures. Comp. Graph. and Image Proc., 9 : 294-300 (1979).

FU, K. S. ; PAVLIDIS, T., Life Sciences Research Report 15. Biomedical Pattern Recognition and Image Processing. K.S. FU and T. PAVLIDIS eds. 441 p. Verlag Chemie (1979).

GARBAY, C., Modélisation de la couleur dans le cadre de l'analyse d'images et de son application à la cytologie automatique. Thèse Ingénieur-Docteur. Institut National Polytechnique de Grenoble, (1979).

GIROUD, F., Effets de la thyroxine exogène sur la cinétique cellulaire chez la larve du triton Pleurodeles waltlii Michah. étudiés dans le cadre du perfectionnement d'un système automatique d'analyse des images microscopiques. Thèse de Spécialité. Université de Grenoble (1979).

GREEN, J. E., A practical application of computer pattern recognition research. The ABBOTT ADC-500 differential classifier. J. Histochem. Cytochem., 27 : 160-173 (1979).

MATHE, G. ; POUILLART, P. ; STERESCU, M. ; AMIEL, J. L. ; SCHWARZENBERG, L. ; SCHNEIDER, M. ; HAYAT, M. ; DE VASSAL, F. ; JASMIN, C. and LAFLEUR, M., Subdivision of classical varieties of acute leukemia. Correlation with prognosis and cure expectancy. Europ. J. Clin. Biol. Res., 16 : 554-560 (1971).

MATHERON, G., Théorie des ensembles aléatoires. Cahiers Centre Morph. Math., ENMP ed.,

Paris (1969).

MERTZ, P. and GRAY, F., A theory of scanning and its relation to the characteristics of the transmitted signal in telephotography and television. Bell System Tech. J., 13 : 464-473 (1934).

MILLER, N. M., Design and clinical results of HEMATRAK : an automated differential counter. IEEE Trans biomed. Eng., 23 : 400 (1976).

MURPHY, S. B. ; BORELLA, L. ; SEN, L. and MAUER, A., Lack of correlation of lymphoblast cell size with presence of T-cell markers with outcome in childhood acute lymphoblastic leukemia. Brit. J. Haemat., 31 : 95 (1975).

NADEL, E. M., Computer Analysis of cytometric fields by the CYDAC and its historical evolution from the CYTOANALYZER. Acta Cytol., 9 : 203 (1965).

NECHELES, T. F. ; BRENNER, J. F. ; BONACOSSA, I. A. ; FRISTENSKY, R. and NEURATH, P. W., The computer-assisted morphological classification of acute leukemia. I-Preliminary results. Biomed. 25 : 241 (1976).

PANTAZOPOULOS, N. and SINKS, L. F., Morphological criteria for prognostication of acute lymphoblastic leukaemia. Brit. J. Haemat., 27 : 25 (1974).

PREWITT, J. M. S. and MÉNDELSOHN, M. L., The analysis of cell images. An. N. Y. Acad. Sci., 128 : 1035-1953 (1966).

ROSENFELD, A., Topics in applied physics. Digital picture analysis. A. ROSENFELD Ed. Springer Verlag, Berlin, 351 p. (1976).

TOLLES, W. E., The CYTOANALYZER, an example of physics on medical research. Trans N. Y. Acad. Sci., 17 : 250-256 (1955).

VEILLON, F., One-pass computation of morphological and geometrical properties of objects in digital pictures. Signal Proc., 1 : 175-189 (1979).

WIED, G. L. ; BARTELS, P. H. ; BAHR, G. F. and OLFIELD, D. G. , Taxonomic intracellular analytic system (TICAS) for cell identification. Acta Cytol., 12 : 180-204 (1968).

YOUNG, I. T., Automated leucocyte recognition. Ph. D. Dissertation. M. I. T. Cambridge, (1969).

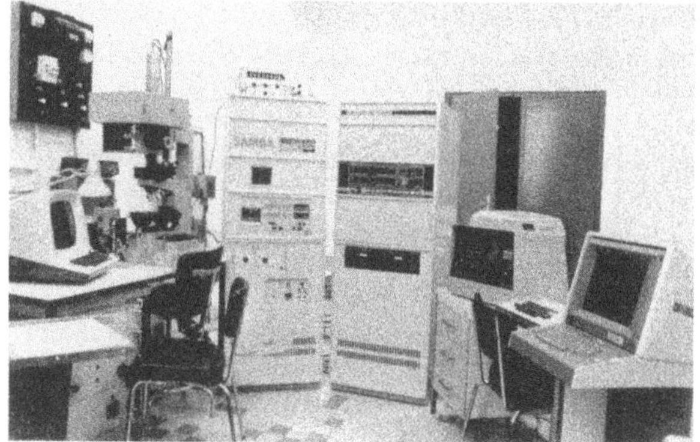

Figure 1 - S.A.M.B.A. (Système d'Analyse Microphotométrique à Balayage Automatique) cell image acquisition and processing system.

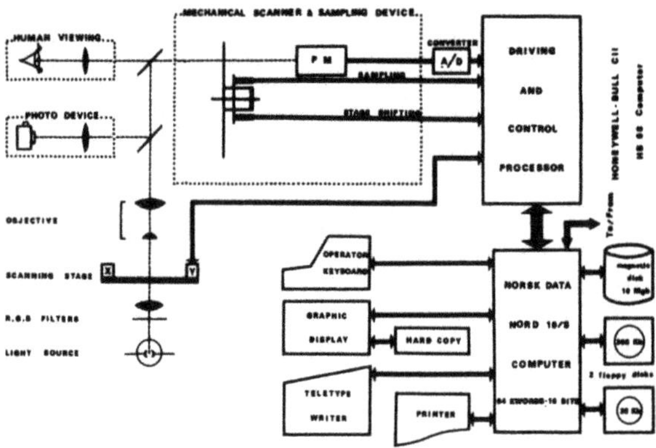

Figure 2 - General schematic organization of the hardware of SAMBA 1 st generation.

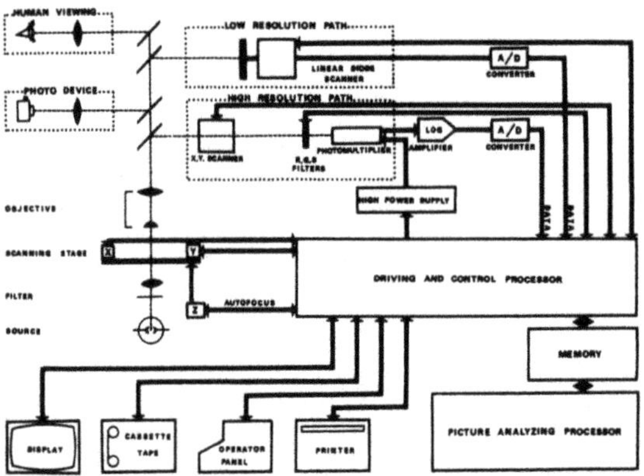

Figure 3 - General schematic organization of the hardware of SAMBA 2 nd generation system.

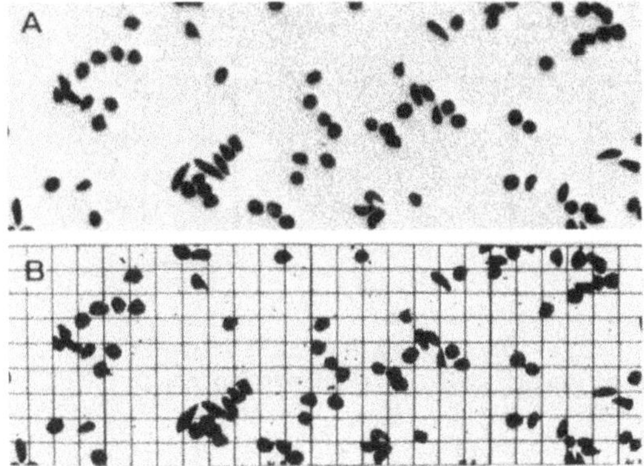

Figure 4 - Comparison between a cell population observed at a low magnification (A) and a graphic binary display of its image (B). The picture B is acquired field after field at the highest magnification of the microscope : each elementary square area corresponds to an elementary field including 1521 digital values. Each elementary field is 16 x 16 µm so that the entire picture is 144 x 400 µm at the object plane.

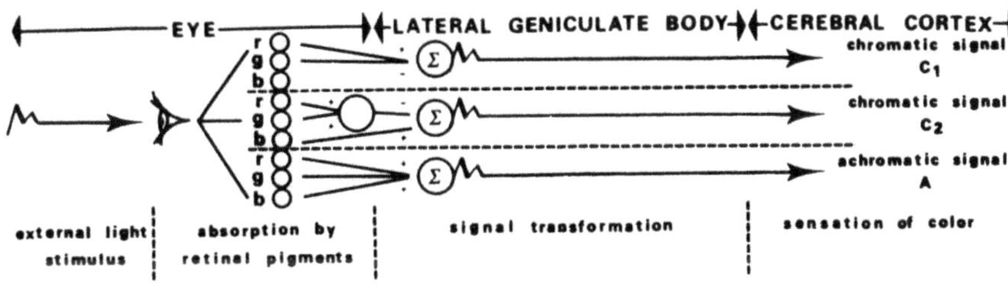

Figure 5 - Human color perception scheme : when absorbed by the retinal pigments, the external light stimulus is converted into 3 R, G, B signals and then transformed into an additive (R+G+B) luminance achromatic signal (A), a differential (R-G) chromatic signal (C_1) and another differential (B-R-G) chromatic signal (C_2). These last 3 signals are responsible for the color sensation.

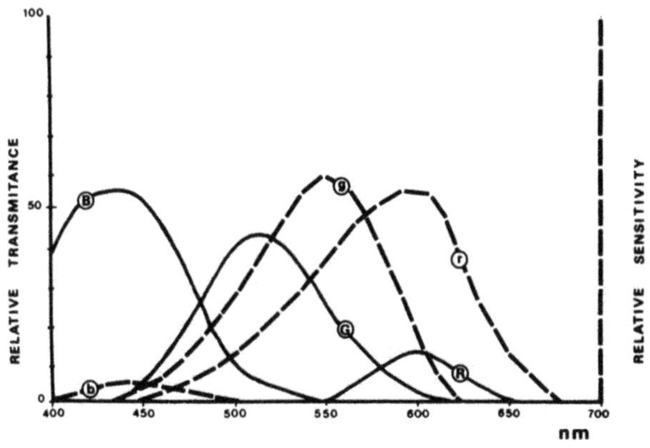

Figure 6 - Red (R), green (G) and blue (B) spectral features of the image acquisition system resulting from the filters, the light source emitting spectrum and the photomultiplier sensitivity. These spectral features have to be compared with the red (r), green (g) and blue (b) absorption curves of the retinal pigments.

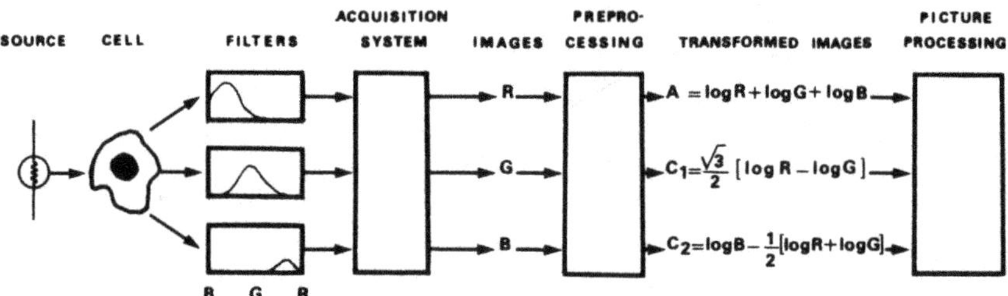

Figure 7 - Acquisition scheme of R, G, B images of bone marrow cells involving a preprocessing compatible with the model of human color vision presented in Figure 5.

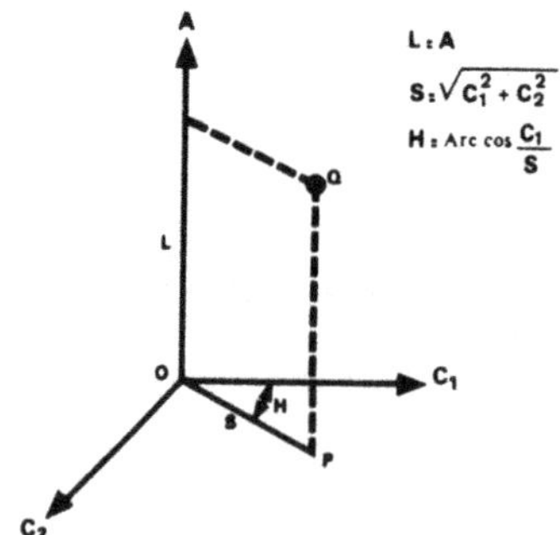

Figure 8 - Color processing. The color of a point Q in the perceptual space (A, C_1, C_2) is reprensed by its luminance L (equal to A), its saturation S (equal to the module of OP, where P is the projection of Q in the C_1, C_2 plane) and its hue H (equal to the angle between C_1 and OP).

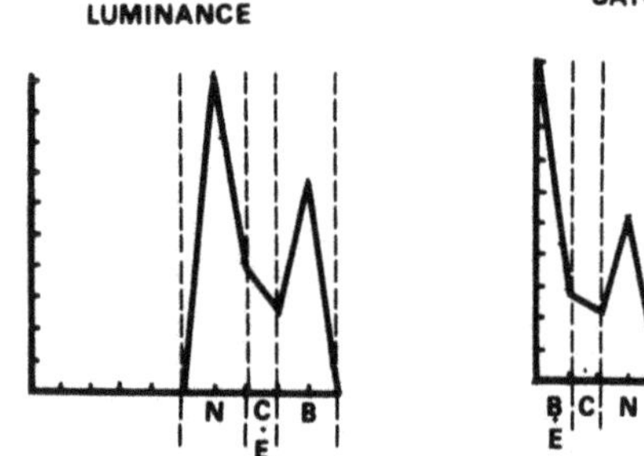

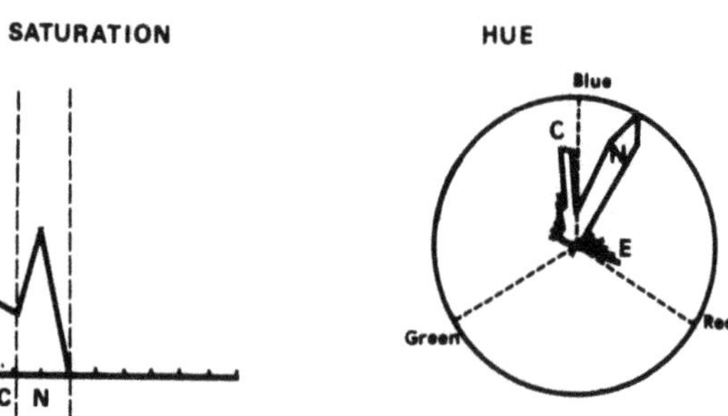

Figure 9 - Histograms of luminance and saturation and clock histogram of hue computed from a cell image. The hue is measured in terms of angle degrees : pure blue = 90°, pure green = 210° and pure red = 330°. The background (B) corresponds to high luminance and high saturation values, the erythrocyte (E) corresponds to intermediate luminance and low saturation values and to an orange-red color ; the cytoplasm (C) corresponds to intermediate luminance and saturation values and to various hues (blue in the case presented here) according to the staining features of the cell type under consideration ; the nucleus (N) corresponds to low luminance, high saturation values and to a purple hue.

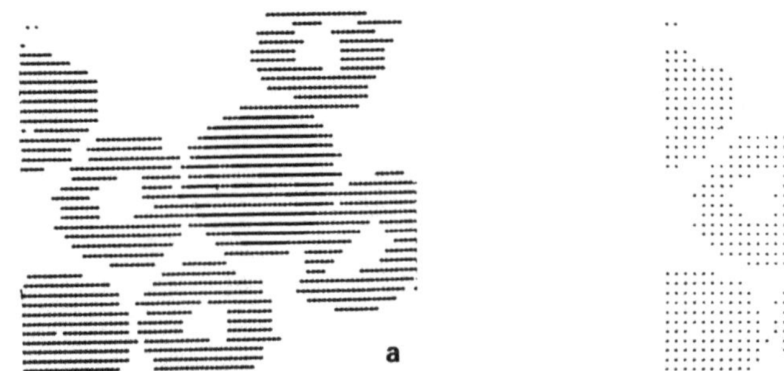

Figure 10 - Segmentation of a microlymphoblast surrounded with several erythrocytes : (a) = segmentation involving a single luminance thresholding ; (b) = segmentation involving a simultaneous luminance, saturation and hue thresholding. The cytoplasm/erythrocyte comfusion which can be noticed in the image (a) is suppressed in the image (b). Nucleus = lines ; Cytoplasm = large dots ; erythrocyte = small dots.

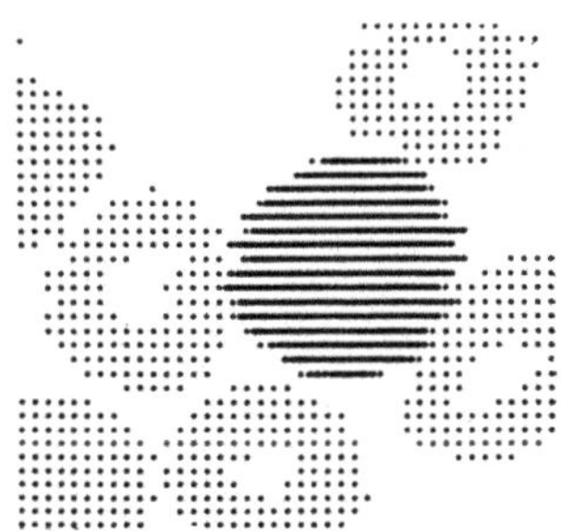

Figure 11 - Segmentation of the same scene as in figure 10 but using a statistically based segmentation algorithm. The results obtained are as suitable as those presented in figure 10, moreover, all the points belonging to the nucleus are correctly detected.

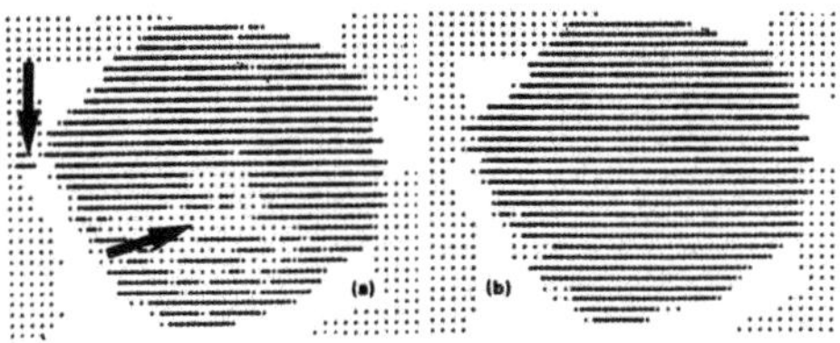

Figure 12 - Neutrophil metamyelocyte isolated using a statistically based segmentation neglecting (a) or involving (b) a contextual information processing. The contextual information suppresses possible confusions between some pale cytoplasmic regions and erythrocyte (arrows).

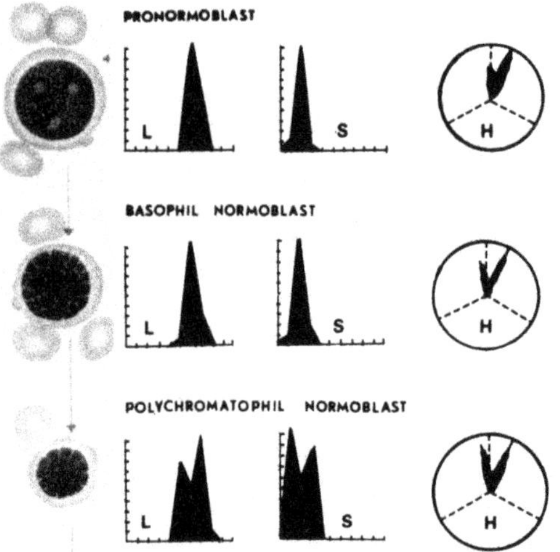

Figure 13A - Evolution of cell luminance (L), saturation (S) and hue (H) histograms during the differentiation of the erythroblastic lineage.

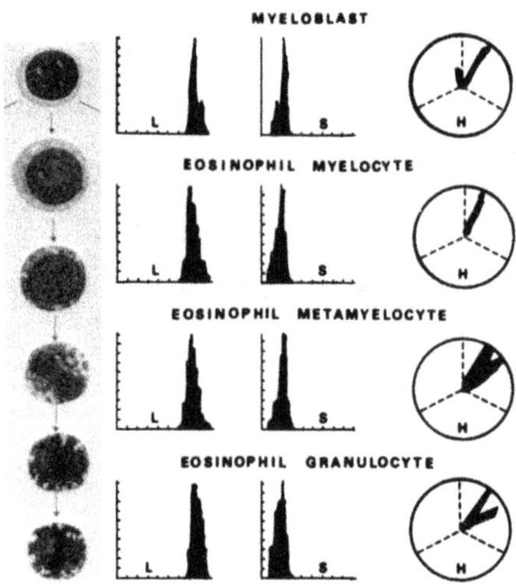

Figure 13B - Evolution of cell luminance (L), saturation (S) and hue (H) histograms during the differentiation of the eosinophil granulocytic lineage.

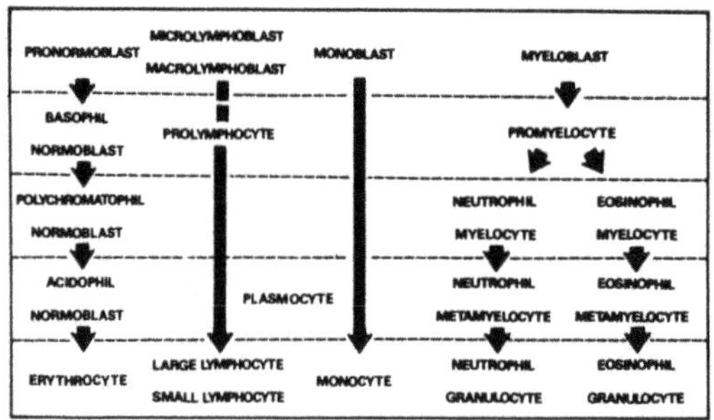

Table 1 - Cell types taken into account in the bone marrow cell analysis.

	LUMINANCE			SATURATION			HUE			GEOMETRY		
	a	v	h	a	v	h	a	v	h	A	P	P²/A
CELL			*			*			*			
CYTOPLASM	*	*		*	*		*	*		*	*	*
NUCLEUS	*	*		*	*		*	*		*	*	*

Table 2 - Color and geometrical parameters computed respectively on the nucleus, the cytoplasm or the entire cell for bone marrow cell type recognition. a = average ; v = variance ; h = histogram ; A = area; P = perimeter ; P^2/A = curvature.

Table 3 - The ten most discriminating parameters in descending order.

1 : HUE CLOCK HISTOGRAM (60°-65°) - 2 : INTEGRATED NUCLEAR LUMINANCE - 3 : AVERAGE CYTOPLASM SATURATION - 4 : AVERAGE CYTOPLASM HUE - 5 : SATURATION HISTOGRAM (0.1-0.2) - 6 : CYTOPLASM AREA - 7 : HUE CLOCK HISTOGRAM (100°-105°) - 8 : HUE CLOCK HISTOGRAM (90°-95°) - 9 : HUE CLOCK HISTOGRAM (65°-70°) - 10 : SATURATION HISTOGRAM (0.2-0.3),

Table 4 - Bone marrow cell cytotechnologist versus computer diagnostics presented according to a confusion matrix.

MAN \ MACHINE	PRN	BAN	PLN	ACN	MNB	MNC	PRL	MIB	MAB	LLC	SMC	PLA	MYE	PRM	NMY	EMY	NME	EME	NGR	EGR
pronormo.	18	1											1							
baso. normo.	2	16											2							
poly. normo.			18								1									
acid. normo.			7	12							1									
monoblast					19						1									
monocyte						16							1		2		1			
prolympho.							16	1	1	2										
microlymph.								20												
macrolymph.							1		19	1										
large lymph.										22										
small lymph.								2			41									
plasmocyte		4										19								
myeloblast		1						1					17			1				
promyel.														17		3				
neutr. myel.						1									16		1	1	1	
eosin. myel.						1							1			15		2		1
neutr. meta.							1				1				1		17			
eosin. meta.					1					1						1		14		3
neutr. gran.																	2		18	
eosin. gran.																		3	1	16

FEATURE EXTRACTION BY MATHEMATICAL MORPHOLOGY IN THE FIELD OF QUANTITATIVE CYTOLOGY

by
Fernand MEYER
Ecole Nationale Supérieure des Mines de Paris
Centre de Géostatistique et de Morphologie Mathématique
35, rue Saint-Honoré
77305 FONTAINEBLEAU (France)

ABSTRACT

Segmentation, construction and recognition of an image are done simultaneously by sequences of parallel neighborhood-transformations. Feature extraction is particularly easy when the transformations are idempotent. Examples are given. The development of a language and of an apparatus specially devoted to automated cytology are discussed.

1. INTRODUCTION

Fifteen years ago G. Matheron considerably enlarged the notion of particle size by introducting the concept of openings and thus made it possible to describe the granulometry or size distribution of a porous medium in which no particles can be individualised. The idea was to use an image transformation, the opening, before any measurement (ref. 10). An image processor was then designed (ref. 8), based on such image transformations, and was soon commercialised by Leitz. The advantage of that machine was its ability to perform image transformations and measurements at TV speed.

Four years ago the C.M.M. added image memories to the machine for the storage of complete images. This made it possible to iterate image transformations (ref. 4). The result surpassed our hopes. We discovered that with very simple basic neighborhood transformations, we could produce much more complex functions such as skeletons, convex hulls and contrast analysis, and, more generally, solve very complex pattern recognition problems.

In this paper we would like to emphasize the special importance of idempotent image transformations in pattern recognition. These transformations work exactly like sieves, filtering all objects in the field of view at the same time. Segmentation, construction and recognition of the image are done simultaneously by successive filters without intervention by the operator.

These transformations turned out to be particularly well adapted to automated cytology. In this field the collaboration between Leitz, the Laboratory of Histochemistry and Cytochemistry in Leiden (Dr. Ploem) and the C.M.M. (Centre de Morphologie Mathématique) has been particularly fruitful : we managed to develop a new approach to the screening and diagnosis of cervical slides, which has been partly described at this same meeting. This approach opens interesting perspectives for specialised software and hardware for quantitative cytology. The word real-time is no longer utopic since high speeds can be reached.

In the first section we shall watch a bottle washer discover the use of idempotence.

In the second section we will see that image transformations may be classified by their complexity which increases as they become more specialized. By giving names to these transformations, it is thus possible to build an interesting programming language adapted to pattern recognition and image processing, and which contains specialised sublanguages. A few examples from the field of cytology will be given briefly.

Finally the design of an adapted hardware and the problems of cost and speed will be discussed.

2. WHERE A BOTTLE-WASHER DISCOVERS THE VIRTUES OF IDEMPOTENCE

Let's imagine a bottle washer faced with the following problem : he has to wash up plates and dishes. But some of them are clean and others dirty. In order to minimize his work, he would like to be able to recognize which are clean and which he will have to wash up. Is there a sure and universal method for recognizing the clean dishes ?

After a short period of reflexion he comes to a very disappointing conclusion : there is no way to reduce his work and he will have to wash up everything. And indeed the casiest way to find out if the cleaning will change a plate or a glass is to wash it and to see what happens. What else is a clean plate than a plate whose aspect is not changed by cleaning ?

Every other test will work only with a given, well defined, type of dish and will fail with any other type. (the test of transparency would work only for a given type of glass : not every glass is transparent, etc...).

The meaning of that rather simple story is the following.

One cannot base an automatic recognition of patterns on measurements if the objects to analyze don't belong to a relatively well defined class (i.e. transparent glasses in the above example). However, it is possible to make a statement about completely unknown objects by using image transformations. The best test for knowing if a completely unknown object is "clean" consists in "cleaning" it to see if it will be changed.

Let us now analyse the "cleaning" operation

(a) if an object is clean, cleaning will not change it

X clean $T_A(X) = X$ (T_A being the transformation cleaning)

(b) if X is unknown $T_A(X)$ is clean

(c) therefore cleaning an object which has just been cleaned doesn't change the object

$$T_A(T_A(X)) = T_A(X)$$

this last property is called "idempotence"

The mechanism of recognition now appears clearly. The property A (to be clean, for example) is associated with a transformation T_A (to clean).

An unknown object X has the property A if $T_A(X) = X$.

If X does not have property A then $T_A(X) \neq X$, because $T_A(X)$ has the property A.

The transformations T_A also gives meaning to measurements. We can try to quantify the difference between X and $T_A(X)$ and thus measure how $T_{A_i}(X)$ varies when A_i approaches A.

As an illustration let's go back to the washing-up scenario. In order to measure how dirty a plate was, we will measure the difference in weight between X and $T_A(X)$, which is the amount of dirt removed.

One could also imagine a washing-up which becomes more and more energetic and see how $T_{A_i}(X)$ varies, where T_{A_j} represents a more energetic washing-up then T_{A_i} if $j > i$.

3. SOME IMPORTANT TRANSFORMATIONS USED IN QUANTITATIVE CYTOLOGY

(a) Opening : a combination of erosion and dilation

Suppose that in cervical cytology we want to detect enlarged cervical nuclei and eliminate leukocytes. And imagine that the interior of the figure we have to analyse is composed of dry grass and that the exterior or background is composed of unburnable wet grass. Suppose a fire is started simultaneously at all points along the boundary. The fire will propagate at uniform speed toward the middle of the figure. (Fig. 1 shows the successive Fire Fronts at times 0,2,4,...). Obviously all leukocytes will have "burnt out" at a time θ much earlier than enlarged cervical cells. If we stop the fire at time θ, the non-burnt up part of the image is the eroded set of the initial image, by an erosion of size θ, (notation $X \ominus (\theta B)$, where B is a disk of radius 1).

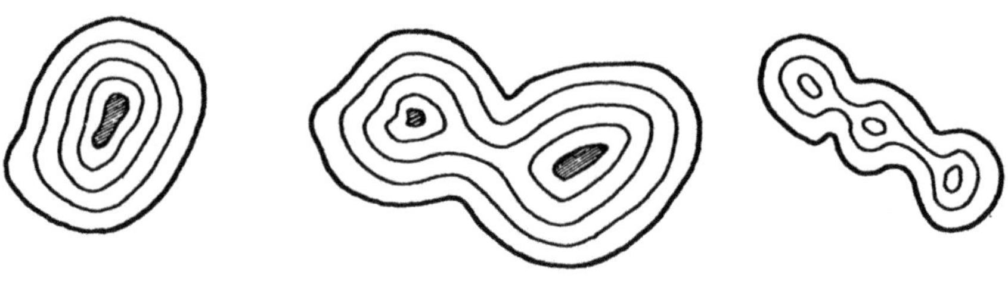

Figure 1 : Successive front lines of the grass fire
Eroded set in grey : $X \ominus (\theta B)$

We note that this operation works even if the cells overlap, for which a test based on the area of cells would fail. This transformation is obviously not idempotent : an erosion of size θ followed by another erosion of size θ is an erosion of size 2θ.

In order to restore the eroded set to it's original size we invert the image and let a fire propagate during the same time θ in the opposite direction. This operation is a dilation of size θ (notation $X \oplus \theta B$) and the erosion of size θ followed by a dilation of same size is an opening of size θ (notation $(X)_{\theta B}$) and now we have an idempotent transformation : $(X)_{\theta B} = [(X)_{\theta B}]_{\theta B}$.

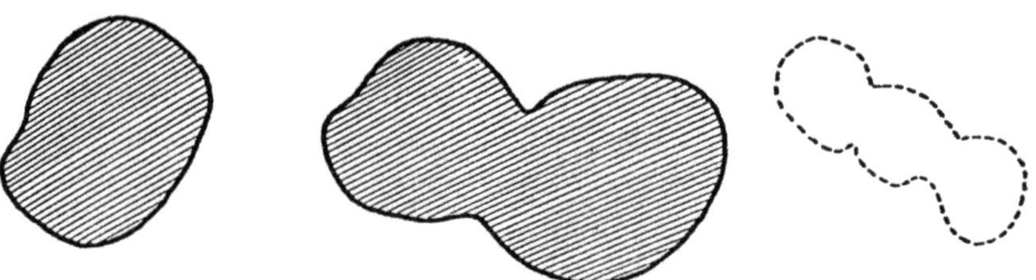

Figure 2 : Opening of X of size θ : $(X)_{\theta B}$

Thus the enlarged cervical cells are simply those which are not changed by an opening of size θ.

ⓑ Reconstruction of grains ; combination of dilations and intersections

Very often it happens that a recognition procedure has detected a subset of all cells of type A in an image and nothing in cells of type B. Starting from this subset as germ, one would like to reconstruct all A cells. This is done by a transformation T called reconstruction of grains. This transformation has two images as input, image X containing all cells and image Y containing the germs. T needs a variable number of steps which depends upon the respective sizes of grains and germs. At each step, T replaces the germs by greater germs. If at step n we had the germs Y_n, at step n+1 they will be replaced by germs $Y_{n+1} = [Y_n \oplus B] \cap X$: the dilation $Y_n \oplus B$ increases the size of Y_n, and the intersection with X ensures that Y_{n+1} is still a subset of X. Finally Y_n fills up all cells A.

Thus T replaces (X,Y) by (X, lim Y_n). T is still an idempotent operation, but the idempotence here is reached only after a variable number of iterations.

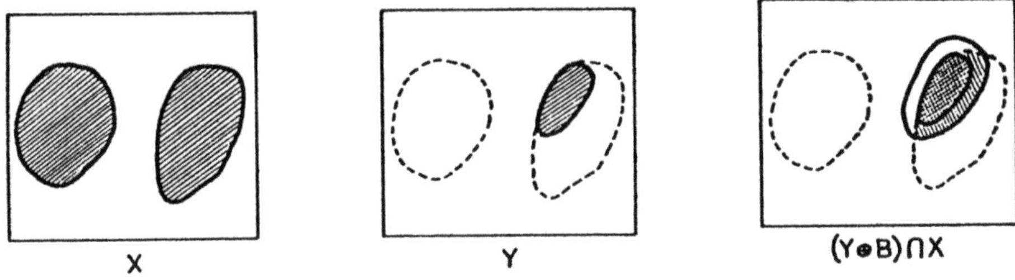

Figure 3 : First step in the reconstruction of grains

ⓒ The use of the grassfire transformation for the separation of overlapping cells

Here we will present a more complex idempotent transformation wich keeps isolated cells unchanged and separates overlapping cells.

For this we will need to introduce the grassfire transformation and the skeleton.

Let's observe the grassfire of section (a) more carefully. The fire propagates toward the middle of the figure with uniform speed ; however, at some points the advancing line of the fire from one region of the boundary intersects with the fire front from another region, and the two fronts will extinguish each other. The points are called quench points of the fire ; the set of quench points defines the skeleton of the figure.

If the speed of the fire is effectively uniform normal to the front of the fire, this is definitely not the case along the skeleton line. If we select all points of the skeleton for which the speed is higher than a given value α , we define the α -conditional bisectrix of the figure. This transformation is particularly interesting since each cell within a cell cluster is transformed into its center (Figure 4b). If we now let a fire spread from these centers toward the border, the quenching lines, on which two fronts starting from two different centers will extinghish each other, will separate the clustered cells in single cells (figure 4c).

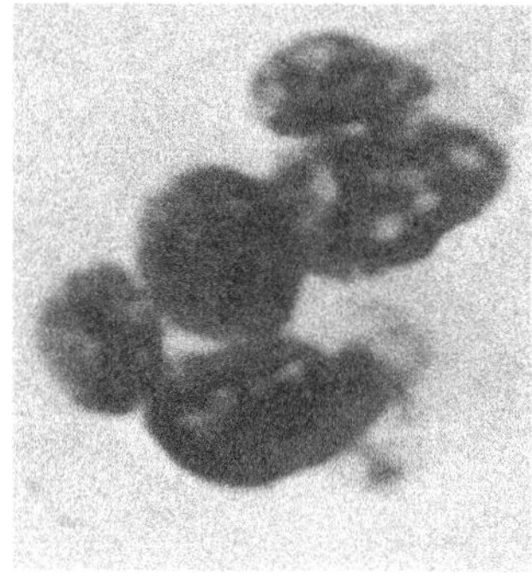

Figure 4A
Original image

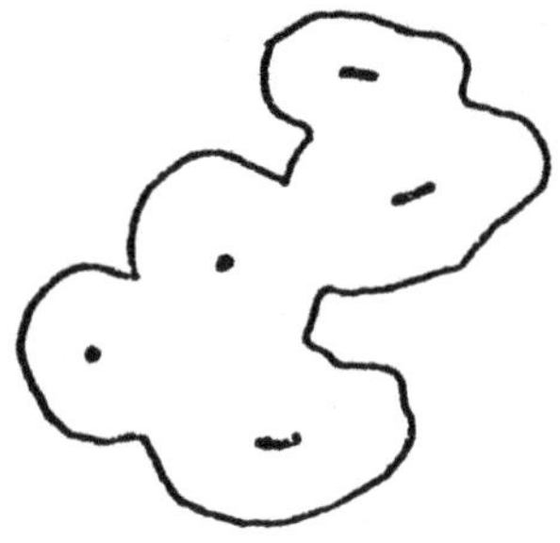

Figure 4B
Threshold and conditional Bisectrix

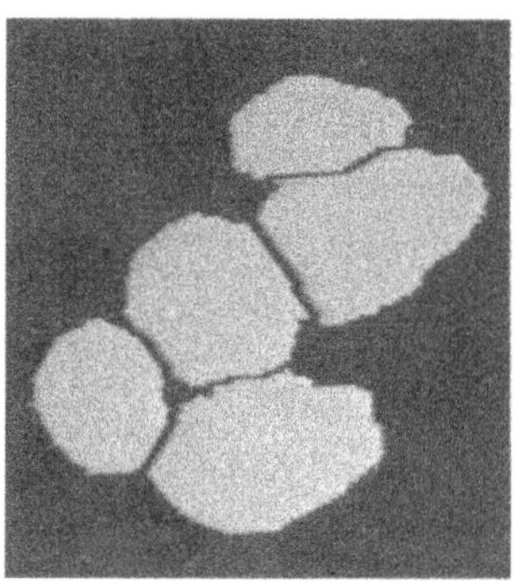

Figure 4C
Séparation

Figure 4 : Automatic separation of clustered cells.

This much more complex transformation is also idempotent, since isolated cells remain unchanged, and clustered cells are separated. The repetition of the transformation will not further modify the image.

(d) Until now we have dealt only with binary images, but in reality we meet only grey tone images. In this last section we will see an application of the opening to contrast analysis in grey tone images. A grey tone image may be represented as a chain of mountains, where the highest points stand for the darkest points and the peaks represent contrast zones in the grey tone image. The discrimination between smooth mountains and peaks may be done with a top-hat. If it is possible to cram the hat on the mountain in such a way that the top of the hat is pierced then the mountain was a peak and otherwise not. This may be clearly understood in figure 5. If we come back to the grey tone image, it means the following: we have detected a peak of contrast when there exists two thresholds h_1 and $h_2 = h_1 + h$ such that :

(a) by the upper threshold something is detected (the hat of height h is pierced

(b) and the lower threshold disappears into an opening of size R. (the peak enters into the hat of radius R).

More details may be found in (13)

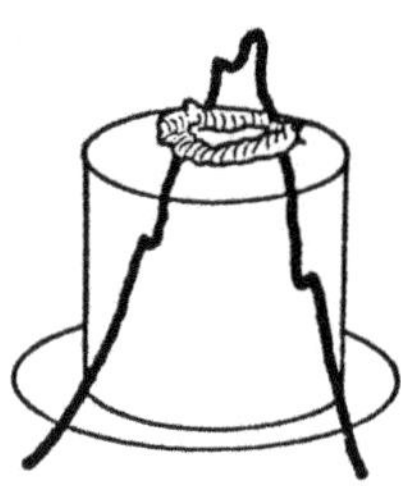

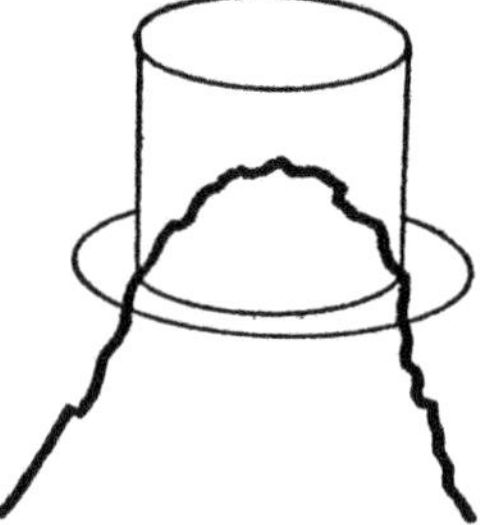

Figure 5 : The top hat transformation.

If represented as a chain of mountains, the chromatin structure would appear as little peaks at various altitudes. The top hat transformation allows us to construct a binary image of the chromatin patterns of the nucleus (Figure 6A and 6B). Further on, this binary image is used for granulometric and densitometric measurements. Obviously the top hat transformation is also idempotent.

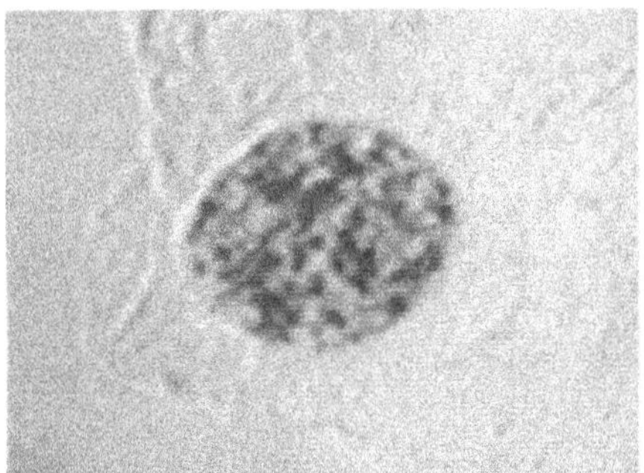

Figure 6A : Original image

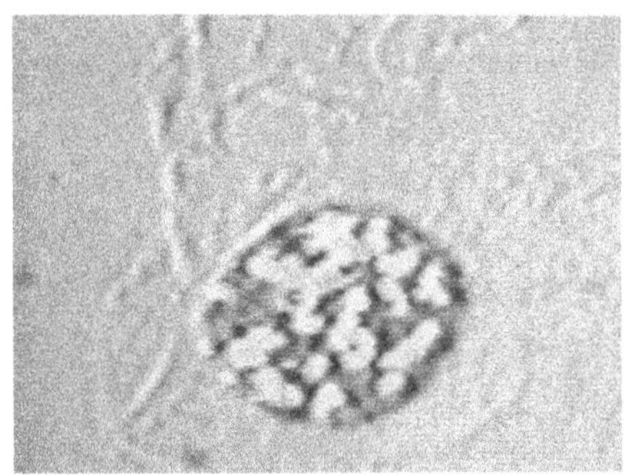

Figure 6B : Binary mask of the chromatin patterns

Figure 6 : Detection of the chromatin

The top-hat transformation turned out to be a particularly flexible instrument in the hands of a cytologist : When he modifies the size of the testing top-hat, he obtains chromatin particles with various degrees of coarseness and contrast. The fact that the top-hat transformation does not depend upon a given threshold makes this transformation particularly valuable : a fluctuation in illumination will not greatly affect the final result.

4. TOWARD A LANGUAGE ADAPTED TO IMAGE ANALYSIS

Throughout the previous examples, we see a hierarchy appearing amont the image transformations. They may be classified according to their complexity. The more complex transformations are combinations of less complex transformations. This appears clearly in the program which performs an automatic diagnosis of cervical slides. It appears that the most complex level is also the most specialized.

Level 4 : The automated diagnosis of cervical slides is a complex and specialized T function which associates each image with the cancerous cervical cells it contains.

Level 3 : T is a succession of less intricate transformations of much wider applicability in cytology, or even in other fields. Some of these functions have been described previously.

$$T(X) = T_n(T_{n-1}(T_{n-2}\dots(T_1(X))) \dots)$$

- T_1 is necessarily an autofocus function.
- T_2 detects particles with increased contrast and eliminates many artefacts (described in reference 14)
- T_3 eliminates strangely shaped artefacts (reference 14)
- T_4 keeps isolated cells unchanged and separates clustered cells into individual cells (as described previously)
- T_n builds a chromatin image.

Level 2 : Each transformation T_i uses the basic tools of image analysis $T_{i,j}$: grassfire transformation, skeleton, gradient, top-hat transformation, opening, etc..

Level 1 : Surprisingly all $T_{i,j}$ are combinations of single neighborhood transformations and of logical combinations between images, and of thesholding.

The following remark is essential to the concept of a programming language adapted to image analysis: the functions of each complexity level may be used without any knowledge of the less complex levels. A cytotechnician, for example may control the performances of the program of automatic cervical cytology without knowing anything about image processing.

Another may use the specialized functions of level 3 for the development of programs in other fields of cytology or histology.

Similarly, it is not necessary to know which sequence of operations is needed to obtain a skeleton or a gradient in order to be able to employ them effectively.

For this very reason, it would be highly desirable to possess a powerful programming language in which each instruction would call a specific image transformation. The cytologist would need only a specialized sublanguage grouping all functions which often occur in automated cytology. The histologist could use another sublanguage. The specialist in image processing would use the universal language of non-specialized functions. The existence of such a language would facilitate the communication between all specialists in natural sciences where image processing problems occur and pattern recognition people. The universality of such a language is well warranted since it is not tied to a particular apparatus. It is possible to compute a skeleton or a gradient in a square or a hexagonal raster, in a specialized image processing device or in many current computers.

Yet, if it is possible to develop a program with several types of hardware, it will not run at the same speed on all these machines. The design of the hardware, so far speed is concerned, becomes very crucial.

5. THE DESIGN OF AN APPARATUS FOR IMAGE PROCESSING

(a) A machine based on neighborhood transformations

A machine specialized in image processing should be able to perform very fast neighborhood transformations ; we hope that the reader is now convinced of the usefulness of such transformations, after having seen such varied applications based on the same elementary transformations. Yet there exists also a theoretical justification for these transformations based on considerations of robustness (for more details see references 12, 16, 17).

(b) The two meanings of parallelism

In order to prevent a confusion which often occurs, we would like to make a little remark about the meaning of parallelism.

Each elementary neighborhood transformation is a parallel transformation, since the neighborhood which characterizes the transformation is the same for each point. A non-parallel transformation would transform each point of a subset Y of X with different rules than those used for the rest of the image. A transformation which gives the mask of the upper left cell of the field is non-parallel and is frequently used for an individual cell-by-cell analysis.

In the next section, we will meet another sense of the word parallel which concerns only the processing unit. A parallel CPU is a processor where each picture point has it's own processing element.

A non-parallel processor like the TAS basically does only parallel transformations and a parallel processor like CLIPP can do non parallel transformations.

Ⓒ Sequential, parallel, semi-parallel, pipe-lined processors

- a sequential machine has one processing unit for each hardwired function and for the whole image. The whole image goes through the processing unit and is transformed point by point. Such a machine is relatively slow. The TAS does the transformations with TV-speed: 20 ms for 10^5 points. The low speed is partially compensated if one multiplies the types of processing units. This has been done in the TAS where more complex functions, such as openings, closings, covariances of various size have been hardwired.

The main advantage of such a machine lies in the independance between the memory size and the number of processing units which reduces the overall cost of the device.

- a parallel machine : each pixel has its own processing unit, and is therefore connected with its neighbour points. For evident reasons of simplicity and feasibility, each point is connected only with its immediate neighbour points. Thus only elementary transformations, those of level 1, can be programmed. This fact is of course compensated by high processing speed. A serious disadvantage is due to the fact that the cost of the machine bound to the number of processors increases with the number of picture points. For this reason the images to be treated are relatively small (96 x 96 in a very interesting machine design by M. Diff, CLIPP 4, see references 6, 9, 20).

The small size of the images has another disadvantage. Many transformations or measurements need edge corrections. Often there exists a dead zone around the image in which the transformed image is unknown ; the size of this zone depends only on the transformation used (see reference 17). For small images the relative area of this dead zone may become extensive giving rise to difficult sampling problems.

- a semi-parallel machine

It would probably be worthwhile to design a machine which would be a compromise between a purely sequential and a purely parallel machine. Such a machine would dispose of on neighborhood processor for each line. It would then be possible with 1000 processors to process an image of 1 million points. Such images already exist in radiography, and could also be furnished with newly designed microscopes and TV cameras or with diode arrays.

For these large images, the edge effects would be essentially negligible.

- pipe-lined machines

Another solution consists in pipelining several processors. The output of each processor serves as input for the next processor. This machine is in fact a sequential machine where the processing unit is a pipe line of elementary processors. The notable machine of this type is the cytocomputer constructed by Sternberg and presented at this meeting. Such a machine is fast with a minor disadvantage : each elementary processor has to be programmed separately and they may all have a different task. Thus the programming time of a long pipe line cannot be discounted anymore when compared to the execution time.

6. CONCLUSION

The various possibilities for the architecture of a machine and the multiplication of available machines has one danger : it may create a Tower of Babel, if we are not able to define a common language devoted to image analysis. And this should not be a difficult task for all the transformations covered by Mathematical Morphology, since these transformations organize themselves in an algebra.

The importance of a well defined and structured language cannot be underestimated.

The trivial interest is to facilitate the exchange of programs. But its major interest lies elsewhere: a language is not a passive expression of our thoughts, the language shapes, initiates, stimulates our thinking. A problem will appear easy to solve if we are able to formulate it in an adequate language and completely impossible in another one.

Please let us avoid the Tower of Babel ...

BIBLIOGRAPHY

1 - BLUM, H. : Biological shape and visual sciences (Part 1) J. of Theor. Biol. 38,2 (1973)

2 - CALABI, L. : On the shape on plane figures. Air Force Cambridte Res. Labs. Res. Rep. (1965)

3 - CALABI, L. : The many face of the skeleton. Air Force Cambridge Res. Labs. Res. Rep. (1969)

4 - DIGABEL H., LANTUEJOUL Ch. : Iterative algorithms, Special Issues of Practical Metallography, Vol. 8, Riederer Verlag Gmbh Stuttgart, 1977.

5 - DUDA Ro, HART E. : Pattern Classification and Scene Analysis, Wiley 1973.

6 - DUFF M.J.B., WATSON D.M., FOUNTAIN T.J. and SHAW G.K. : A cellular logic array for image processing, Pattern recognition, Vol. 5, pp. 229-247 (1973)

7 - GOLAY M.J.E. : Hexagonal Pattern Transforms, IEE Trans on Comp., Vol. C18 n° 8, August 1969.

8 - KLEIN J.C., SERRA J. : The texture analyser, J. of Microscopy, 95 (2) p. 349-356 (1972)

9 - KRUSE B. : A parallel picture processing machine, Trans. IEEE, Vol. C22, n° 2 p. 1075

10 - LANTUEJOUL Ch. : La squelettisation et son application aux mesures topologiques des mosaïques Pollycristallines, Thesis, Ecole des Mines de Paris (1978)

11 - MATHERON G. : Eléments pour une théorie des milieux poreux, Masson, Paris (1967)

12 - MATHERON G. : Random Set and Integral Geometry John Wiley and Sons, (Interscience) New-York (1975)

13 - MEYER F. : Contrast features extraction, Special Issues of Practical Metallography, Vol. 8, Riederer Verlag Gmbh Stuttgart 1977

14 - MEYER F. : Iterative image transformations for an automatic screening of

15 - PRESTON K. Jr : Feature extraction by Golay hexagonal pattern transforms, Trans. IEEE, Vol. C-20, p. 1007.

16 - SERRA J. : One, two, three... Infinity : Special Issues of Practical Metallography, Vol. 8, Roederer Verlag Gmbh Stuttgart (1977)

17 - SERRA J. : Image analysis by Mathematical Morphology Acc. Press (in press)

18 - STERNBERG S.R. : Language and architecture for parallel image processing, Proceedings of the Conference on Pattern Recognition in Practice, 1980 North Holland Publishing Company.

19 - VROLIJK J. : A real time TV image analysis system for automated Cytology, J. of Histoch. and Cytoch. Vol. 27, n° 1 (1979)

20 - WATSON D.M. : The application of cellular logic to image processing, Ph. D. Thesis, University of London.

AUTOMATION IN CYTOGENETICS
AT : C.E.A. PARIS

by
R.J.P. Le Gô, M.D., Ph. D

Commissariat à l'Energie Atomique
Centre d'Etudes Nucléaires. P.o. Box 6
Fontenay-aux-Roses, France, 92260

ABSTRACT

In order to facilitate the task of cytogeneticists two systems have been built: 1. A metaphase finder, called EIDOMAT which can scan a slide at high speed and locate the correct metaphases with a rate of success of about 60%. 2. An image analysis assembly, using interactive data treatment after numerization of the microscopic image, to clear the memory of the improper images or from overlaps. After a propositional karyotype has been displayed a second interactive phase allows operator to correct the karyotype. 3. The future use of a parallel computer PROPAL 2 will enhance the speed of treatment by an important factor.

1. INTRODUCTION

The importance of Chromosome Analysis (C.A.) in different domains of Biological Sciences is increasing. In the particular field of Radiation Protection,C.A. is a precious and reliable tool for biological damage assessment in cases of accidental human irradiation.Whatever the application the needs for automation is evident if one is to perform the number of C.A. that circumstances demand and which presently cannot be achieved.

C.A. by human Cytogeticist implies several distinct phases: a) biological phase : culture, specimen treatment, slide staining by various techniques (Standard Giemsa, banding). b) scanning of slides by the microscope, to locate the metaphases of sufficient quality to be karyotyped. c) metaphase analysis, at high magnification, to : identify individual chromosomes, reconstruct the cytologic "anatomy" of the cell by the establishment of its karyogram. d) diagnosis phase, in which : individual abnormalities are when present, scored within a single cell, a global diagnosis then is set, for the whole sample of the studied cells. Each of these phases can be considered as appropriate for automation. But they have not elicited the same degree of interest.

Automation of lymphocyte culture has not really been extensively studied. Some attemps have been made to automate staining procedures for chromosome smears [1] . This particular aspect of automation certainly is of great importance, not only to speed up the procedures but also to achieve a standardization of the staining techniques. As a matter of fact the subsequent phases of automation (metaphase finding, recognition of chromosomes) are strongly dependant on the good quality of the stained objects submitted to treatment. Conversely, the other phases of C.A. have elicited considerable effort in a number of groups, in the States, in European countries and more recently (but not less intensively) in Japan. [2] - [15] .

In this paper we shall deal essentially with the automatic selection of good metaphases on the one hand and with the pattern recognition of chromosome images and karyotyping by machine, on the other.

2. METAPHASE FINDING

It is common knowledge that the number of "good metaphases" differs from slide to slide. Rich slides can offer several hundreds of correct images and as few as ten metaphasic cells can be scored on other samples. Such a paucity is especially common in accidentally irradiated patients in whom the number of circulating lymphocytes falls to very low levels in a few days. Therefore the usefulness of metaphase finders is evident in such situations. Furthermore if a machine can rapidly scan the slide and find the good cells without missing a noticeable proportion of them, it will be of general interest. The problem of metaphase finding can be summarized as follows on a slide surface of 8 square centimeters, detect objects of a mean size of 2000 square microns, with a "circular" area of dispersion, from a field containing other circular objects (nuclei or bad mitoses) which are a little smaller and hundreds of times more numerous, plus some other artitacts, debris, stain blobs, glass micro-bubbles, etc.

2.1 The experimental metaphase finders.

A small number of Metaphase Finders have been built for experimental purposes but at present to my knowledge, none have been released. These machines are based upon different physical principles and devices.

T-V based Systems.

In the T-V based systems the microscope field is scanned by a vidicon camera and the video signal is processed to detect objects of interest in the field. If no such object is present the associated computer shifts the motorized stage to scan the next field.
If a potentially interesting object is present, the system runs algorithms to detect some features characteristic of a metaphase. The metaphase finders based on this principle are : the Jet Propulsion Laboratory system, built by K. CASTLEMAN [10] , the Leuven system, described by OOSTERLINCK [11] , the first Edinburgh system, built by GREEN and D. RUTOWITZ [12] .

In the first Edinburgh system, for instance, the computer has to detect a so-called double humped signal. The underlying assumption is that in a metaphase a number of the randomly oriented chromosomes are vertically oriented. These chromosomes will give a pair of closely connected pulses when intersected by the scan.

In the Leuven approach a connexity algorithm permits the detection of the "ends" of objects. Their number and clustering within the area of a metaphase diameter is estimated. A similar approach has been described by the Leiden group (J.VROLIJK, R. PEARSON, Inge AL) using the "erosion-dilatation" operation from J. SERRA which is used in the Texture Analysis System (T.A.S.)of LEITZ. The main difficulty in such systems lies in the necessity of stopping the stage over each microscope field to allow TV scanning and signal processing. Thus the scanning time for a slide is in the range of 20 minutes, or longer.

Optical Fourier Transform Systems.

An Optical Fourier Transform system first described by Niel WALD and also by NORGREN [13] requires the use of a laser beam.The FOURIER transform of the image can then be processed at high speed and the energy level in the high frequencies versus the energy in lower frequencies can optimally characterize the dispersion of the chromosomes in a metaphasic cell. A similar approach by HUTZLER is in development at Neuherberg (München) The system is attempting to detect the presence of two separate chromatids for each chromosome. These may not always be present.

Linear arrays of sensors and continuous scanning.

The use of linear arrays of sensors allows a large strip of the microscope field to be scanned at once in the Y-direction (vertical diameter of the field), the X-axis being scanned by the continuous displacement of the motorized stage. Such was the approach in our labs, during the years 68-70. First we use a simulation program that ran on large IBM computers. Then a first prototype was developed in Grenoble

(L.E.T.I.) in 1973 and called the EIDOMAT [14] . This approach was also adopted for the second generation of Metaphase Finder by RUTOWITZ and GREEN, and later by the TUFT'S Hospital group in Boston, Massachussets. Since then a second and a third version of our EIDOMAT have been built. These last versions will be described now.

2.2 The EIDOMAT system.

The EIDOMAT system comprises :
A ZEISS photomicroscope, whose stage is motorized in X,Y and Z directions. The Z-motor is a step motor. The X - and Y- motors move on a continuous mode. Both movements are quantified.

A linear array of 512 (EIDOMAT-2) or 1024 (EIDOMAT-3) CCD sensors which scan a "vertical" diameter of the microscope field.

A microprocessored logic which selects the candidate objects.
A computer program which monitors the system and allows interaction with the operator.

1. The microscope is standard and required no modification to access the three manual knobs of the stage.

2. The photo-sensor array has a hardware shading correction which is operated once only at the beginning of the session by using a dark field and an blank one to set the min and max responses for each sensor.

3. The microprocessor is a bit-slice processor which continuously performs a "connexity algorithm" on the sensor signals between two steps of the system clock. The signals are submitted to a double threshold: a "black" threshold to eliminate the darker signals generally coming from nuclei, a "white" threshold to eliminate the background. The microprocessor algorithms calculate a number of parameters on line for each object : area, perimeter, circular index P2/S, number of internal holes. These parameters together with the X-Y coordinates of the stage are sent to the computer which selects those images whose parameter values lay between two preset values chosen by the operator.

4. The computer is a mini 32 K (MULTI-6: INTERTECHNIQUE).

Procedure.

The operating procedure is sequenced as follows :

1. Setting the parameters.

A number of questions are asked of the operator which allow him to indicate :
. the origins X-zero and Y-zero of the area to be scanned
. the X and Y dimensions of this area
. the min and max values for each parameter : area, perimeter, etc..

2. Phase 1

The Phase 1 can then be activated by pressing the appropriate switch on the Command Box. The stage is moved at the X-zero, Y-zero point and then scanned continuously according to a "greek key pattern" until the prescribed aread is scanned in totality. During this phase 1, the X-Y coordinates of the candidate objects are picked up on line on the moving stage and stored in the computer memory. At the end of the Phase 1 the program prints the number of candidate objects which have been memorized. This allows the detection of missetting of parameters if for instance the number of objects is very low.

3. Phase 2

Among the memorized objects :
part are irrelevant, or false positive
part are metaphases but of poor quality
other are good metaphases.

The Phase 2 is designed to select only good metaphases among these objects. It is an interactive phase activated by pressing the appropriate switch on the command box. The computer pilots the stage on the first memorized address and waits for an operator command. After examining the image under the objective, the operator may choose to press either the switch "rejection" or the switch "next object". In case of rejection the object is flagged in memory as irrelevant but not erased. If "next object" switch is pressed the stage moves immediatly to the next address. This displacement between objects is very fast (mean 0.3 second). Thus the total time for this phase is less than five minutes for about a hundred objects.

4. Outputs.

At the end of Phase 2, the computer prints the number of good metaphases. The results can then be edited on a printer and/or punched on a paper tape, using appropriate commands of the monitor.

5. Commands.

The operator can interact with the program monitor through a number of three - character commands. For instance :

"LIS" causes the list of the objects to be edited on the printer. This list contains for each object :

The X-Y coordinates, the values of the parameters for this object : area, perimeter, P2/S, etc. The objects which have been rejected during the Phase 2 are marked with an asterix if the "COM" command (for compression) has not yet eliminated the improper objects. If the appropriate key on the front panel is in down position, the program allows the operator to type a comment for the object just listed on the same line. This feature is useful for a systematic test of the machine.

The command "HIS" gives a histogram of the objects for the area and a histogram for the perimeter.

The commande "GDT" calculates the speed of the X-motor as a function of the objective magnification and the scan time for one line.

The command "CHE",n causes the object number n, to be presented. "CHE",o sets the stage at the origin.

There is a total of 26 such ergonomic commands.

6. Manual Operation.

A special feature has been implemented which allows the operator to substitute himself for the machine. In this manual procedure the stage is moved very slowly so as to allow the operator to watch the moving microscope field attentively. When a good metaphase crosses the vertical diameter of the field the operator presses a switch to memorize the object. This allows the scanning of very poor slides for which none of the metaphases should be lost. It also allows the comparison of the results of scans of the same slide by the operator and by the machine.

7. Results.

Because the stage displacement need not be stopped during the scan in the x-direction the speed of the machine is good. It scans at the rate of about 30 seconds per square centimeter. This speed can be increased : the electronic data processing is actually not limitative for the speed of data acquisition. The rate of success, as for other types of such machines depends of a number of factors.

1. Some are linked to the operator choice of the set of parameters for a particular slide. For a large window the number of good metaphases detected is maximum. But the number of irrelevant images increased and the rejection rate during Phase 2 can be high, in the 60 per cent range. For a narrow window a percentage of correct metaphases is lost but the rate of rejection of irrelevant objects is decreased. This balance between the rate of false positive and the rate of false negative has to

be chosen according to the quality of the slide as regards to the number of available metaphases and the number needed to complete the chromosome analysis of the sample.

2. Other factors which influence the success rate are linked to the quality of the preparation and staining. In this respect, homogeneously GIEMSA stained slides give better results than slides treated by banding techniques, the contrast of which is generally poor.

Typical values for the two types of staining are :

about 60 per cent good metaphases for Giemsa staining
about 40 per cent for banded chromosomes.

2.3 Digitizing function of EIDOMAT 2/3.

The two versions 2 and 3 of EIDOMAT have a digitizing function. EIDOMAT-2 gives a raster of 512 x 512 pixels. EIDOMAT-3 gives a raster of 1024 x 1024 pixels.

To use this function a metaphase is centered under the objective lens at high magnification and the command for digitizing is sent to the computer. The stage first backs up at a distance,then runs towards the metaphase. The analog signals from the CCD are taken into account from a step which is at half a raster behind the centering point to a symmetric point at half a raster past this point. The conversion is made on 8 bits.

A pair of buffers in flip-flop mode is fed with the data corresponding to a step for the whole CCD array and the buffer contents are transferred to a magnetic disk where they constitute the data sets for further treatment.

3. COMPUTERIZED KARYOTYPING.

Our attemps to computerized karyotyping were developped in two phases : first, a simulation program using an IBM-360-91 in Saclay, Atomic Energy Commission Center; second, an application program using a local minicomputer.

The simulation program allowed us to write a number of segmentation and pattern description algorithms. Starting from a low speed drum digitizer (giving a data set of 200 000 pixels on 4 bits) the segmentation program gave the 46 "vignettes" on a magnetic tape. From this tape, the second package gave the computer determination for arm tips and centromeres and presented these results as marks on the contour of each chromosome displayed on an IBM-2250 facility. An interactive program allowed some false determinations for the characteristic points of the image to be corrected.

This simulation program showed :

first,that pattern recognition algorithms ran correctly.
second, that the operator interaction at the level of an individual chromosome was much too slow.
third, that the use of a large computer with graphic unit was much too costly for biologists.

Thus we decided to build a system around a mini computer and to reduce the interaction at the two ends of the processing : data acquisition and data output.

The PARIS system comprises :

3.1 A T-V camera coupled to a ZEISS photomicroscope and to an A to D converter with thresholding.

3.2 The digitized data are packed and fed into a 32-K 8 bits MOS memory. Symmetrically the memory contents can be unpacked and fed through a D to A converter into a

T-V monitor and displayed on a screen. The conversion speed allows the numerical image to be displayed on line. Thus an optical adjustment on the microscope is made possible (focusing, centering...) under numerization process.

3.3 An automaton named A.S.T.I. (Automaton Specialized for Treatment of Images) allows the operator to interact with the memory content through a small dark index appearing on the screen which can be moved by a joy-stick . This index can be put in contact with one of dark images. The operator selects an appropriate operation by depressing one of the control function buttons of the ASTI. This function acts on the selected image.

The A.S.T.I. is implemented with the following functions :

1. Transferring the image into memory. It required 150 milliseconds from a T-V frame.

2. Automatic segmentation of the memory content ; this function requires about 1.5 second for the 40-50 images.

3. By using the joy-stick, the following treatments can be applied to a particular image :

3.1 marking of a particular image to be treated by other functions.

3.2 erasing a blob (for instance a nucleus image present among the chromosomes).

3.3 cutting the contact area of two touching chromosomes or dissecting two overlapping images.

3.4 applying a "logical level" to a particular image or to a collection of images which are logically linked by this function. They can appear together by twinckling on the screen. Thus for instance the marked images for the A-group will twinckle for logical level 1,those for the B-group for logical level 2 and so on. These different functions are designed to clean up the digitized image before computer treatment.

The last function of the automaton is the transfer of isolated images to the mini computer on its request by an interrupt signal. In this case each vignette containing one chromosome is sent to the computer on its request until the entire set of images is analysed.

3.4. The computer is a mini 32K (MULTI-6 INTERTECHNIQUE) with a 5 megaoctet disk. It is coupled to a 4015 TEKTRONIX graphic unit, plus hard copy.

The pattern recognition algorithms which we have programmed on this computer system are : clockwise contouring, rotation, transversal cutting, median axis or parabola axis and density profile, etc ... [15] [19] [16].

3.5. The outputs are as follows :

A "fac simile" of the microscopic image, in which each chromosome is drawn by its contours in a position homothetic to its position in the metaphase under the microscope.

A "propositional" karyogram in which the chromosomes are vertically oriented and classified according the DENVER/PARIS groups.

An interactive program then allows the operator to introduce corrections in this karyogram : for instance EXCHANGE chromosomes i and j, or : put the chromosome k into the group n ...so that the karyogram is correct according to the operators judgment.

3.6 Operation time.

The time required to obtain a definitive karyogram from a cell located under the objective is approximately eight to ten minutes, allocated as follows:

Optical adjustements : 1 minute
Digitization-memorization : 150 milliseconds
Interactive cleaning up of the memorized image : 2 minutes
Transfer of the 46 vignettes, calculations, drawing the fac simile : 30 seconds
Recognition, grouping, drawing the propositional karyogram : 50 seconds
Interactive corrections of the misclassifications : variable time: 1 to 4 minutes.

This running time is obviously too long for the system to be qualified as operational. Therefore we are presently modifying the structure of the system along two lines.

1. The 32 K-octects MULTI-6 will be replaced by a 192 K-words MITRA-125 (S.E.M.S.). We are presently re-writing the algorithms for this machine.

2. As in other group conception (GRANLUND [20]), a large part of the algorithms will be transferred to a Parallel Processor: PROPAL-2. In our actual configuration PROPAL-2 is a set of 64 Elementary Processors (P.E.) which are under the control of a Master Processor.

Each of the E.P. has its own memory space, divided into two parts:
operational fast memory (256 bits) and
extension memory (16 K bits)

The extension memory can be functionally divided into zones. Each zone is a least one pixel wide. Thus a total image field of 64 × 2 K pixels can be stored in the parallel memory.

Arithmetic or Boolean operations can be applied at once to a whole column of pixels. This reduces drastically the processing time. A test program to demonstrate the speed of treatment by PROPAL-2 was based upon a comparison of the treatment time for the same algorithm (skeletonisation of five chromosome images) ran on PROPAL-2 on the one hand and on the MITRA-125 sequential minicomputer : (116 -words) on the other.

The Figure 1 shows the configuration of the demonstration: each of the phases of skeletonization on both computers was displayed simultaneously on the same video screen, showing the very fast evolution of the successive images from the PROPAL output, compared to the MITRA output.

The Figure 2 shows the visualization diagram of display in which the same time processing of 4 milliseconds was regularly allocated to the two machines, between periods of 350 miliseconds allowing the display.

The Figure 3 shows the time diagram of the processing for skeletonization in four phases.

It shows that the four phases for the total set of five different chromosomes are terminated on PROPAL whereas the first phase on the first chromosome is far from being terminated on MITRA. A magnification of the PROPAL diagram shows that the processing time rate is of 500/ u:125 times faster for this test.

4. CONCLUDING REMARKS.

We have just begun to use this machine which needs special training to be efficiently programmed.

With such a facility at our disposal, we hope that a lot of redundant algorithms can be added to the actual set of morphognostic algorithms leading to a reduced number of misclassifications.

This will considerably shorten that portion of time presently devoted to the operator interaction on the propositional karyogram. The automated or semiautomated karyotyping is still not solved in the sense of a really fast operational tool. The introduction of parallel processing in the conception of the whole system certainly is a step forward this goal.

ACKNOWLEDGMENTS.

We are indebted to many persons for the research reported here, in particular : C. Richalet, Th. Pichon, Suyama (Adersa-Gerbios), Y. Cassin, R. Boudarel (L.E.T.I. Grenoble) B. De Cosnac, A. Spywack (S.E.S. Saclay).

This resarch was supported by the Commissariat à l'Energie Atomique, Institut de Protection de Sûreté Nucléaire.

REFERENCES.

1. J. Melnyk, G. Persinger, B. Moun, K.R. Castelman, "A semi automated specimen preparation system for cytogenetis", J. Reproductive Med. Vol. 17,1976, pp. 59-67.

2. C.W. Gilbert, S. Muldal, " Measurement and computer system for karyotyping human and other cells"., Nature New Biol., Vol. 230, 1977, pp. 203-207.

3. N. Wald, R.W. Ranshan , J.M. Herron , J.G. Castle, "Progress of an automatic system for cytogenetic analysis" Human population cytogenetics. Jacobs, Price & Law , Eds. University of Edinbourg press, Edimburg, 1970.

4. J. Piper, E. Granum, D. Rutovitz D., H. Ruttledge, " Automation of chromosome analysis".

5. M.E. Drets, " Bandscan, a computer program for on line linear scanning of human banded chromosomes " Comput. Programs Biomed. Vol. 8 , 1978, pp. 283-294.

6. S.W. Wright , B.F. Crandall, L. Boyer, " Perspectives in Cytogenetics, Ch. C. Thomas, Springfield, Illinois.

7. K. Castleman, J. Melnyk, H.J. Frieden, G.W. Persinger, R.J. Wall, " Karyotype analysis by computer and its application to mutagenicity testing of environmental chemicals" Mutation Research, Vol. 41, 1976, pp. 153-162

8. S. Wakazono, N. Ichihara, K. Hibi, T. Ariga, " The development of chromosome image data processing and executer system", Proceedings of the International Symposium on Medical Information Systems" Osaka, 2-6 Oct. 1978 (Medis 78) pp. 174-176.

9. T. Sekiya, M. Saito, " Automatic system for identifying banded human chromosomes", Proceedings of the International Symposium on medical information Systems, Osaka, 2-6 Oct. 1978, (Medis 78) pp. 176-178.

10. K. R. Castleman, J.H. Melnyk, " An automated system for chromosome analysis" Final Report J P L 5040-30, Pasadena , July 4, 1976.

11. A. OOTERLINCK, J. Van Dayle, "Computer assited karyotyping with human interaction", J. Histochem Cytochem., Vol. 25, 1977, 754-762.

12. D. Rutowitz, Personal communication.

13. P.E. Norgren, " High speed automatic laser beam detection of chromosome speads" Ann. N.Y. Acad. Sci. Vol. 157, 1969, 514-524.

14. R. Le Gô, "Un système de sélection automatique des métaphases", C.R. Acad. Sci. Vol. 274, 1972, pp. 108-111.

15. H. Van den Berg, J. Habbema, H. De France, H. Bakker, G. De Vries, " On the use of distribution function to describe and classify chromosome density profils" , Comput. Biol. Med. , Vol. 9, 1979, pp. 11-20.

16. G.L. Carayannopoulos, E.A. Patrick, " An algorithm for segmentation of metaphase speads ", Pattern Recognition, Vol. 8, 1976, pp. 151, 161.

17. M.L. Mendelsohn, D.A. Hungerford, B.H. Mayal, B.H. Perry, T. Conway, J.M.S. Prewitt, " Computer oriented analysis of human chromosomes" Ann. N.Y. Acad. Sci. Vol. 157, 1969, 375.

18. N. Wald, S.F. Fatora, J.M. Herron, K. Preston, CC. Li, L. Davis " Status report on automated chromosome aberration detection", J. Histochem. Cytochem. Vol. 24, 1976, pp. 156-159.

19. R.K. Aggarwal, K.S. Fu, " Automatic recognition of irradiated chromosomes", J. Histochem. Cytochem. Vol. 22, 1974, pp. 561-568.

20. D.K. Green, J. Cameron, "Metaphase finding by machine", Cytogenetics Vol. 11 1972, pp. 475-487.

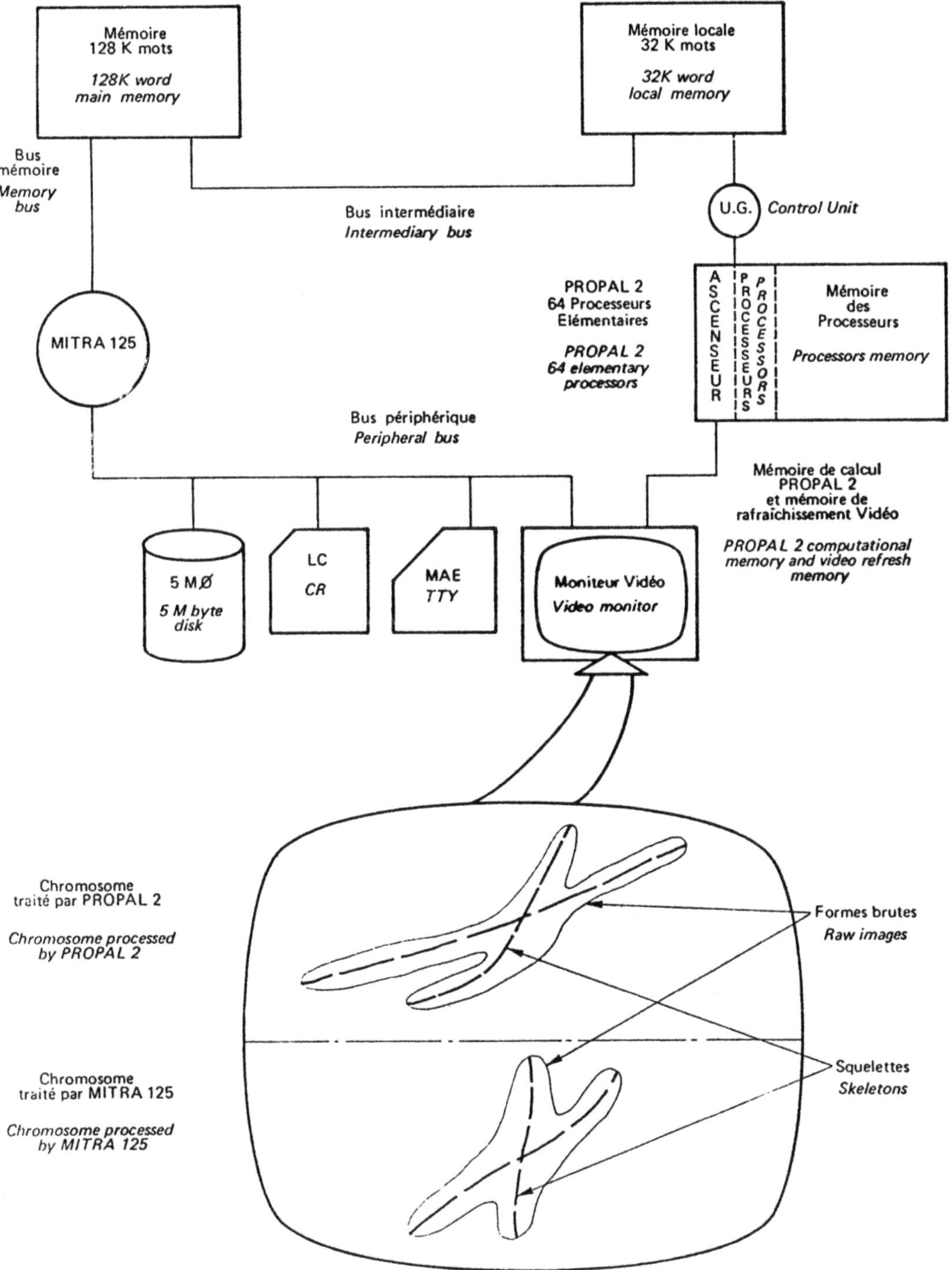

Figure 1. Comparison between the time processing ran on the two machines : PROPAL-2, MITRA-125. Configuration of the test desmonstration.

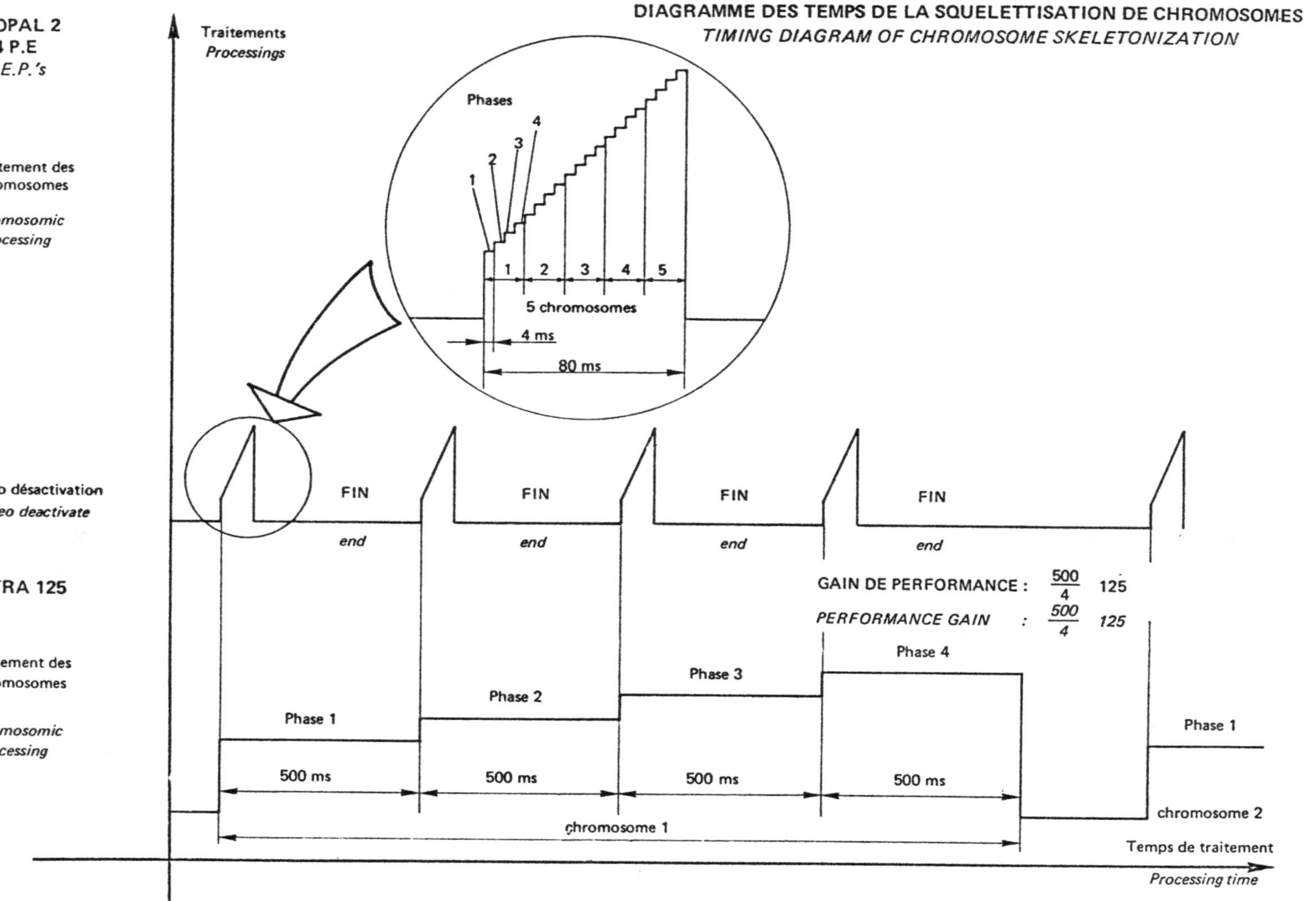

Figure 2. Visualization diagram of the test demonstration.

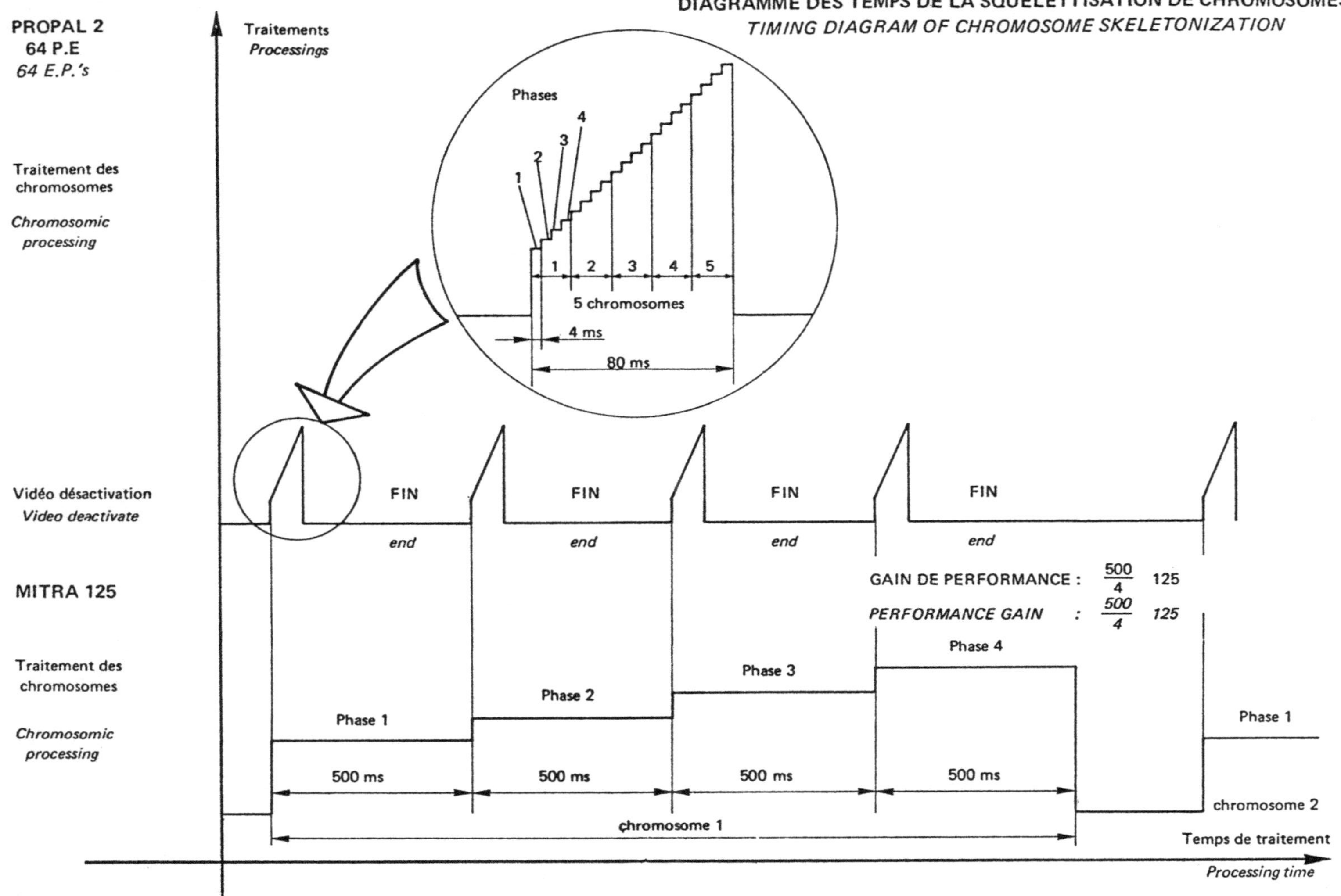

Figure 3. Time diagram of the test demonstration.

Image Processing In Acoustic Microscopy

by
R. C. Eggleton and F. S. Vinson
Ultrasound Research Division of the
Indianapolis Center for Advanced Research, Inc.
Indianapolis, Indiana 46202 U.S.A.

Abstract

The term "image processing" has become synonymous with computer processing because of the immense power and versatility of computer processing methods. There is a tendency, therefore, to overlook optical and analog electronic processing methods. In the field of acoustic microscopy with its high frequencies and wide bandwidth requirements, it is still attractive to consider some of the older methods of image processing, even though these methods may not offer the same flexibility and versatility of the processing software. Eight bit video digitizers operating at 30 MHz are available at nominal cost, and can be readily used for low resolution image processing; however, the 100 or 200 MHz digitizers required for higher resolution are still very costly. The optical and analog electronic processing methods offer a much higher data rate than present day digital systems can handle. It is therefore cost effective to utilize analog image processing systems in acoustic microscopy.

In this paper we will be considering various means of data presentation such as optical or acoustic spatial domain imaging in register with parametric mapping. Frequency domain imaging may be achieved using Fourier optics to characterize the spatial frequency of scatterers within the specimen. Time domain imaging is used to visualize events taking place on a time scale which is short compared to a television frame rate. The time domain imaging can be combined with time varying parametric recording. These multi-parameter imaging techniques can be of immense value in appreciating and understanding dynamic biological events.

1. INTRODUCTION: ACOUSTIC MICROSCOPES

1.1 The Sokolov Acoustic Microscope

The very concept of acoustic microscopy is intriguing. Acoustic microscopy offers the possibility of examining optically opaque specimens. In 1949 Sokolov [1] described an ultrasonic microscope which he had patented in 1936 [2]. This instrument makes use of two electron beam tubes (see Fig. 1). The first is the acoustic field sensor, and in this device the tube is terminated with a piezoelectric window, and the secondary electrons from the scanning electron beam impinging on the window vary in accordance with the local sound pressure and are used to modulate the beam current of the display tube. A raster generator causes the electron beam in each tube to move in synchronism. The system resolution is limited by the spot size of the pickup tube or the resonant frequency of the pickup window. Although this first instrument was not of practical design for a microscope, it did represent the beginning for the field of acoustic microscopy.

The use of sound to produce magnified images of objects promises from the outset to provide new and different information about the form and structure of objects. The image displays the viscoelastic properties of material in contrast to optical or electron density, as is the case with light or electron microscopes. Moreover, the acoustic waves may propagate freely through some materials which are opaque to both light and electron beams, allowing examination of the internal microstructures which were previously inaccessible.

Inasmuch as sound is a wave phenomenon which obeys the laws common to any type of propagating wave, it is possible to form images with acoustic lenses analogous to image formation in optical systems. A simple acoustic lens can be used to form a magnified image of the acoustic field propagating in a material. It is not necessary, however, to produce magnified acoustic images analogous to the light microscope in order to obtain enlarged displays of the acoustic field.

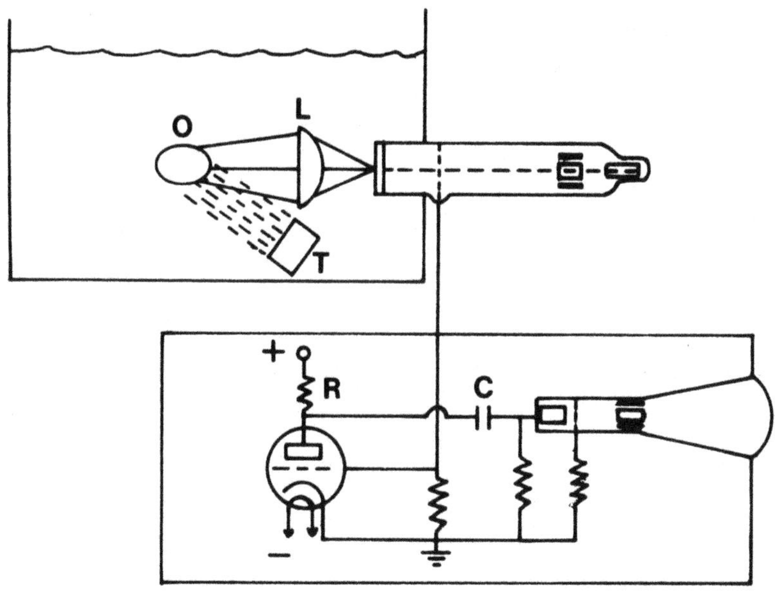

Figure 1. The first acoustic microscope was developed by Sokolov in 1949.

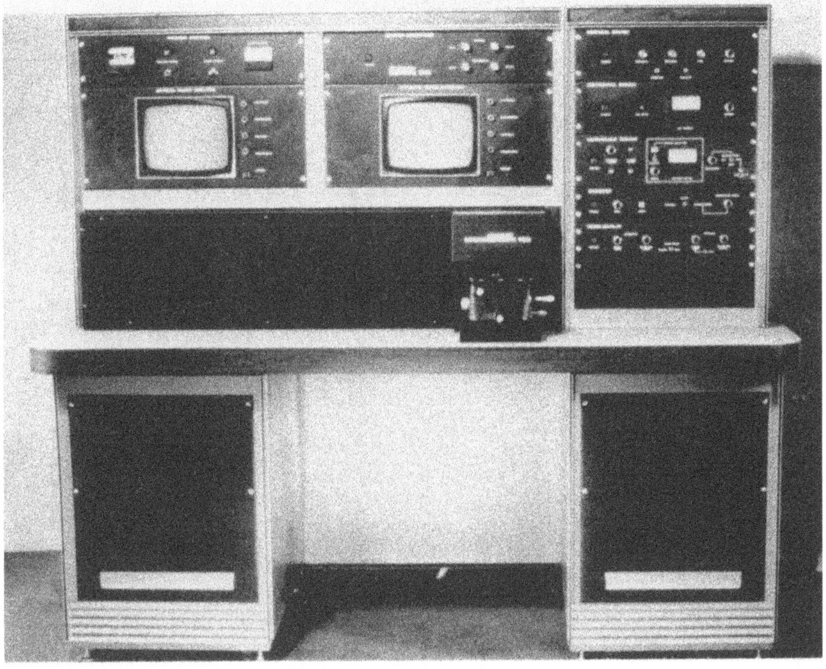

Figure 2. The Scanning Laser Acoustic Microscope is the first commercial instrument and has stimulated wide interest in the field of acoustic microscopy, for both biomedical and material science applications.

1.2 The Kessler Microscope

At present there are two types of acoustic microscopes in general use. The first type, called the SLAM, (Scanning Laser Acoustic Microscope) operates by detecting the distortion of a mirrored plastic surface produced by the sound field emerging from the specimen (see Figs. 2 and 3). The plastic mirror has an image of the specimen impressed on its surface by the sound field. This image is detected by a microspot laser system in which the scanning laser beam is reflected from the mirror surface and converted to an electrical signal with a photocell. The angle of the reflected laser beam is modulated by the local sound pressure amplitude which distorts the mirror surface. This angular modulation is converted to an intensity modulation by passing the beam over a knife edge so that varying amounts of light are received by the photocell.

The image on the mirror is the same size as the object and the magnification of this system corresponds to the ratio of the size of the laser raster to the display raster.

The SLAM system was developed by Kessler et al. [3] and manufactured by Sonoscan, Inc. This microscope has been operated in the frequency range from 100 kHz to 500 MHz. In the 100 MHz instrument the wavelength of sound in water is 15μ. The laser spot is about the same size as the ripples on the mirror surface, i.e., one wavelength.

The surface distortion method of sound field detection is capable of responding to the minute particle displacements of the propagating wave. The sound field in the microscope is typically on the order of 25 $mWcm^{-2}$. A portion of this sound is absorbed by the specimen and perhaps 10 mW impinges on the mirror surface. This local field intensity will cause a displacement of the mirror of less than 1Å, which is smaller than the interatomic spacing.

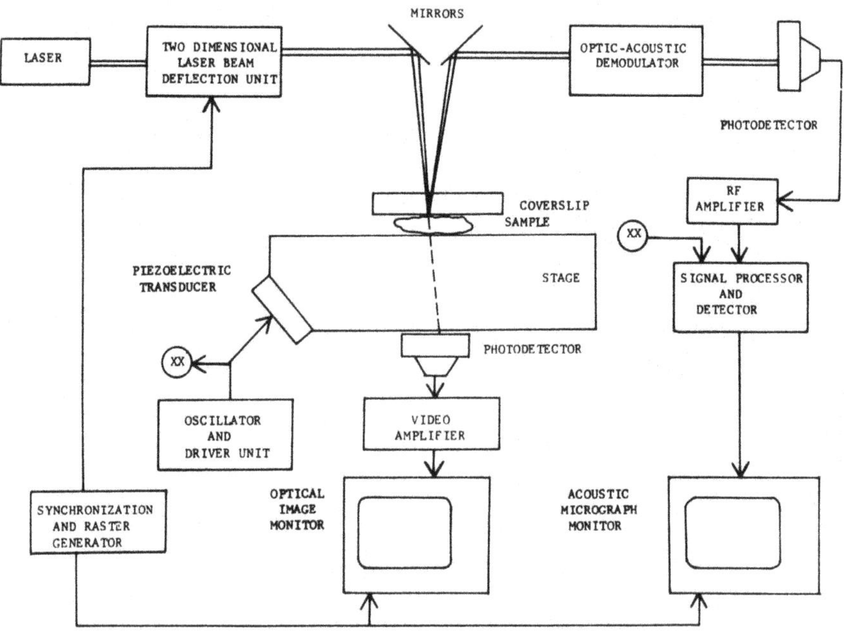

Figure 3. The Sonoscan SLAM utilizes a scanning laser detection system.

Typical Values

Sound in water		(20°C)
Frequency	f	= 100 MHz
Intensity	I	= 1 Wcm^{-2}
Density	ρ_0	= 998 kg/m^3
Particle Displacement		= 1.85Å
Sound Pressure Amplitude	P_0	= 1.8 atm

The distortions which the sound wave imparts to the optically reflective surface are not visible to the naked eye. The pattern impressed on the surface is an optical phase replica of the sound field, but despite these small amplitude changes, the angular changes of the reflected light are sufficient to result in a useful electrical signal from the photocell.

1.3 The Quate Microscope

A second system, developed by Lemons and Quate [4], utilizes acoustic lenses to focus the sound field to a beam of very small cross sectional area. The transmitted acoustic wave is picked up on a second transducer and converted back to an electrical signal (see Fig. 4 and 5). The specimen is scanned through a stationary sound field to develop a raster, thus the name Scanning Acoustic Microscope (SAM). Here, as in the case of the SLAM, the magnification corresponds to the relative size of the objective and display rasters. The Stanford microscope typically operates at 1 GHz and at a sound intensity of the order of one Wcm^{-2}. The particle displacement amplitude is only 0.18Å. This, however, is ample to produce a useable signal amplitude in the piezoelectric detector. However, the frame rate is slower in the SAM than in the SLAM.

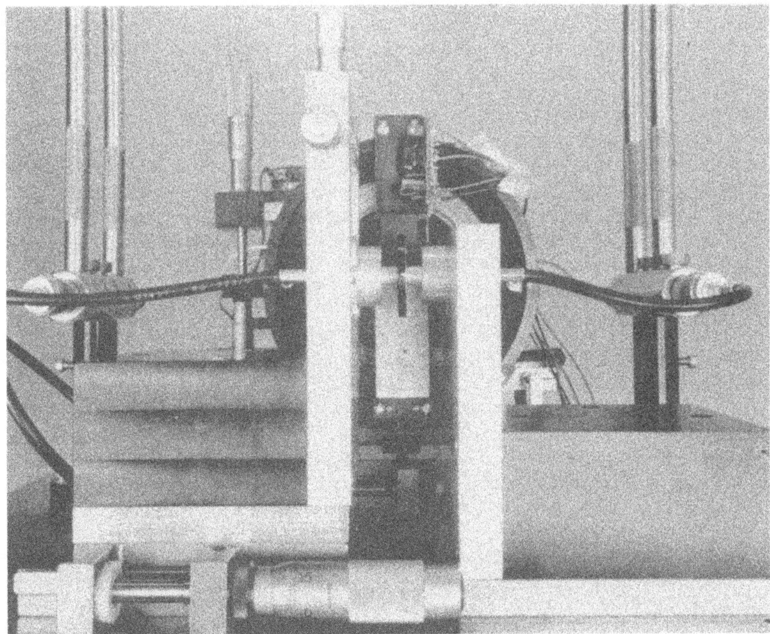

Figure 4. The Stanford acoustic microscope utilizes a speaker cone with a horizontal sweep and a small motor for the vertical sweep. The specimen is mounted on a thin mylar film stretched between the fixed transmitting and receiving transducers. Tuning stubs are used to match the electrical impedance of the transducers to the driver and receiver. Micrometer adjustments are utilized to insure reproducibility of transducer positioning. (Photo provided by Dr. C. F. Quate.)

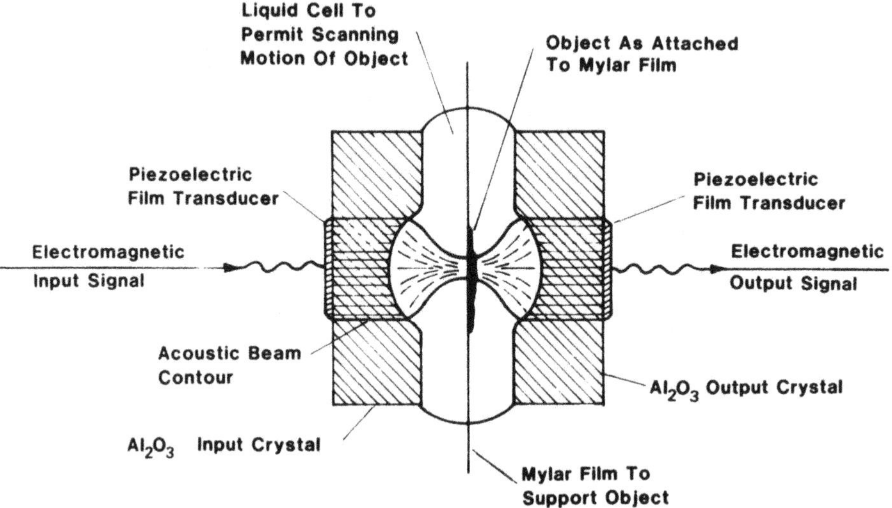

Figure 5. Specimen support membrane is scanned through the stationary sound field in the SAM. Sapphire lenses are used to focus the sound field in the plane of the specimen. Water is used as the transmitting medium.

1.4 Comparison of Acoustic, Light and Electron Microscopes

The acoustic microscope is capable of operating at wavelengths where the resolution is comparable to that of the light microscope. Quate [5] has operated this instrument at frequencies above 2 GHz, and have achieved a resolving power of better than 0.5μ. The images obtained from biological specimens are comparable to black and white photomicrographs taken with the light microscope except image detail is based on viscoelastic properties (see Fig. 6). The acoustic microscope does not require staining in order to visualize structure because the transmission properties of biological specimens produce ample contrast. In the light microscope, light is more or less uniformly transmitted through the specimen, but phase shifts occur which make phase contrast imaging able to display unstained material. Acoustic microscopy can also benefit from phase contrast imaging in a manner analogous to the light microscope technique (see Fig. 7). Most biological specimens prepared for the light microscope are fixed, dehydrated, embedded, sectioned and stained. These steps are unnecessary in the preparation of a specimen for the acoustic microscope.

The electron microscope specimen likewise requires special preparation because the vacuum environment and lack of specimen contrast precludes the examination of fresh specimens. The poor penetrating power of the electron beam requires that the specimen be cut in ultra-thin sections.

The acoustic microscope is capable of visualizing structure through greater tissue thicknesses than either the light or electron microscopes. This is frequently an advantage in appreciating the three-dimensional organization of biological systems. For example, we have utilized the acoustic microscope to study the fetal mouse heart supported in organ culture in a viable, functioning state (see Fig. 8). This one mm thick specimen is opaque to the light microscope. The acoustic microscope is capable of transmission imaging of the heart making it possible to visualize internal activity such as valve motion, ventricular chambers, etc. The time at which contraction occurs in various parts of the heart can be determined with a light pen technique (Fig. 9). Small photocells mounted in suction

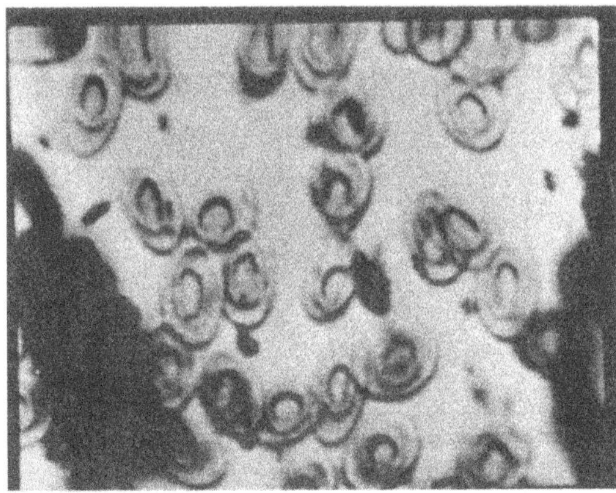

Figure 6. An acoustic microgram of erythrocytes is shown at a magnification of 1000X. The blood smear was unstained but yet shows good cellular detail. The image was produced on the SAM instrument and is comparable to the quality of image obtainable with the light microscope. (Photo provided by Dr. C. F. Quate.)

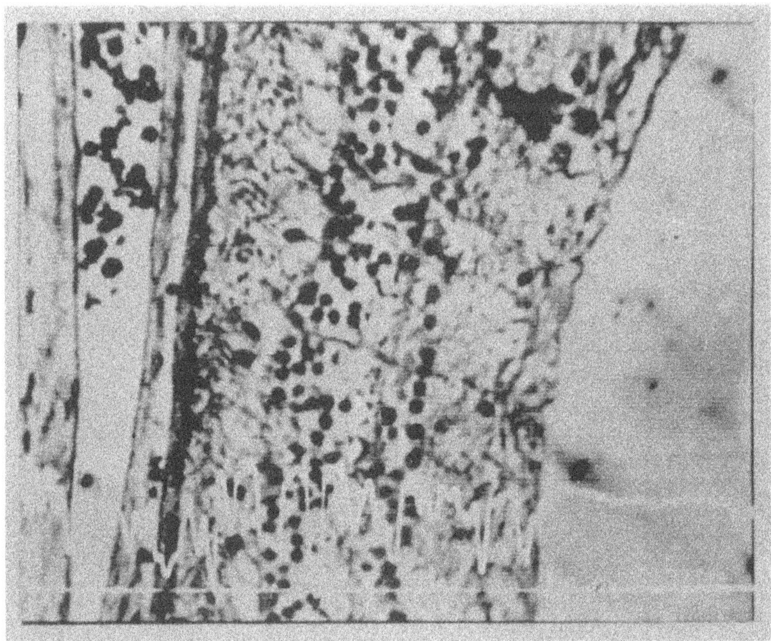

Figure 7. A phase contrast image produced on the SAM instrument showing a cross section of an unstained retina. The image quality produced by the phase contrast method compares favorably with a stained optical micrograph made on a light microscope. The acoustic transmission data is shown near the bottom of the micrograph. (Photo provided by Dr. C. F. Quate.)

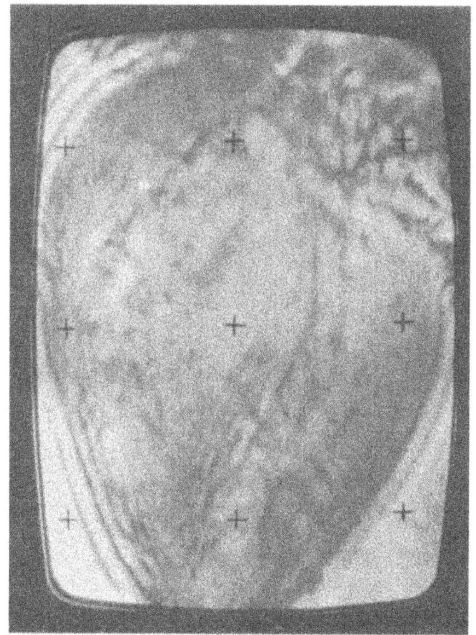

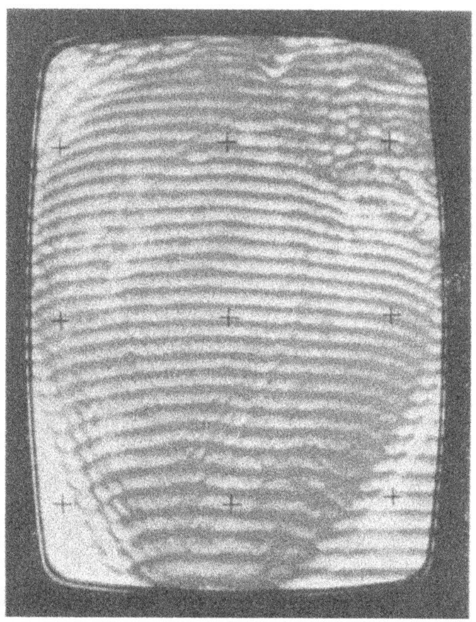

Figure 8. An acoustic micrograph is shown of an excised, functioning fetal mouse heart supported in organ culture. The frame on the left shows a transmission image, and the frame on the right shows an interferogram of the same field. The interferogram provides a map of the speed of sound by displaying lines of constant phase.

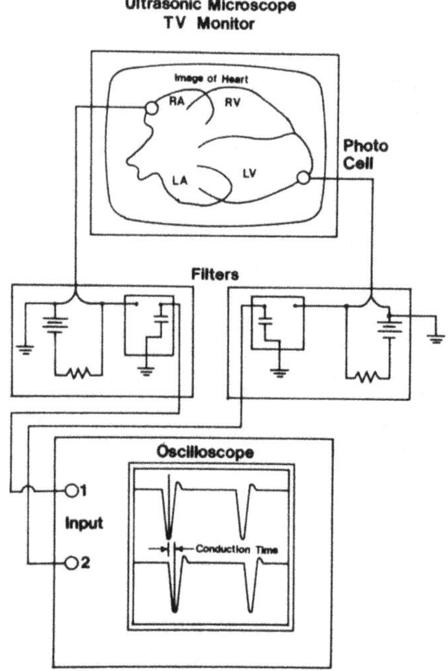

Figure 9. Contractile activity is recorded at two points in the image of the heart. The relative phase of contraction of these two points can be recorded on the tv monitor and displayed on an oscilloscope, and can be used to obtain the approximate conduction time of the action potential.

cups can be applied to various parts of the display. For example, such a pickup applied over the pacemaker records the modulation in light level associated with activity at the pacemaker. A second pickup can be placed over the apex of the ventricle. The time delay between contractile activity at the pacemaker and at the apex is approximately equal to the propagation time of the action potential between these two points. Thus, an important functional parameter can be investigated in the intact functioning mammalian organ free of extrinsic controls. Further, by using an appropriate mixer, these two contracted waveforms can be superimposed on the image. There is an obvious advantage in combining into one display format the contractile activity and the propagation velocity of the action potential through the bundle of Hiss. A similar technique has been utilized to record valve motion and blood flow.

The SLAM operates at a frame rate of 30 per second, each frame being comprised of two interlaced fields as per television format. Therefore, events occurring more rapidly than this may be outside of the time resolution capability of the spatial domain imaging of this instrument. The SAM operates at a slower frame rate (approximately one per second) and a scan converter is used to store the data as well as providing a means of continuous viewing or photographing a single frame.

2. PHYSICAL BASIS FOR ACOUSTIC IMAGING

In propagating through tissue, sound is subjected to various perturbations based upon the local properties of the tissue. Some energy is transmitted and some is absorbed due to internal friction and converted to heat. Another portion of the sound is reflected due to variations in acoustic impedance along the path of propagation. The sound power reflection coefficient is expressed as:

$$\alpha_r = \left(\frac{Z_2 \cos \theta_1 - Z_1 \cos \theta_2}{Z_2 \cos \theta_1 + Z_1 \cos \theta_2}\right)^2$$

where Z_1 and Z_2 are impedances along the path, θ_1 and θ_2 are the angles of the incident and reflected wave. Refraction of sound waves is produced by the specimen when the beam encounters regions exhibiting a different acoustic index of refraction (speed of sound). Acoustic refraction obeys Snell's Law which is expressed as:

$$\frac{\sin \theta_1}{\sin \theta_2} = \frac{C_1}{C_2}$$

Small discontinuities in the acoustic properties of the specimen can produce scattering of the acoustic beam. Scattering is one of the important components of attenuation in biological tissue. Where this scattering is produced by an ordered structure, diffraction of the acoustic beam can be detected, i.e., order can be seen in the frequency domain which may not be recognizable is the spatial domain (see Fig. 10). The diffraction angles θ_0, θ_1, θ_2, etc. are given by the expression:

$$\sin \theta = m \frac{\lambda}{d}$$

where d is the spacing between scattering elements, λ is the wavelength, and m is an integer. The diffraction pattern can, therefore, be used to infer information concerning the characteristic spatial frequency of the scatterers. The speed of sound in the medium is given by the expression:

$$C = K_a/\rho_0$$

where C is the speed of propagation, K_a is the adiabatic bulk modulus of elasticity, and ρ_0 is the equilibrium density. The elastic modulus, (K), or its reciprocal compressibility, (β), is an important parameter in describing the mechanical properties of a specimen. The properties are determined by the molecular makeup of this multiphase medium. In a biological specimen, the medium is largely water with various molecules in solution in a network of membranes. The molecular weights of the materials in solution range from tens in the case of salts up to millions in the case of some of the larger molecules of the cell. Although the speed of sound is dominated by water, the other molecular species present in tissue have an important influence and are responsible for the acoustic image contrast. Because the average speed of sound varies from one tissue to another, the measurement of this parameter can be useful in discriminating between tissue types.

Tissue	Speed of Sound (Ms^{-1})
Fat	1450
Muscle	1585
Blood	1570
Skin	1700
Pure Collagen	2000

3. IMAGE FORMATS

3.1 Spatial Domain Imaging with Parametric Mapping

In an anisotropic medium such as muscle, the speed of sound is found to be dependent upon the direction of propagation. We have developed means of recording the acoustic parameters of muscle as a function of angle, while at the same time recording the stimulation and force developed by the muscle in contraction. Figure 10 shows the muscle holder, electrodes and force transducer built into a circular lucite plate. The force transducer consists of a photodiode mounted in a hypodermic needle. Light from the diode is picked up by two photocells whose output is applied to the input of a differential amplifier. The shaft of the needle is the spring member of the force transducer. A transducer similar to this was described by Meiss [5].

The circular lucite plate is held on the stage of the microscope by a second lucite plate having a hole cut with a diameter that matches the outside diameter of the muscle holder. This outside plate is secured to the stage of the microscope in a position that places the center of rotation in the center of the microscope field (see Fig. 11). The monitor then contains a protractor which can be used for determining the alignment of the muscle fibers in the sound field (see Fig. 12).

The equipment is instrumented to implement the recording of two images in quick succession (Fig. 13). The top portion of the frame shows the muscle in the relaxed state, whereas the bottom portion is in the contracted state. The microscope is used in the interference mode to display phase as well as spatial information. The interference mode provides a map of the relative speed of sound as a function of position. Displacement of the interference lines to the right occurs when the phase of the arriving wave is earlier than the surrounding medium, and a line deflected to the left signifies a slower speed of sound. The pattern of interference lines maps the local fluctuations in the transit time of the sound through the specimen. By combining the interference pattern with the image data, it is then possible to identify which features of the specimen produce an increase or decrease in the speed of sound. In some instances, it is advantageous to combine the interference data with the optical image. In other instances, there is an advantage of combining it with the acoustic image.

Attenuation by the specimen is directly visualized in the acoustic image. As noted above, attenuation is contributed by several sources including reflection, refraction and scattering, all of which are due to the non-homogeneous character of a material. Attenuation also results from absorption due to the internal friction

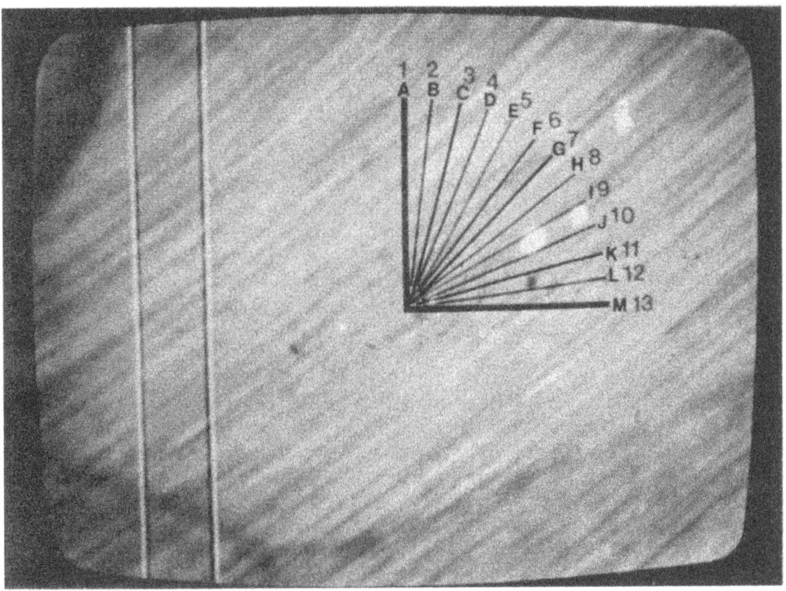

Figure 12. A protractor shows the alignment of the muscle fibers with respect to the sound field (H8, 50.5°). The parallel lines on the left side of the picture are channels to display excitation and muscle tension.

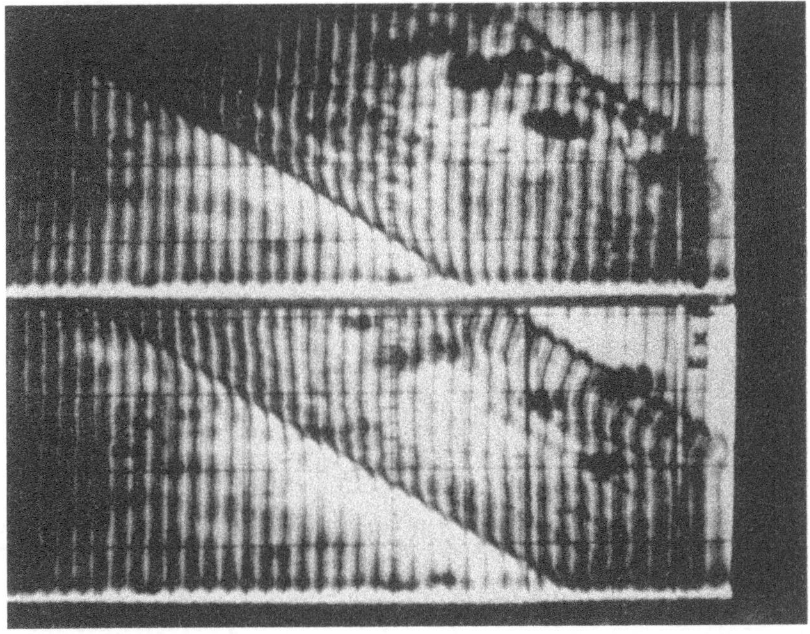

Figure 13. Two images are recorded in quick succession. The upper image is of the muscle in the relaxed state; the muscle in the lower image is in tetanus.

of the medium, and can occur in homogeneous media. Changes in absorption along a given tissue path as a function of time may indicate changes, such as changes in molecular properties.

3.2 Time Domain Imaging

Time domain imaging may be particularly important where events are occurring at a rate which is high compared to the frame rate of the microscope. Figure 14 shows a line-scan interferogram [6] in which distance along a muscle is plotted against time. (The horizontal sweep is 15,750 lines per second.) The interference lines show changes in the speed of sound as a function of muscle contraction. The picture also illustrates changes in transmission as a function of time. This image is produced by disabling the vertical sweep and plotting the horizontal scan as a function of time, and is a useful mode for displaying time-dependent specimen changes.

While acoustic microscopic interferometry is equivalent to phase contrast optical microscopy, other electronic methods can be used to extract phase information from acoustic signals. In particular, a phase-locked loop can be used to retrieve the carrier signal, free of amplitude information, but retaining the phase information imparted to the traveling acoustic wave by the specimen. This information can be used to construct a phase map which offers a greater degree of precision that that obtained using the interference method. Further, the phase information can be readily digitized for computer analysis of variations in the speed of sound within a specimen. In the case of anisotropic specimens, for example, an elasticity tensor can be computed for each specimen, as a function of varying conditions.

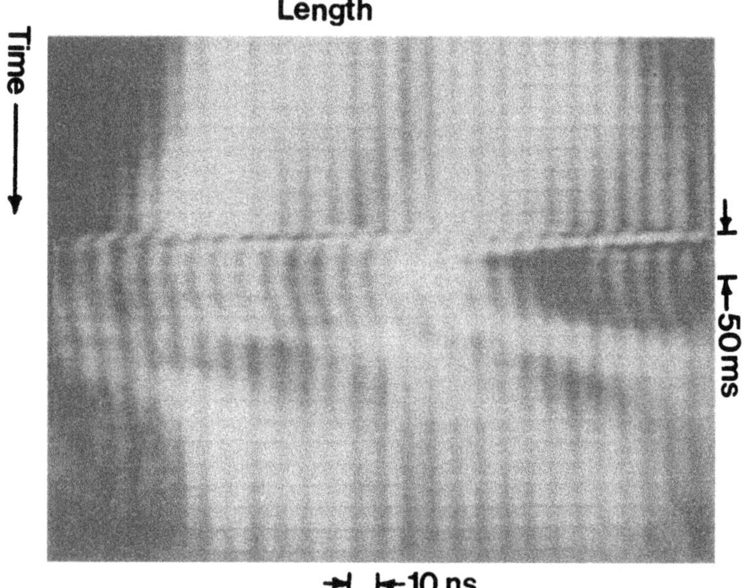

Figure 14. The line scan interferogram shows a change in transit time of sound through muscle as a function of contraction. It also shows changes in transmission.

Kessler [8] has demonstrated the utility of combining acoustic and optical data on a color monitor using one color (blue) to represent the sound transmission, and another color (yellow) to represent light transmission. The combined images contain more information than either of the images taken independently.

3.3 Frequency Domain Imaging

One of the most remarkable and useful properties of a converging lens is its inherent ability to perform two-dimensional Fourier transformations (see Fig. 15). The Fourier transforming operation is one which is generally associated with electronic spectrum analyzers or the fast Fourier transform operations performed in complex computer systems. This complex analog operation can be performed by a simple lens function of an acoustic system [9]. An experiment was performed at low frequencies (2.5 MHz) visualizing the Fourier plane (diffraction plane) using an acoustic lens to display the image of a grating in the frequency domain (see Fig. 16). The specimen consisted of wires spaced 2 mm apart and the image shows zero, first and second order diffraction using the RCA Ultrasonovision system to visualize the sound field. Frequency domain imaging is particularly useful for recognizing order in the specimen. Figure 17 shows a random array of scatterers in a rectangular block (top left). The diffraction image of this specimen is shown below in the circular field. A second specimen produced by making a double exposure with a 2.5 mm displacement of the first set is shown at the top right. The diffraction image displays the order in the double exposure as a series of parallel lines. The characteristic spatial frequency associated with the scattering pairs is directly measureable using the diffraction image.

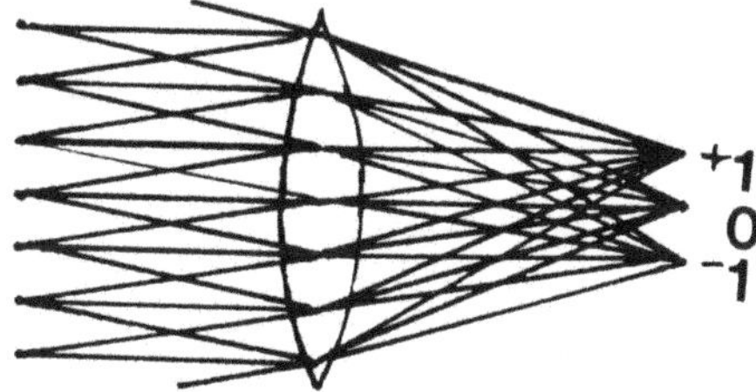

Figure 15. The Fourier transform of f(x,y) is:

$$F(\omega_x,\omega_y) = \int_{-\infty}^{\infty}\int_{-\infty}^{\infty} e^{2\pi j(\omega_x x+\omega_y y)} f(x,y)dx\,dy$$

The inverse Fourier transform of $F(\omega_x,\omega_y)$ is the complex conjugate of its Fourier transform. Both are performed in two dimensions by this lens.

4. CONCLUSIONS

Until rather recently, it was widely accepted that diffraction effects represented the fundamental limits to optical system performance. Resolution beyond the classical diffraction limit was believed hopeless. Even an infinitely large lens would be limited by the ever-present wave phenomenon which would have resolution limits in the order of a wavelength. J. L. Harris [10] has demonstrated resolving power well below the so-called diffraction limits. Likewise, C. W. Barnes [11] extends the resolution limits of imaging systems. The history of Fourier synthesis techniques can be traced to experiments by Abbey in 1893 [12] in which he performed intentional manipulations of the spectrum of the image by filtering in the frequency domain. Abbey and Porter [13] both demonstrated considerable insight into image processing through controlling the frequency distribution of image signals. Their experiments provided a powerful demonstration of the detailed mechanism by which coherent images are formed and, indeed, the most basic principles of Fourier analysis itself.

Position invariant linear operations on images can be implemented by optical means in a more cost-effective way than via digital computers. However, as computers grow in size and capability for handling complex calculations, there is a tendency for computer oriented image researchers to ignore the strength of the optical methods. The utility of the optical processing techniques in the formation of images from synthetic aperture data lies in the extreme simplicity with which the optical system performs the rather complex and intricate linear transformations required to obtain these images. This simplicity is due, to a large extent, to the

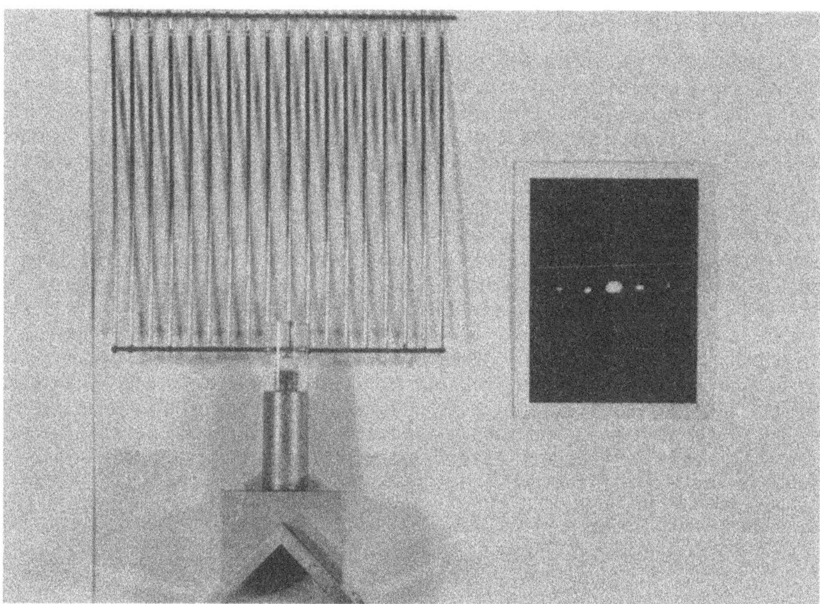

Figure 16. The acoustic diffraction image of the target shown above is pictured at the right showing the zero, first and second order diffraction. This image was produced at 2.5 MHz on the RCA Ultrasonovision system.

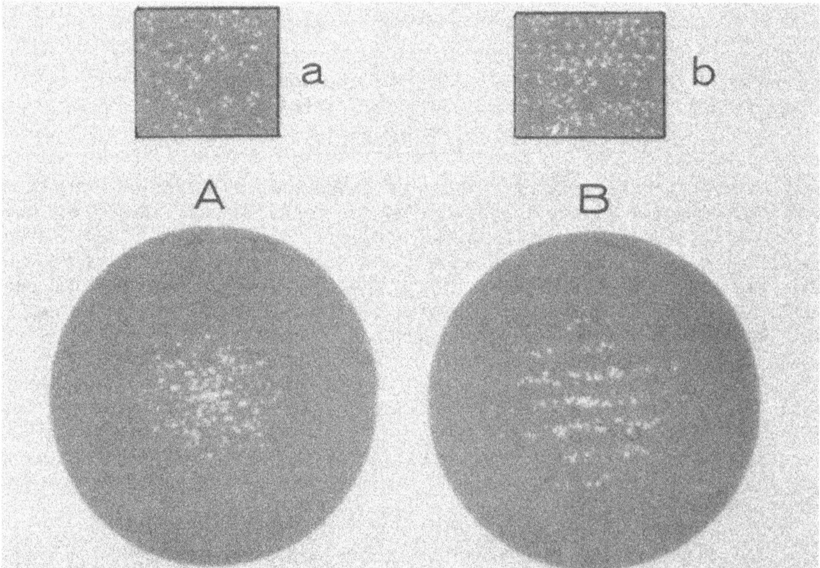

Figure 17. A diffraction image of a random array of scatterers shown as A on the left. A double exposure of the scatterers displaced by 2.5 mm is shown on the right (b) and its diffraction image (B) is shown below. Note that the order in the second array is easily detected in the diffraction image.

identical nature of the laws governing the propagation of acoustic and electromagnetic waves. Likewise, the use of spatial frequency filters can function in a miraculous way to enhance images by eliminating undesirable interference of a periodic nature.

Functions have their equivalents in optical systems. Any position in variant linear operation is determined by specifying its point spread function. The point spread function is the two-dimensional analog of the impulse response in electronics, the green structure in photography, or the spot produced by the electron beam in the television tube. The integral of the point spread function of θ, taken from $-\infty$ to ∞ is a measure of the effect of θ on the constant functions. It is often convenient to describe θ in terms of its effect on some other simple input function rather than on a one point function.

The two-dimensional treatment in computer processing can be demanding in terms of both software and hardware, but not so in optical processing. The modulation transfer function corresponds to the frequency response in electronics. It can be thought of as describing how θ attenuates the sinusoidal input as a function of the spatial frequency. In optics, the finite aperture of the exit pupil sets the spatial frequency cutoff, but within the pass band of the optical system the response can be essentially flat.

It is straightforward to convolve two digital pictures in a computer; however, the number of manipulations grows rapidly with the number of picture elements because computers are basically sequential processors. In optics these operations take place in parallel, i.e., simultaneously. Conventional digital computers with sequential processing have the capability of simultaneously performing simple logical and shifting operations on each binary digit of a word. If digital circuitry is used to perform operations in parallel, a large network of individual components is required.

In order to deal with images of living systems where dynamics of the image are important, it is necessary for digital circuitry to perform operations in parallel. There are, however, logical operations involving position invariant linear operations. In this instance, electrooptical or electroacoustic implementations of these operations becomes practical. Examples of this are phase contrast microscopy, which has been implemented by Quate. Reversing contrast, that is, displaying a negative image as opposed to a positive image, is readily achieved in either the SLAM or SAM instruments.

To multiply a picture by a positive or negative constant can be a simple electronic operation. One can perform arbitrary position invariant linear operations on a sequentially generated picture. Non-linear operations can also be performed by using the appropriate non-linear elements in the circuitry, but these are not under operational or software control. Position invariant linear operations on images can be implemented simply using optical means. Persons involved in image processing should therefore be versed in both optical and computer methods capable of designing hybrid optical-digital computational methods.

ACKNOWLEDGMENT

This work was supported in part by the National Science Foundation, Grant APR-75-15908 and by the Indianapolis Center for Advanced Research, Inc. The work on the RCA Ultrasonovision system was performed by W. D. McNeely, Jose Keuwez and J. A. Whitcomb.

REFERENCES

1. Sokolov, S., "The Ultrasonic Microscope", Akadema Nauk SSSR, Doklady 64, pp. 333-345, 1949.

2. Sokolov, S.: USSR Patent No. 49 (31 Aug. 1936); British Patent No. 477,139 (1937); and U.S. Patent No. 21,64,125 (1939).

3. Kessler, L.W., Korpel, A. and Palermo, P.R.. "Characteristics of Scanning Laser Acoustic Microscope," J. Opt. Soc. Amer., Vol. 61A, p. 1573, 1971.

4. Lemons, R.A. and Quate, C.F.. "Integrated Circuits as Viewed with an Acoustic Microscope," Appl. Phys. Letters, Vol. 25, pp. 251-253, 1974.

5. Quate, C.F., "Acoustic Microscopy," Microscopy, An Introduction to Microscopy by Means of Light, Electrons, Ionis, X-rays, and Ultrasound, (E.G. Rochow and T.G. Rochow, eds.), Plenum Pub. Corp., New York, 1978.

6. Meiss, R.A., "An Isometric Muscle Force Transducer," J. Appl. Physiol., Vol. 30, No. 1, pp. 158-160, January 1971.

7. Eggleton, R.C. and Vinson, F.S., "Heart Model Supported in Organ Culture and Analyzed by Acoustic Microscopy," Acoustical Holography, Vol. 7, (L.W. Kessler, ed.), Plenum Pub. Corp., New York, 1977, pp. 21-35.

8. Kessler, L.W.. "High Resolution Visualization of Tissue with Acoustic Microscopy," Proceedings of the Second World Congress on Ultrasonics in Medicine, (deVlieger, M., White, D.N. and McCready, V.R., eds.), American Elsevier Pub. Co., Inc., New York, 1974.

9. Goodman, J.W., Introduction to Fourier Optics, McGraw-Hill Book Co., San Francisco, 1968.

10. J.L. Harris, "Resolving Power Decision Theory," J. Opt. Soc. Amer., Vol. 54, pp. 606-611, May 1964.

11. G.H. Barnes, R.M. Brown, M. Kato, D.J. Kuck, D.L. Slotnick and R.A. Stokes, "The ILLIAC IV Computer." IEEE Trans. Computers, Vol. C-17, pp. 746-575, August 1968.

12. Abbey, E., Archiv. Mikroskopische Anat., Vol. 9, p. 413, 1873.

13. Porter, A.B., "On the Diffraction Theory of Microscope Vision," Phil. Mag. (6), Vol. 11, p. 154, 1906.

DIGITAL IMAGE PROCESSING OF ELECTRON MICROGRAPHS

by
P.W. Hawkes
Laboratoire d'Optique Electronique du C.N.R.S.
B.P. 4347, F-31055 Toulouse Cedex

ABSTRACT

A general account of the reasons why digital processing of electron microscope images is of interest is given, with references to a wide range of specific applications. Emphasis is placed on the stimulus provided by the radiation damage problem. Some brief comments on image readout in TEM and STEM are included.

1. INTRODUCTION

Modern commercial electron microscopes are capable of real point-to-point resolutions of the order of a few ångströms, although it is rare for genuine structure to be preserved at this level in biological and medical material, whether embedded and sectioned or negatively stained or frozen. Nevertheless, it is certainly true that fine structure often survives the various processes of specimen preparation but is destroyed by the beam before a usable image can be recorded. This problem can be alleviated to some extent by so-called "minimum exposure" techniques, in which such destructive operations as focusing and adjusting the microscope use a specimen region adjoining that containing the structure of interest, and the latter is irradiated only for the time necessary to record an image. Such techniques can hardly be used routinely for they require not only considerable skill and a particularly good microscope but a good measure of luck as well - and even given all these, the minimum dose may still be too high. It is therefore most desirable to be able to record images with a very small number of electrons indeed (as low as an electron or a few electrons per Å^2 at the specimen) and treat the resulting pictures digitally in a separate step, in order to obtain a usable composite image.

The problem of *radiation damage* is not the only reason for computer processing, nor indeed was it the earliest. The most striking successes of digital processing have been in the field of *three-dimensional reconstruction*, which has been applied to a range of specimens exhibiting some natural symmetry, so that a single picture effectively contains several views of the specimen. Several structures, including numerous viruses, have been reconstructed in three-dimensions by these methods. Attempts are now being made to extend this work to non-periodic specimens, and although a certain measure of success has been achieved, it is clear that this requires complicated modifications to the microscope as well as a massive computing effort.

The other developments in image processing, which we describe briefly in Section 4, are concerned with image filtering to reduce the effect of the resolution-limiting aberrations of the microscope and with phase determination. Neither of these groups of methods has had much impact on biological or medical electron microscopy as yet, though the situation is likely to change as the methods are perfected and made easier to use.

The foregoing remarks have been made with the traditional "conventional" electron microscope in mind, in which the electrons are shone on the specimen, deflected within the latter, and proceed along the microscope to form an essentially phase-contrast image at the screen.

This image is recorded on a photographic emulsion and in order to perform any processing, it must first be measured with the aid of a microdensitometer, which furnishes its measurements either direct to a computer, or in a computer-readable form (magnetic tape, magnetic disc, etc...). Only after this time-consuming step, which requires access to a very expensive measuring instrument, can any processing commence. An alternative type of microscope is, however, gradually finding its way into the laboratory, which avoids this photography-microdensitometry stage completely : this is the scanning transmission electron microscope (STEM, or "Crewe" microscope). The STEM image is formed point-by-point, like a television image, and generates signals that can be sent straight to the computer, by means of readily available circuitry. Several types of processing can therefore be performed immediately, while the image is being formed or very shortly after, so that the user can examine a processed image of the specimen in the microscope. We have therefore devoted a separate section to this type of instrument.

It is only fair to add that strenuous efforts are being made to interface conventional (static-beam) microscopes to computers ; highly sensitive and sophisticated readout units have been built for this purpose, though none is so far commercially available. Nevertheless, such links add a major degree of complication to the instrument, which a STEM avoids, though the latter is more technologically demanding than the conventional microscope in other respects (gun design, vacuum requirements and specimen handling in particular).

The publications referred to in this paper have been selected to be comprehensible to readers with comparatively little mathematical background, wherever possible, though most of the literature is written by and for physicists or computer scientists. We also draw attention to a number of review articles addressed primarily to biologists : Horne and Markham [30], Frank [12], Hawkes [17,18,19], Misell [37], and Baumeister [3] .

2. RADIATION DAMAGE

We begin with the problem of forming a usable image of very beam-sensitive specimens, for research into this question has become particularly active in the last few years. For a good idea of the present state of the subject, we refer to the proceedings of a meeting on structure determination and assembly of regular two-dimensional arrays of macromolecules (Baumeister, [3]). The various methods that are under investigation are governed by one imperious constraint : the electron dose (number of electrons per $Å^2$) at the specimen must not exceed some destruction threshold, which varies from specimen to specimen and may be as low as 1 electron/$Å^2$. Such doses are thus often too low to produce a usable image and we are therefore driven to obtain several low-dose images of different examples of the same specimen and combine these to give a legible picture. This can be done either by contriving to organize a large number of identical specimen structures into a regular array or by superposing all the individual images, using the computer to ensure good alignment.

The first technique has been used by Unwin and Henderson [46], in a celebrated series of experiments and calculations, to determine the structure of the purple membrane of *Halobacterium halobium*. These authors then went on to perform a three-dimensional reconstruction of the structure of this membrane (Henderson and Unwin, [23]). For a more recent application of these techniques, to tubulin, see Amos and Baker [1,2].

The second method, superposition of individual images, requires very precise alignment of the pictures to be superposed, which must be as nearly identical as possible, as the final result will obviously be unacceptably blurred otherwise. Simple though the principle seems, there are numerous practical difficulties : the task of aligning the separate low-dose images in both position and orientation is not straightforward and becomes even less so if the magnifications are not all exactly the same. Furthermore, it is clearly only worth including "good" images, in which the structure in question has not suffered any obvious misfortune in the complex process of specimen preparation or of course during microscopy ; this is a subjective choice and attempts are being made to establish objective criteria that will permit us decide quantitatively to what extent an image resembles those with which it is to be combined. For a full account of the correlation methods that are used for alignment, see Frank [13] and for a preliminary allusion to a method of comparing the resemblance between images, see Hawkes in Baumeister [3] : this latter volume includes numerous examples of the successful use of superposition to render low-dose images interpretable. Further examples are the study of acetylcholine receptors by Zingsheim *et al.* [52] and by Wade *et al.* [50].

We cannot however leave the topic of radiation damage without referring to some very recent experiments that suggest that the problem may after all be overcome without recourse to processing - or more realistically, that the images to be processed may be obtained with doses considerably above the apparent damage threshold. It has long been suspected that cooling the specimen should provide "cryoprotection" against damage, but although the relatively few experimental results were mildly encouraging, they were far from proving that low temperature is a universal panacea against beam damage. Very recently, however, using a superconducting lens microscope, in which the entire specimen environment is at liquid helium temperature (∿ 4K), rather than an ordinary microscope with a liquid helium stage where the actual specimen temperature is rather uncertain and probably a little above 4K, Dietrich *et al.* [9] of Siemens (Munich) and Dubochet and Knapek [10] of the EMBO Laboratory (Heidelberg) have found that fragile specimens survive very considerable doses at a low enough temperature. If this proves to be a general result, it remains to be seen whether the technological problems of low temperature can be made less intimidating than those of digital processing.

For general surveys of radiation damage in electron microscopy, see Cosslett [6].

3. THREE-DIMENSIONAL RECONSTRUCTION

The computer was already being used to reconstruct three-dimensional images of objects with internal symmetry, especially viruses, long before other types of digital image processing became at all common in electron microscopy. It is no coincidence that those concerned with developing the techniques were already familiar with related crystallographic methods of structure determination and it remains true that many (though not all) of the major centres concerned with this problem have a considerable crystallographic bias.

The subject has been extensively reviewed, notably by Crowther and Klug [8] who, with D.J. de Rosier and L. Amos, introduced the technique, Vainshtein [47], Klug [33] and by Mellema [36], and we therefore confine the present account to the essential ideas. Numerous types of biological specimen exhibit a certain measure of natural symmetry or regularity, with the result that a single view in the electron microscope contains information corresponding to several other sections through the object. After digitization, this can be used either alone or more realistically in conjunction with other independent views of the same specimen (or of specimens of the same type, if radiation damage is a problem) to reconstruct a three-dimensional model of the structure. Numerous examples of the type of information that can be extracted by exploiting the internal symmetry of biological material are to be found in the reviews already cited, to which we may add [1,2].

Not all specimens are naturally regular or can be coaxed to form crystalline arrays, however, and it is therefore of considerable interest to develop methods applicable to objects with little or no symmetry. Two groups have been particularly active here : the M.R.C. Laboratory of Molecular Biology in Cambridge (Amos, Crowther, Klug, Unwin), where the techniques already developed have been applied to material with less and less symmetry ; and the Structure Determination Unit in the Max-Planck-Institute of Biochemistry near Munich, led by W. Hoppe, who is developing a suitably modified microscope as well as elaborate software for data handling. The latter approach and preliminary results obtained are described very fully in surveys by Hoppe and Hegerl [28], Hoppe [27] and Hoppe and Typke [29].

4. OTHER TYPES OF PROCESSING

In this section, we mention a number of methods ranging from very simple image cleaning or "cosmetic" processing to the much more difficult, non-linear problem of determining the phase and amplitude of the electron wave function.

We first list the various procedures used to improve the appearance and facilitate visual appreciation of an image : such techniques are by no means confined to electron microscopy, however, and are fully described in general texts on image processing such as Rosenfeld and Kak [40] or Pratt [39] to which we refer for details. Image granularity may be reduced, with care, by low-pass filtering the image - the fine granularity is assumed to be smaller than any useful specimen detail, so that by suppressing the appropriate ("high-frequency") part of the Fourier transform of the image, a smoothed, less grainy image will be seen. If the transform consists of isolated spots, the remainder can be set rigorously to zero after which a strictly periodic specimen with no irregularities can be reconstructed - any real departures from regularity are of course inevitably lost in this way. If the spots indicate that the specimen has n-fold rotational symmetry, for example, the image can be superposed after appropriate rotation to create an improved version. Other techniques that are almost trivial with the computer involve the removal of any unevenness of the background (or ramp), redistribution of the grey-level histogram to suit the response of the eye, and removal of any implausible variations of intensity (dust).

We now turn to linear filtering of images, which is necessary to render high-resolutic detail faithful to the specimen. In order to understand this, we must explain that at high resolution, the image in an electron microscope is essentially a phase contrast image formed not with a true phase-plate, as in the optical phase-contrast microscope, but with the very crude analogue furnished by a combination of the defocusing and spherical aberration of the instrument. The latter is fixed by the design but the defocus can be varied at will by the user, who can therefore create the desired phase shift, for a range of spacings only, by balancing aberration against defocus. For the class of specimens that scatters only weakly (weak phase, weak amplitude objects), this effect can be described by a transfer function : the contrast (C) of the image is *linearly* related to the phase (ϕ) and amplitude (s) components of the specimen transparency and more simply still, the Fourier transform (or spatial frequency spectrum) of the image contrast is equal to the sum of the transforms of these phase and amplitude components, each weighted with an appropriate transfer function. These two transfer functions are of the form 2 sin γ and - 2 cos γ, in which the angle γ is determined by the electron wavelength (i.e. by the accelerating voltage of the microscope), the coefficient of spherical aberration, C_s, the defocus Δ and the spatia frequency, t. Thus denoting Fourier transforms $\bar{C}$, etc.., we have :

$$\bar{C} = 2 \sin \gamma(t) \;\; \bar{\phi}\;(t) - 2 \cos \gamma\;(t)\; \bar{s}\;(t)$$

where the specimen transparency is $1 - s + i\,\phi,\ s,\ \phi <<1$. In order to determine ϕ and s separately and to cancel the effects of the transfer functions as far as possible, we need several micrographs taken at different values of defocus. Suitably composed weighted sums of these yield optimum estimates of $\bar{\phi}$ and $\bar{s}$ and hence of ϕ and s. The one-dimensional case of this problem is very well-known and has been thoroughly explored ; the extension to two dimensions and two types of "signal" is not difficult. In reality, however, the expressions sin γ and cos γ are only a first approximation to the true transfer functions, since in deriving them, the finite energ spread of the electron beam and the fact the electron source is not strictly a point have been neglected. These two factors can be taken into account by multiplying sin γ (or cos γ) by appropriate modulating functions, the main effect of which is to attenuate the basic transfer function as the spacing gets smaller. In other words, unless the beam is very monochromatic and the spread of angles very narrow, high resolution information will be irretrievably lost. For more information about such filtering procedures, see Kübler *et al.* [34], Kübler [34a], Welton [51], Erickson [10a] and a review by Hawkes [21].

Finally, we do no more than draw attention to methods of extracting s and ϕ from micrographs when one or both is not small compared with unity. In practice, the conditions in which ϕ <<1 are very rarely satisfied, whereas s << 1 is a much more reasonable requirement. It is therefore of interest to enquire how s and ϕ can be derived : given an intensity distribution on the photographic plate, can we calculate the amplitude and phase of the wave that produces it ? Holographic methods of doing this are known but are not easy to implement with electrons (see Wade, [49] for a review). The information can in principle be extracted from various pairs or sets of electron micrographs, as Gerchberg and Saxton [15,16] showed, but the practical difficulties and uncertainties are so considerable that the methods have not been much used, except to study the properties of magnetic materials (Chapman, [5]. The question is treated very fully in Saxton [41, 42], Misell [38] and Ferwerda [11]. For a recent practical application, see Saxton [43].

5. DIRECT IMAGE READOUT : STEMs AND INTERFACES FOR STATIC-BEAM MICROSCOPES

In the preceding sections we have described the procedures used or planned for processing electron microscope images but we have said very little about the hardware involved, apart from a passing allusion to microdensitometry. Clearly, if photographic recording, development and microdensitometry must precede any computer processing, the whole operation becomes relatively slow and very off-line. This is tolerable though inconvenient for elaborate types of processing, such as three-dimensional reconstruction, but is highly unsatisfactory for the simpler manipulations. Even for the more complex operations, it is likely to be found more inconvenient in the future, as processing software becomes more sophisticated and dedicated computers more powerful.

For these reasons, direct microscope-computer links have been studied for some years for static-beam electron microscopes but the advent of the STEM and the gradual appearance of commercial models in the laboratories of Europe, the United States and Japan has changed the situation abruptly. As we have already mentioned, this type of microscope provides point-by-point information about the image in analogue form, which can readily be converted into a digital record for the computer and all the simpler types of processing can, or could in principle, be performed directly on line : the user can see pictures before and after processing on two adjacent monitors, for example, or in different colours on a single colour screen; see Isaacson *et al.*[31], for a review of the possibilities in STEM. Such processing has been routinely associated with the reflection scanning instrument (SEM) for many years and incorporated into commercial equipment ; for a general account, see Jones and Smith, [32], and for a particular example, see Vicario *et al.*, [48]. Furthermore, certain types of "processing" can be included in the microscope design itself - by choosing the geometry of the detector that collects the electrons used to generate the image appropriately, several interesting types of information can be generated immediately (see Hawkes, [22], for a survey).

For the needs of image processing, therefore, the STEM is clearly a particularly suitable instrument. It is nevertheless still a very rare one and in view of its technological sophistication (and its price) it is likely to remain so and many microscopists will hence wish to process static-beam microscope images. No straightforward interface for reading the image into a computer is as yet on the market, though it seems reasonable to expect that this will be remedied fairly soon (at a price !). Conversely, several research laboratories in the U.S.A., France and Germany have built their own systems, for on-line processing, which fall into two broad categories : those that connect the electron microscope to an optical bench, for simple analogue processing, and those that convert the image into digital form for computer processing. We shall not consider the first category here, since it falls outside our terms of reference ; for details, see Beorchia *et al.* [4], Herrmann and Krahl [25], Herrmann [24], Laberrigue *et al.*[35], Colin *et al.*[7]. Of the second category, systems have been developed primarily in the U.S.A. and Germany (see Hawkes, [21] for references) ; the most highly perfected is that described by Herrmann and colleagues in a series of papers, of which Herrmann *et al.*[26] give a clear account. This consists of an image intensifier chain connected to the screen of the electron microscope by a fibre-optics link ; the intensified image is read-off by an EBS camera tube at a rate of fifty 312-line frames/s (non-interlaced) after which an analogue-digital converter transforms the picture into digital form.

6. CONCLUDING REMARKS AND PREDICTIONS FOR THE FUTURE

In this account, we have tried to show what digital processing of electron micrographs has to offer biological and medical research. Although image processing is passing through a phase in which only a few new results are being obtained, since the techniques are naturally developed on reasonably well-known material, this situation will soon alter and image processing equipment will become as indispensable as the unadorned electron microscope is today. For this to come about, it is essential that both hardware and software are easy to use and reliable, which is not yet the case. The situation is already changing rapidly, however : STEMs are now available ; interfaces for fixed-beam instruments must surely soon come on the market. Program packages for the tasks described above are already on sale and some have been particularly designed for use by those with little familiarity with the computer (Smith, [45]; Saxton *et al.* [44] ; Frank and Shimkin [14] ; Kübler [34a]). Intensive courses on three-dimensional reconstruction are regularly provided by the M.R.C. Laboratory of Molecular Biology in Cambridge under the auspices of the EMBO. It is safe to predict that, financial constraints permitting, digital processing of electron images will expand rapidly during the coming years, in the life sciences in particular.

Moreover, with some pooling of resources, digital electron image processing need not be unduly difficult. A call for collaboration has been made by Burge (see *Scanning Electron Microscopy*, 1980) and attempts to develop it further are being made in the U.K. (private communication; see *Proc. R. Microsc. Soc. 15*, 1980, 267-269).

In the life sciences, the advantages of image processing are clear for three purposes observation of easily damaged material ; three-dimensional reconstruction from thin specimens ; improvement of the visual appearance of micrographs from difficult material. We have considered all of these above and there is no doubt that either of the first two would alone justify all the effort that is currently being devoted to electron image processing. There is, however, one major problem that we have not raised - that of the relation between stain and structure or in other words, the fidelity of the electron image to the structure under investigation. Electron microscope specimens are stained in a host of different ways but the various techniques may be classified essentially as *positive staining*, in which, crudely speaking, the stain is assumed to cling to the ultrastructural detail and hence provide contrast, and *negative staining*, in which the image consists of zones from which stain is absent In both cases, and particularly in the former, the risk of artefact is ever-present and a means of studying unstained material would therefore be extremely welcome. Digital processing of the very low-contrast image formed by an unstained specimen is one of the ways in which this aim may be achieved and is indeed one of the main incentives in some processing centres.

In view of this, it is safe to predict that the next few years will see steady progres in the treatment of images exhibiting very little contrast, because a low dose has been used or because the specimen is unstained or both. Progress is not likely to be rapid, however, for the example of electrical engineering shows that there are no easy solutions to problems involving weak signals in noise in one dimension, and here we are inevitably concerned with two-dimensional signals. The methods are likely to be non-linear, since phase determination is the ultimate aim, with all the attendant complications. At the same time, and if possible in combination with this low-contrast work, three-dimensional reconstruction will be extended to specimens with little or no symmetry. This requires not only sophisticated data handling but also quite difficult modifications to the objective area of the microscope, to obtain the necessary views of the specimen. Such modifications are being undertaken only in W. Hoppe's laboratory, so far as we are aware. For all these developments, and others that will emerge as the work proceeds, we shall need suitable microscopes ; suitable image read-out equipment for static-beam instruments ; adequate computing facilities and personnel ; high-level and preferably portable software or a centralized facility with easy on-line access, ample file space, straightforward editing, etc... At the same time, extensive cross-fertilization between microscope users and computer scientists is essential, so that the former know what the computer can offer them and understand what kind of image they must provide and so that the latter realise what are the problems to be solved and how they can be translated into algorithms.

REFERENCES

1. L.A. Amos and T.S. Baker (1979) : "Three-dimensional image of tubulin in zinc-induced sheets, reconstructed from electron micrographs", Int. J. Biol. Macromol. 1, 146-156.

2. L.A. Amos and T.S. Baker (1979) : "The three-dimensional structure of tubulin protofilaments", Nature (London) 279, 607-612.

3. W. Baumeister, ed. (1980) : Electron Microscopy in Molecular Dimensions. State of the Art and Strategies for the Future. Springer, Berlin and New York.

4. A. Beorchia, P. Bonhomme and N. Bonnet (1980) : "Modulation transfer function and detective quantum efficiency of Electrotitus", Optik 55, 11-22.

5. J.N. Chapman (1975) : "The application of iterative techniques to the investigation of strong phase objects in the electron microscope", Phil. Mag. 32, 527-540 and 541-552.

6. V.E. Cosslett (1978) : "Contrast and radiation damage in biological specimens : an introduction", J. Microsc. Spectrosc. Electron. 3, 551-562 ; (1979) : "Radiation damage : experimental work", Adv. Structure Res. Diffraction Methods 7, 81-99.

7. P. Colin, B. Keith, P.L. Wendel and P. Oudet (1980): "Traitement en ligne d'images de matériel biologique en microscopie électronique conventionnelle", J. Microsc. Spectrosc. Electron. 5, 555-564.

8. A.C. Crowther and A. Klug (1975) : "Structural analysis of macromolecular assemblies by image reconstruction from electron micrographs", Ann. Rev. Biochem. 44, 161-182.

9. I. Dietrich, H. Formanek, F. Fox, E. Knapek and R. Weyl (1979) : "Reduction of radiation damage in an electron microscope with a superconducting lens system", Nature 277, 380-381.

10. J. Dubochet and E. Knapek (1979) : "Use of very low temperature to reduce electron beam damage in biological specimens", Chemica Scripta 14, 267-269.

10a. H.P. Erickson (1973) : "The Fourier transform of an electron micrograph - first order and second order theory of image formation", Adv. Opt. Electron Microsc. 5, 163-199.

11. H.A. Ferwerda (1978) : "The phase reconstruction problem for wave amplitudes and coherence functions", in Inverse Source Problems in Optics (H.P. Baltes, ed.), pp. 13-39. Springer, Berlin and New York.

12. J. Frank (1973) : "Computer processing of electron micrographs", in Advanced Techniques in Electron Microscopy (J.K. Koehler, ed.), pp. 215-274. Springer, Berlin and New York.

13. J. Frank (1980) : "The role of correlation techniques in computer image processing", in Hawkes [20], pp. 187-222.

14. J. Frank and B. Shimkin (1978) : "A new image processing software system for structural analysis and contrast enhancement", Proc. 9th Int. Cong. Electron Microscopy, Toronto, vol. 1, pp. 210-211.

15. R.W. Gerchberg and W.O. Saxton (1972) : "A practical algorithm for the determination of phase from image and diffraction plane pictures", Optik 35, 237-246.

16. R.W. Gerchberg and W.O. Saxton (1973) : "Wave phase from image and diffraction plane pictures", in Image Processing and Computer-aided Design in Electron Optics (P.W. Hawkes, ed.), pp. 66-81. Academic Press, London and New York.

17. P.W. Hawkes (1975) : "Computer processing of electron micrographs : a nonmathematical account", Int. Rev. Cytol. 43, 102-126.

18. P.W. Hawkes (1977) : "Electron image processing and improvement", J. Microsc. Spectrosc. Electron. 2, 437-449.

19. P.W. Hawkes (1978) : "Computer processing of electron micrographs", in Principles and Techniques of Electron Microscopy (M.A. Hayat, ed.), vol. 8, pp. 262-306. Van Nostrand-Reinhold, Princeton and London.

20. P.W. Hawkes, ed. (1980) : Computer Processing of Electron Microscope Images, Springer, Berlin and New York.

21. P.W. Hawkes (1980) : "Image processing based on the linear theory of image formation", in Hawkes [20], pp. 1-33.

22. P.W. Hawkes (1980) : "Improvements in STEM imaging by special probe and detector shaping techniques", Scanning Electron Microscopy, vol. I, pp. 93-98.

23. R. Henderson and P.N.T. Unwin (1975) : "Three-dimensional model of purple membrane obtained by electron microscopy", Nature 257, 28-32.

24. K.H. Herrmann (1978) : "The present state of instrumentation in high-resolution electron microscopy", J. Phys. E : Sci. Instrum. 11, 1076-1091.

25. K.H. Herrmann and D. Krahl (1976) : ""Real-time" - Elektronenbildwandlung mit Thermoplastschichten", Optik 45, 231-247.

26. K.H. Herrmann, D. Krahl and H.P. Rust (1978) : "A TV system for image recording and processing in conventional transmission electron microscopy", Ultramicroscopy 3, 227-235 ; (1980) : "Electronic recording and processing of CTEM images", J. Microsc. Spectrosc. Electron. 5, 639-653.

27. W. Hoppe (1979) : "Three-dimensional low dose reconstruction of periodical aggregates", Adv. Structure Res. Diffraction Methods 7, 191-220.

28. W. Hoppe and R. Hegerl (1980) : "Three-dimensional structure determination by electron microscopy (non-periodic specimens)" in Hawkes [20], pp. 127-185.

29. W. Hoppe and D. Typke (1979) : "Three-dimensional reconstruction of aperiodic objects in electron microscopy", Adv. Structure Res. Diffraction Methods 7, 137-190.

30. R.W. Horne and R. Markham (1972) : "Application of optical diffraction and image reconstruction techniques to electron micrographs", in Practical Methods in Electro Microscopy (A.M. Glauert, ed.), vol. 1, pp. 327-440. North Holland, Amsterdam and London.

31. M. Isaacson, M. Utlaut and D. Kopf (1980) : "Analog computer processing of scanning transmission electron microscope images", in Hawkes [20], pp. 257-283.

32. A.V. Jones and K.C.A. Smith (1978) : "Image processing for scanning microscopists", Scanning Electron Microscopy, vol. I, pp. 13-26.

33. A. Klug (1979) : "Image analysis and reconstruction in the electron microscopy of biological macromolecules", Chemica Scripta 14, 245-256.

34. O. Kübler, M. Hahn and J. Seredynski (1978) : "Optical and digital spatial frequenc filtering of electron micrographs", Optik 51, 171-188 and 235-256.

34a. O. Kübler (1980) : "Unified processing for periodic and non-periodic specimens", J. Microsc. Spectrosc. Electron. 5, 565-579.

35. A. Laberrigue, G. Balossier, A. Beorchia, P. Bonhomme, N. Bonnet and M. Troyon (1980) : "Traitement direct en m.e.t., déconvolution holographique à l'aide de l'Electrotitus. Utilisation d'un diaphragme de phase de type électrostatique", J. Microsc. Spectrosc. Electron. 5, 655-664.

36. J.E. Mellema (1980) : "Computer reconstruction of regular biological objects" in Hawkes [20], pp. 89-126 ; (1980) : "3-D structure of biological objects by electron microscopy. Methods, results and fidelity", J. Microsc. Spectrosc. Electron 5, 611-62

37. D.L. Misell (1978) : Image Analysis, Enhancement and Interpretation, Practical Methods in Electron Microscopy (A.M. Glauert, ed.), vol. 7, North Holland, Amsterdam, New York and Oxford.

38. D.L. Misell (1978) : "The phase problem in electron microscopy", Adv. Opt. Electron Microsc. 7, 185-279.

39. W.K. Pratt (1978) : Digital Image Processing. Wiley, New York and Chichester.

40. A. Rosenfeld and A.C. Kak (1976) : Digital Picture Processing. Academic Press, New York and London.

41. W.O. Saxton (1978) : Computer Techniques for Image Processing in Electron Microscopy. Academic Press, New York and London.

42. W.O. Saxton (1980) : "Recovery of specimen information for strongly scattering objects", in Hawkes [20], pp. 35-87.

43. W.O. Saxton (1980) : "Correction of artefacts in linear and nonlinear high resolution electron micrographs", J. Microsc. Spectrosc. Electron. 5, 665-674.

44. W.O. Saxton, T.J. Pitt and M. Horner (1979) : "Digital image processing : the SEMPER system", Ultramicroscopy 4, 343-354.

45. P.R. Smith (1978) : "An integrated set of computer programs for processing electron micrographs of biological structures", Ultramicroscopy 3, 153-160.

46. P.N.T. Unwin and R. Henderson (1975) : "Molecular structure determination by electron microscopy of unstained crystalline specimens", J. Mol. Biol. 94, 425-440.

47. B.K. Vainshtein (1978) : "Electron microscopical analysis of the three-dimensional structure of biological macromolecules", Adv. Opt. Electron Microsc. 7, 281-377.

48. E. Vicario, B. Escudie and A. Hellion (1979) : "Essai de traitement du signal en microscopie électronique à balayage", J. Microsc. Spectrosc. Electron. 4, 341-350.

49. R.H. Wade (1980) : "Holographic methods in electron microscopy", in Hawkes [20], pp.223-255

50. R.H. Wade, A. Brisson, L. Tranqui (1980) : "The application of image treatment to structural analysis in biology", J. Microsc. Spectrosc. Electron. 5, 699-715.

51. T.A. Welton (1979) : "A computational critique of an algorithm for image enhancement in bright field electron microscopy", Adv. Electron. Electron Phys. 48, 37-101.

52. H.P. Zingsheim, D.Ch. Neugebauer, F.J. Barrantes and J. Frank (1980) : "Structural details of membrane-bound acetylcholine receptor from Torpedo marmorata", Proc. Natl. Acad. Sci. USA. 77, 952-956.

COMPUTER-ASSISTED MEASUREMENT OF CORONARY ARTERIES FROM CINEANGIOGRAMS: PRESENT TECHNOLOGIES AND CLINICAL APPLICATIONS.

by
B. Greg Brown, M.D.,Ph.D., Robert B.
Petersen Ph.D., Cynthia D. Pierce, B.S.,
Wadsworth VA Hospital
Los Angeles, California 90073

and
Edward L. Bolson, MS, Harold T. Dodge, M.D.
Cardiovascular Computation Laboratory
University of Washington School of Medicine
Seattle, Washington 98195
U.S.A.

ABSTRACT

The need for an objective method for analysis of coronary cineangiograms is described. The current alternative, visual estimates of "percent stenosis", is entirely too variable for use in objective studies of short-term and long-term interventions in coronary disease. A number of other, more precise, methods for analysis of coronary angiograms are described. In particular, a digital computer-based method for true-scale, three-dimensional characterization of the diseased coronary lumen is described in some detail. Clinical applications of this method are described. Examples of the tabular, statistical, and graphical outputs of the three related programs (ARTERY, ARTDATA, and HISTORAT) are given. This method has already provided substantial insight into mechanisms of coronary vasomobility and flow limitation; it promises to be a valuable tool in the assessment of interventions designed to retard or reverse progressive coronary atherosclerosis.

1. INTRODUCTION

Atherosclerotic narrowing in the coronary arteries is presently the single greatest health problem in technologically advanced western cultures. Clinical investigation of coronary artery disease has attempted to determine the effects of certain risk factors (smoking, cholesterol, hypertension, diabetes) on its symptomatic progression, and to determine the effect of certain treatments (drugs, diet, exercise) on relief of symptoms.

Until recently, there has been no objective, quantitative way to characterize coronary atherosclerosis. Arterial disease is commonly visualized with the coronary cineangiogram, as illustrated in Figure 1. These x-ray cine-films are made during the direct injection of an iodinated radioopaque solution (Renografin 76) into the coronary arteries through a catheter entering the arterial circulation via the brachial or the femoral artery. Images of the quality shown in Figure 1 are readily available. The accepted clinical method for analysis of these images is, at present, a simple visual estimate of the "percent stenosis" (percent diameter reduction) of the narrowed region. For example, the narrowing in Figure 1 would be called a 56% stenosis. Treatment decisions are made on the basis of these estimates. Evaluation of new diagnostic techniques in cardiology is also based on the angiographic visual estimate, which has been the only "gold standard" of disease severity.

How valuable is this visual estimate? The standard deviation of the "% stenosis" estimate is 15 to 30% [1-4]. Thus individual estimates of disease severity for a 50% narrowed vessel may easily range from 20% to 80%. Furthermore, the visual estimate tends to overstate disease severity in the narrower vessels [1,5]. Since the resistance to blood flow through an arterial stenosis is inversely proportional to the fourth power of lumen diameter, the minimum diameter of the arterial lumen at the point of greatest narrowing may be a more useful estimate of disease severity. Because of the strong dependence of flow resistance on the absolute lumen diameter, the complete spectrum of clinical episodes in coronary disease occurs over a range of

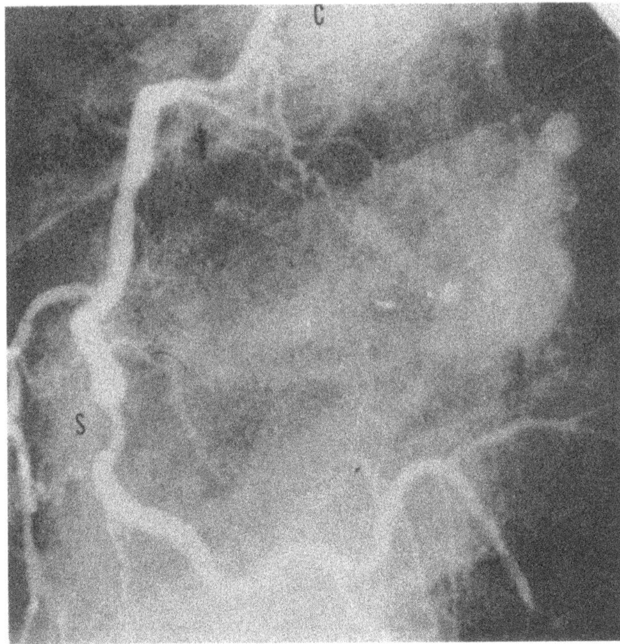

Figure 1: Example of a cineangiogram of a human right coronary artery. The catheter (C) is positioned in the origin of the artery. Several atherosclerotic narrowings are seen; the most prominent stenosis (S) is a 56% narrowing.

arterial narrowing from 1.5 mm (mild) to 0.5 mm (very severe). The visual estimate of percent stenosis, in addition to its great variability, does not provide dimensional information.

Thus a more precise and appropriate characterization of coronary disease would assist clinical decision-making and would facilitate the clinical investigation of treatments which may have beneficial short-term or long-term effects on coronary narrowing. Several such approaches are described below, including the digital-computer-based method for true-scale, three-dimensional characterization of a coronary stenosis which we have developed in the Cardiovascular Computation Laboratory of Dr. Harold Dodge at the University of Washington, Seattle [6,7].

2. Present Technologies for Measuring Coronary Disease

2.1 The Visual Estimate

As mentioned above, the variability of the visual estimate of angiographic disease severity makes it undesirable for objective analysis of coronary disease. Figure 2 illustrates the variability of this method. The upper error curve is for the visual method.

2.2 Caliper Measurement of Arteries

Rafflenbeul et al [8] and Feldman et al [9] have used vernier calipers to estimate the % stenosis from projected cineangiographic frames. The latter reported an edge detection accuracy of ±0.5 mm on the projected surface, or about ±0.25 mm in absolute dimensions. These workers do not attempt a three-dimensional characterization, or to determine true dimensions using the catheter as a scaling factor. Their methods are considerably more accurate than the visual approach, and are relatively easily used. A similar approach using an optical digitizer has been reported by Gensini [10] and used to demonstrate dilation by the coronary arteries following nitroglycerin.

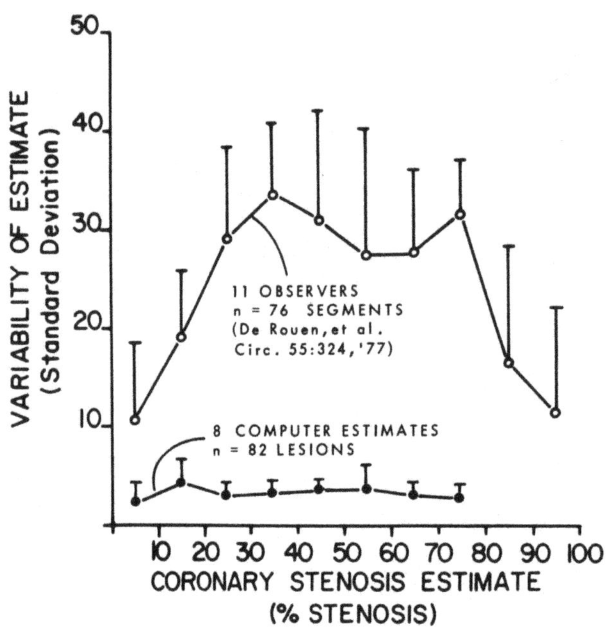

Figure 2: Comparison of the variability (standard deviation of the estimate) of the estimation of coronary artery "percent stenosis" by two different methods. Upper curve eleven observers; lower curve 8 different computer-based estimates. The computer estimates are about 10 times less variable.

2.3 Photodensitometry

Paulin et al [11] and Crawford et al [12] have used photodensitometry of coronary and femoral arteries to estimate the degree of lumenal narrowing from single angiographic projections. This method requires special care to avoid saturating the film exposure; if done properly, it will provide three-dimensional information from an apparently two-dimensional image. The third dimension is derived from the optical density of the exposed film, which is proportional to the thickness of the dye column in the dimension perpendicular to the image. The technique has greater application to peripheral arteries, where cut-film angiograms and a perpendicular orientation to the vessel axis can be obtained, than it does to the coronaries. Geometric constraints and the need for specialized film processing make this novel approach relatively impractical for coronary vessels. Absolute dimensions are not obtained in the coronary method [11].

2.4 Edge Irregularity Detection

Blankenhorn et al [13] have reported the use of scanning photodensitometry to detect the borders of angiographic images. Coronary and femoral arteries have been studied although the approach has been applied to the latter only, in clinical studies [14].

2.5 Computer-Assisted Coronary Angiometry

In response to the need for accurate methods to characterize coronary lesions, our group developed a digital-computer based method for measurement and computation of a number of dimensional parameters in diseased coronary arterial segments [6,7]. Briefly, coronary arteriograms are performed in routine fashion using Judkin's technique in multiple projections including cranially angulated views. For each left oblique (LAO) projection, a perpendicular right oblique (RAO) projection was filmed. Our General Electric Fluoricon 300 system operates at less than 7 msec/frame with 70-120 kV maximum. A six-inch angiographic field is used. Individually adjusted film processing results in consistently high quality images. Cine frames are selected from the pair of perpendicular views which shows a particular diseased arterial segment nost clearly. Each cine frame is projected at about five-fold magnification of true vessel dimensions and the borders of the arterial lesion are digitized along with a segment of the catheter (a known dimension) used as an internal scaling factor. The border data are digitized from a Tektronixs #4953 Digitizing Tablet and # 4012 Video Display Terminal by means of a Vadic #3400 modem through standard telephone lines at 1200 baud. Transmission is presently successfully accomplished from Ann Arbor, Michigan and Los Angeles, California to the digital computer in Seattle, Washington. The computer is a DEC PDP 11/45 with 124 K memory. The operating system is DEC IAS version 3.0. Disc storage is 17 megabytes. Computer time is shared between up to 3 local users and 3 telephone users at once. There is a direct link to a DEC KL 10 at 4800 baud for access to additional statistical and graphics display programs.

The computer program ARTERY processes this border data to eliminate the effects on the image of pincushion distortion, x-ray beam divergence, and optical magnification. The result is a true-scale, three-dimensional characterization of the diseased arterial lumen in a form suitable for calculation of a number of potentially important lesion parameters. Figures 3 and 4 illustrate the geometrical steps. A report is generated, as illustrated in Figure 4, which provides a true scale visual representation of each of the perpendicular views of the diseased arterial segment, mathematically stretches these two views out to true length to eliminate the effects of foreshortening, and tabulates over 50 different computed lesion parameters. Of particular interest are: diameter and cross-sectional area in the "normal" portion of the vessel segment and at the point of greatest narrowing; percent diameter and area reduction; atheroma length and volume; stenosis flow resistance (R_1) calculated from fluid mechanics theory at an assumed flow of 1 ml/sec; maximum angles of lumen convergence and divergence. The method is accurate to within ±0.035-0.080 mm (SD) of known dimensions [1,6,10]. Reported multi-observer variability is ±0.105-0.150 mm (SD) on estimates of human stenosis minimum diameter and ±3% on estimates of "percent stenosis" [1,6,16]. Figure 2 suggests that this method has only about one-tenth the variability of conventional visual interpretation of the coronary angiogram. It has been very precise in predicting the cross-sectional area of diseased human coronaries from post mortem hearts [6].

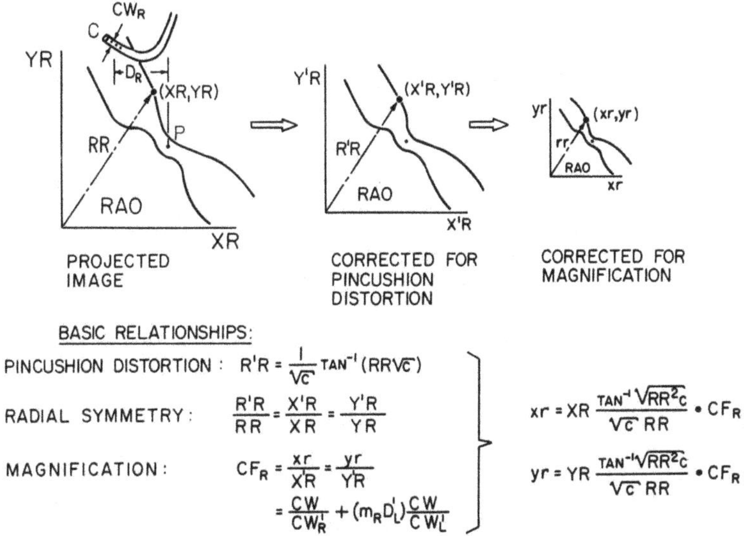

Figure 3: Pictorial display of coordinate transformations in the steps of image processing. The important mathematical relationships are given below.

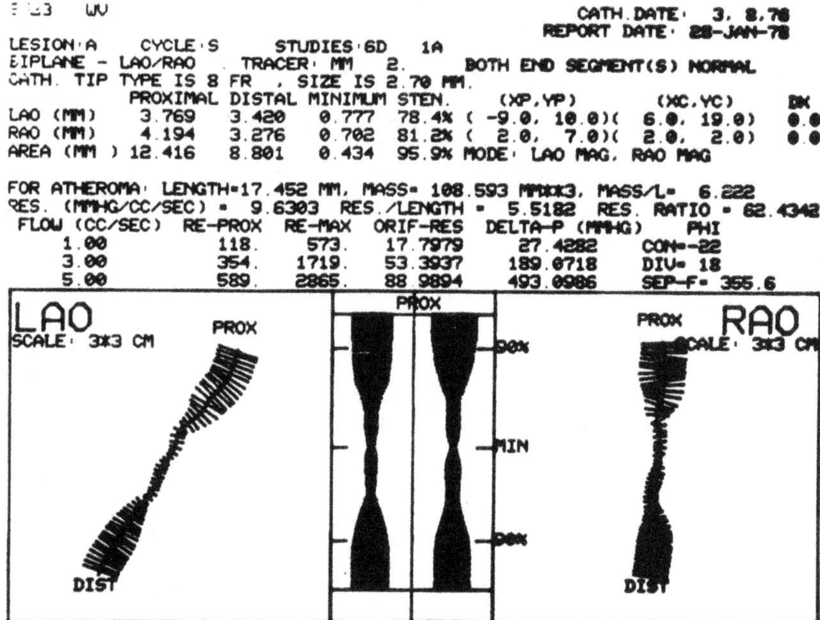

Figure 4: Example of the computer print-out of the report of an individual arterial segment analysis.

3. Applications of the Computer Angiometric Method.

3.1 The "Critical" Human Stenosis

McMahon et al [16] measured the stenosis present in 10 patients with single vessel coronary disease, intractable angina pectoris occurring intermittently at bed rest, and no collateral vessels. Unstable angina in these patients was associated with minimum lumen diameters averaging 0.88 mm, an area of 0.63 mm^2, representing 72% diameter and 92% area stenosis. Subendocardial myocardial infarction was found in 5 similar patients in association with lumen diameters averaging 0.64 mm, an area of 0.35 mm^2, a 78% diameter and 95% area stenosis. These measurements bracket the "critical" human coronary artery stenosis in a proximal major branch.

3.2 Coronary Vasodilation with Cardiovascular Drugs:

Doerner et al [17] demonstrated a 27% increase in normal lumen area and 24% increase in minimum area in coronary disease patients following sublingual nitroglycerin. This resulted in an average 26% reduction in stenosis flow resistance in all coronary lesions greater than 50% stenosis. Nitroprusside, i.v. had a comparable effect. Chew et al [18] demonstrated that verapamil was only about 60% as potent as nitroglycerin as a dilator of large coronary arteries.

3.3 Coronary Constriction with Isometric Handgrip:

The hemodynamic and coronary caliber response to isometric handgrip was studied [19] in twelve patients with coronary disease. In spite of a 25% increase in blood pressure, the coronary arteries constricted about 17% in "normal" cross-sectional area, and stenosis flow resistance increased 29%. This is a response mediated by a generalized sympathetic nervous system activation. Thus sympathetic nervous activity will constrict the large coronary arteries.

The computer has a graphics program for displaying individual patient (ARTDATA) and patient group (HISTORAT) data. The use of HISTORAT in the display of the nitroglycerin and handgrip response is illustrated in Figure 5. The ratio of normal lu-

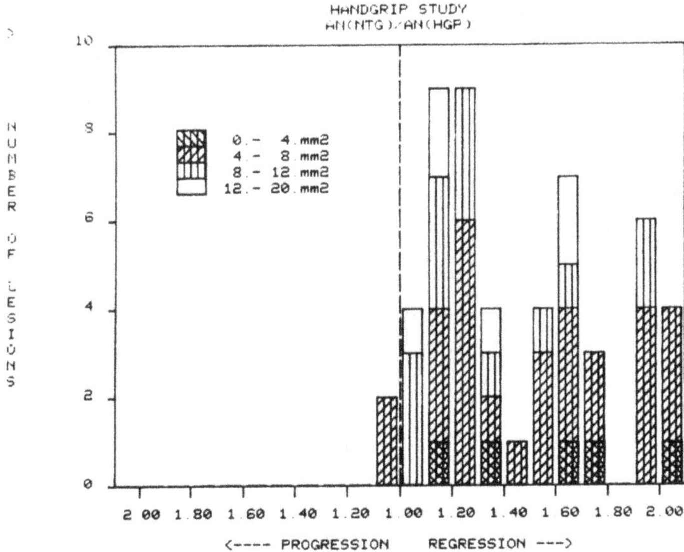

Figure 5: Graphical output of the HISTORAT program. Here, the ratio of normal lumen area following nitroglycerin to that during handgrip in the same arterial segment is computed. The frequency distribution of different values of the ratio are displayed, for four different ranges of normal lumen area.

men area following nitroglycerin to area during isometric handgrip is plotted in Figure 5 as a frequency distribution for all lesions which were studied sequentially with handgrip and nitroglycerin. From this figure, one can see that normal coronary arteries undergo up to two-fold inducible variation in lumen area with these simple maneuvers. In addition, vessels of smaller caliber have more vasomobility.

3.4 Progression of Coronary Atherosclerosis

We are presently nearing completion of a prospective, randomized, double-blind study of the effect of aspirin and dipyridamole on the progression of coronary atherosclerosis over an 18-month interval. The first catheterization was performed for clinical indications in symptomatic patients; the second is done electively after 18 months of either drug or placebo. Angiograms are performed in identical projections in both studies. The same views of a given lesion are analyzed from both studies. Each patient averages 11 lesions (mild to severe).

The first 260 lesions for which measurements were completed were analyzed as group data [20,21] without breaking the drug code. Figures 6,7,8, and 9 illustrate the power of the computer method for compiling, statistically analyzing, and displaying group data.

Each of the more than 50 parameters calculated for each analysis of a lesion are stored on magnetic discs. Each lesion is analyzed from six different cine frames in each of the two angiograms. The accumulated data for 5 selected parameters (normal area, minimum area, predicted pressure drop, Poiseuille resistance, and equivalent length) is tabulated in Figure 6 for each of the two studies, averaged, compared as a ratio and by paired-t statistics, and assigned a p-value for the null hypothesis.

WU ,CA-M43 ROBINSON,ROBERT 01-MAY-80
Data for study Coronary Disease Progression
comparing Initial, medically treated, (1A) on 13-OCT-78
versus Final study, n years interval, (1B) on 11-APR-80

S TRC CYC	NORM A		MIN A		DELTAP 1		POISEUIL		EQ LEN	
M CPRP1 D	5.41	5.25	1.56	1.90	1.83	1.26	1.45	0.97	3.0	2.8
M GBGB1 D	5.48	5.35	1.59	2.02	1.78	1.19	1.36	0.92	2.9	3.3
M CPRP2 D	5.79	5.81	1.59	1.77	1.76	1.37	1.37	1.04	3.0	2.8
M GBGB2 D	5.65	5.95	1.49	1.69	1.79	1.57	1.21	1.12	2.3	2.8
M CPRP3 D	5.11	5.21	1.59	1.52	1.73	1.84	1.33	1.23	2.9	2.5
M GBGB3 D	5.99	5.35	1.84	1.62	1.31	1.62	1.04	1.13	3.0	2.6
AVERAGES	5.57	5.49	1.61	1.75	1.70	1.48	1.29	1.07	2.9	2.8
ST. DEV.	0.31	0.31	0.12	0.18	0.19	0.25	0.15	0.11	0.3	0.3
RATIOS	0.98		1.09		0.87		0.82		0.97	
PAIRED T	0.65	5	-1.41	5	1.48	5	2.47	5	0.47	5
P-VALUES	1.000		0.500		0.200		0.100		1.000	
N CPRP1 D	2.55	2.73	1.31	1.02	3.18	3.86	2.70	2.97	4.1	2.8
N GBGB1 D	2.73	2.94	1.41	1.22	1.82	2.43	1.44	1.84	2.5	2.4
N CPRP2 D	2.60	2.80	1.12	1.00	3.08	3.49	2.42	2.31	2.7	2.1
N GBGB2 D	2.51	2.95	1.42	1.02	1.76	3.16	1.41	2.00	2.5	1.9
N CPRP3 D	2.66	2.83	1.00	1.16	3.73	2.95	2.74	2.25	2.4	2.7
N GBGB3 D	2.98	3.04	1.29	1.28	2.45	2.28	2.00	1.74	3.0	2.5
AVERAGES	2.67	2.88	1.26	1.12	2.67	3.03	2.12	2.18	2.9	2.4
ST. DEV.	0.17	0.11	0.17	0.12	0.79	0.61	0.60	0.44	0.6	0.4
RATIOS	1.08		0.89		1.13		1.03		0.83	
PAIRED T	-4.16	5	1.68	5	-1.17	5	-0.38	5	2.11	5
P-VALUES	0.010		0.200		0.500		1.000		0.100	

Figure 6: Tabular output of the ARTDATA program. See text for description.

Figure 7 shows the computer-generated graphical display of the tabular display data of Figure 6. Here, each of eight lesions has an assigned letter name. The

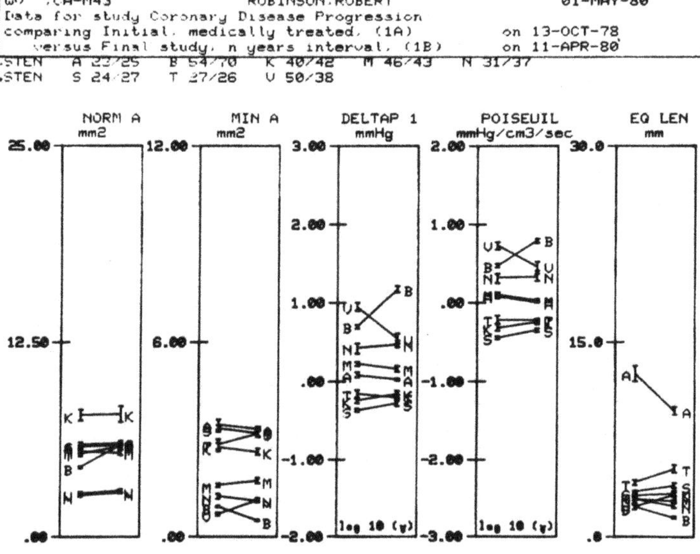

Figure 7: Graphical output of the ARTDATA program. See text for description. Here, the average change in 5 different lesion parameters is displayed for 8 different lesions characterized from the initial clinical angiogram, and from an elective angiogram done 18 months later.

mean and standard deviation of the initial (left) and 18-month (right) value of each of the 5 parameters is plotted. Lesion B has had a significant worsening, while lesion V has significantly improved. The remaining 6 lesions have not changed in any of the important parameters.

Display of group data for all 260 lesions so stored on magnetic disc is shown in Figure 5, 8, and 9. In Figure 8, the difference in percent stenosis between the two studies (%S2-%S1) is plotted, coded for four different levels of lesion severity.

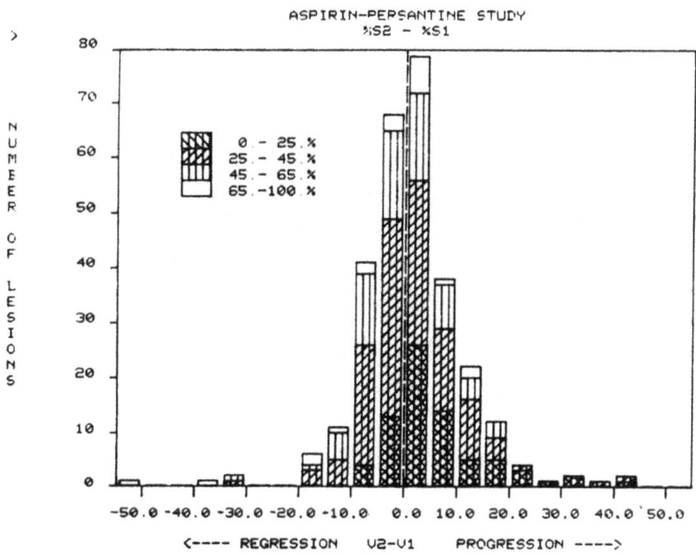

Figure 8: Graphical output of the HISTORAT program. Here, the frequency distribution of the change in "percent stenosis" (%S2-%S1) is plotted for 260 lesions analyzed from 24 patients who had angiograms separated by 18 months. Considerable progression and regression are documented.

The frequency distribution of this population of 260 lesions of all degrees of severity from 24 coronary disease patients centers about zero (no change in % stenosis). The 99.9% confidence value for this difference to represent "true" change is 10.6%. Thus by this criterion 12% of all lesions progress and 5% regress in 18 months. Figure 9 displays the frequency distribution of the transformation of the ratios of flow resistance for the two studies ($\log_{10} \frac{R2}{R1}$). Again, there is little increase, on the average, in stenosis severity. By this parameter, at the 99.9% confidence level, 17% of all lesions show "true" progression and 11%, regression.

4. CONCLUSIONS

A method for computer-based measurement of coronary artery caliber is described. This is presently the only such method, employing a digital computer, which is actively used for clinical evaluation of coronary disease. This method has an application in three important clinical areas: 1.) precise evaluation of coronary stenosis severity, 2.) assessment of the immediate effect of drugs and other short-term interventions on lumen caliber, and 3.) measurement of the progression (and regression) of coronary atherosclerosis. These three applications are briefly illustrated in this report.

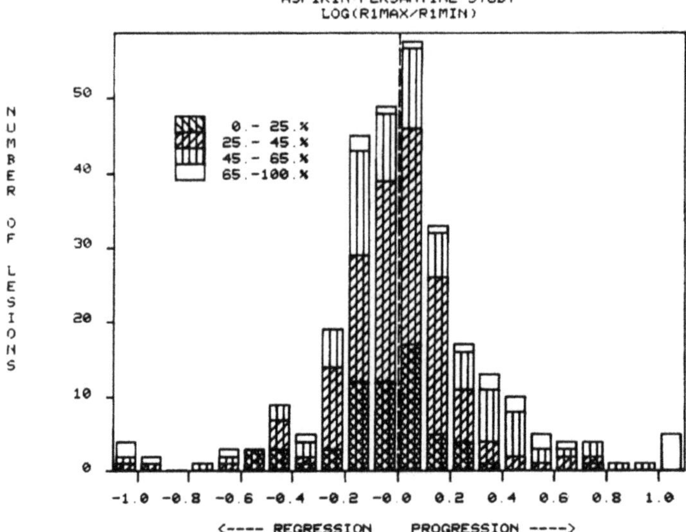

Figure 9: Graphical output of the HISTORAT program. Here, the logarithmic transformation of the flow resistance ratio (R_2/R_1) is plotted as a frequency distribution. Again, considerable progression and regression are noted.

ACKNOWLEDGMENTS

The manuscript was prepared by Lacy Goede, whose skill and assistance are greatly appreciated.

REFERENCES

1. D. Koh, S. Mitten, D. Stewart, E. Bolson, H.T. Dodge, Comparison between computerized quantitative coronary angiography and clinical interpretation. Circulation 60: (Suppl II) 1979, p. 160.
2. K.M. Detre, E. Wright, M.L. Murphy, T. Takaro, Observer agreement in evaluating coronary angiograms. Circulation 52: 1975, p. 979.
3. L.M. Zir, S.W. Miller, R.E. Dinsmore, J.P. Gilbert, J.W. Harthorne, Inter-observer variability in coronary angiography. Circulation 53: 1976, p. 627.
4. T.A. DeRouen, J.A. Murray, W. Owen, Variability in the analysis of coronary arteriograms. Circulation 55: 1977, p. 324.
5. M.M. McMahon, B.G. Brown, R. Cukingnan, E.L. Bolson, E.L. Rolett, H.T. Dodge, Quantitative coronary angiography: Measurement of the "critical" stenosis in patients with unstable angina and single-vessel disease without collaterals. Circulation 60: 1979, p. 106.
6. B.G. Brown, E.L. Bolson, M. Frimer, H.T. Dodge, Quantitative coronary arteriography. Estimation of dimensions, hemodynamic resistance, and atheroma mass of coronary artery lesions using the arteriogram and digital computation. Circulation 55: 1977, p. 329.
7. E. Bolson, B.G. Brown, H.T. Dodge, M. Frimer, Computer analysis of coronary lesions. Proceedings of the Digital Equipment Users Society. 1: 1977, p. 453.
8. W. Rafflenbeul, R. Heim, M. Dzuiba, B. Henkel, P. Lichtlen, Morphometric analysis of coronary arteries. In Coronary Angiography and Angina Pectoris. Symposium of the European Society of Cardiology, edited by P.R. Lichtlen, Stuttgart,

Georg Thiene, 1976, pp. 255-265.
9. R.L. Feldman, C.J. Pepine, R.C. Curry, C.R. Conti, Coronary arterial responses to graded doses of nitroglycerin. Am. J. Cardiol. 43: 1979, pp. 91-97.
10. G.G. Gensini, A.E. Kelly, DaCosta B.C.B., P.P. Huntington, Quantitative angiography: The measurement of coronary vasomobility in the intact animal and man. Chest 60: 1971, pp. 522-530.
11. S. Paulin, T. Sandor, Densitometric assessment of stenosès in coronary arteries. S.P.I.E. (MED-IV) 70: 1975, pp. 337-340.
12. D.W. Crawford, S.H. Brooks, R. Barndt, Jr., D.H. Blankenhorn, Measurement of Atherosclerotic Luminal Irregularity and Obstruction by Radiographic Densitometry. Investigative Radiology 12: 1977, p. 307.
13. D.H. Blankenhorn, S.H. Brooks, R.H. Selzer, D.W. Crawford, H.P. Chin, Assessment of Atherosclerosis from Angiographic Images. Proc Soc Exp Biol Med 145: 1974, pp. 1298-1300.
14. R. Barndt, Jr., D.H. Blankenhorn, D.W. Crawford, S.H. Brooks, Regression and progression of early femoral atherosclerosis in treated hyperlipoproteinemic patients. Ann. Int. Med. 86: 1977, pp. 139-146.
15. W. Kato, M. Wong, Optimizing cinefilm. Cathet. Cardiovasc. Diag. 1: 1975, pp. 97-106.
16. MM McMahon, B.G. Brown, R. Cukingnan, E.L. Rolett, E. Bolson, M. Frimer, H.T. Dodge, Quantitative coronary angiography: Measurement of the "critical" stenosis in patients with unstable angina and single-vessel disease without collaterals. Circulation 60: 1979, pp. 106-113.
17. T.C. Doerner, B.G. Brown, E. Bolson, M. Frimer, H.T. Dodge, Vasodilatory effects of nitroglycerin and nitroprusside in coronary arteries - a comparative analysis. Amer. J. Cardiol. 43: 1979, p. 416.
18. C.Y.C. Chew, B.G. Brown, M. Wong, P.M. Shah, B.N. Singh, E. Bolson, H.T. Dodge, The effects of verapamil on coronary hemodynamics and vasomobility in patients with coronary artery disease. Amer. J. Cardiol. 45: 1980, p. 389.
19. B.G. Brown, R.B. Petersen, C.D. Pierce, M. Wong, E. Bolson, H.T. Dodge, Coronary artery constriction and hemodynamic responses during isometric handgrip in patients with coronary artery disease. Amer. J. Cardiol. 45: 1980, p. 431.
20. B.G. Brown, C.D. Pierce, R.B. Petersen, E. Bolson, H.T. Dodge, The natural history of a coronary lesion: A new quantitative approach to the clinical investigation of coronary atherosclerosis. Proceedings, 5th International Symposium on Atherosclerosis, Houston, November, 1979.
21. B.G. Brown, C.D. Pierce, R.B. Petersen, E. Bolson, H.T. Dodge, A new approach to clinical investigation of progressive coronary atherosclerosis. Circulation 60: II, 1979, p. 66.

IMAGE ANALYSIS IN X-RAY RADIOGRAPHY

by

M. Laval-Jeantet, M. D'Haenens and J. Klausz
Hopital Saint-Louis - Place due Dr. A. Fournier
75010 PARIS

ABSTRACT

Radiologic analysis, like everything, has limitations imposed by the physical and psychological principles. New technologic advances, and computer's use could improve image analysis but it remains very difficult to say what could be the place of automatic image analysis and treatment in a near future. In all radiologic systems, four main processes are involved;

- physical process: creatuion of the roentgen radiation pattern its detection and transformation.
- imaging process: specification of the X-ray image by the luminance, the contrast, the unsharpness; the noise (and signal/noise ratio).
- psychological process with comparison to previous impressions obtained by training.
- diagnosis.

Analysis of "diagnostic" quality is seemingly most important than analysis of "physical" quality, but these components are not independent. Physical quality could be insufficient for diagnosis, but, conversely, the question arises very often whether too much information may be present or not.

ANALYSIS OF IMAGE QUALITY

The quality of a radiographic image may be defined as the ability of the film to record each point in the object as a point on the film. The radiologic reproduction is never perfect, and quality analysis show three main causes of image degradation:

Radiographic mottle
Unsharpness
Loss of contrast

A good radiographic image is able to detect small contrast, as the fractional intensity change required to just recognize a change in intensity. The resolution is the reciprocal of minimal resolvable distance in cm between two lines.

Two methods give a synthetic approach of image quality analysis, the line spread function and the modulation transfer function. They give an evaluation of unsharpness cuased by light spreading in the screen film system, or by focal spot dimensions of X-ray tubes, and an associate evaluation of loss of contrast in the system.

The line spread function is determined by analysis of the image of a 10 microns slit with a microdensitometer. The shape of the curves allows us to predict the sharpness of the image boundaries. The modulation in the image is a result of the convolution of the line spread function of the imaging device with the input distribution.

The modulation transfer function is an attempt to analyze the amount of information transferred from the X-ray image to the detecting system.

$$\text{MTF} = \frac{\text{Information recorded}}{\text{Information available}}$$

The MTF plays an important role in evaluating a complex imaging system (16). The total MTF of the entire system may be obtained by multiplying the MTF's of each of the components. But the practical use of MTF measurements, as of many other methods of analysis in radiology, is still being evaluated.

Line spread and MTF analysis are a very good approach of "physical" image quality, but if we consider a complex image as a whole we must introduce, with Cleare (2), the bandwidth-gain concept. A radiographic image is made only by a small part of the modulation of intensity of the X-ray beam. The gain of a system could be defined as the useful absorption in the primary conversion element for typical X-ray spectra. Bandwidth is the range of spatial frequency from zero to the frequency at which the MTF drops to the 4 percent level. The higher is the gain-bandwidth product, the higher is the objective quality of the image. This method of analysis introduces the speed of system, and the dose to the patient. From such studies, exact indications for use of direct magnification techniques can be calculated, and an adaptation of radiographic technique to the nature of the object examined can be developed.

Analysis of image quality in Computerized Tomography and Digital Radiography introduces another limit.

The properties of these Digital images are the result of a compromise between a relatively low spatial resolution, a high contrast detection, and the necessary lowest possible dose to the patient.

Computerized Tomography is the result of the reconstruction by computer of a tomographic plane of an object. It is developed from multiple X-ray absorption measurements made in different angulations of tube and detectors.

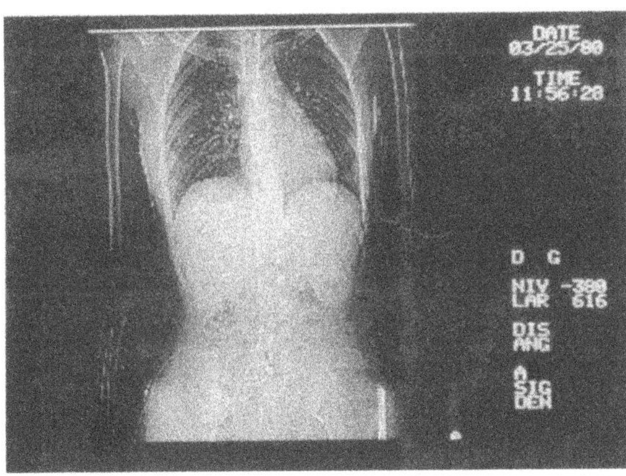

Figure 1. Direct Digital Radiography obtained on C.T. Scanner (C.G.R. C.T. 10000)

Direct Digital Radiography can be obtained with a scanographic system derived from a CT scanner (9). The basic hardware of the detector system is used, with the X-ray tube and detectors kept fixed, and the patient translated at a constant speed through the gantry.

In C.T. and D.D.R., the narrow X-ray beam reduces the scattered radiation. The high signal/noise ratio and the high gain of detectors give a good detection of smaller contrasts in soft tissues. The digitalization of image data allows immediate analysis and enhancement.

Image analysis of "physical" quality of digital radiography employs the usual parameters of spatial resolution and contrast detection, but with different conditions:

The determination of spatial resolution of CT is more complicated than of film-screen radiography, because there are four intrinsic elementary sizes which determine the resolution in the image: (1) the width of the detector element aperture, (2) the distance between sampling points (3) the form of the convolution filter and (4) the display picture element size (the pixel).

The contrast resolution analysis is simple: low contrast test objects could be evaluated, and a contrast-detail diagram describes the ability of the system to detect small contrasts. (Figure 2)

In practice, it is possible to define a MTF curve for digital radiography, exactly like in screen film systems.

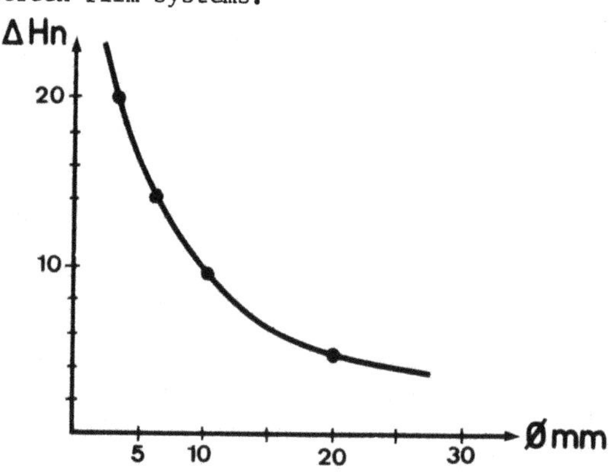

Figure 2.
Contrast-detail
for a C.T.Scanner

DIAGNOSTIC ANALYSIS

Diagnosis quality of a radiographic image is a very complicated concept, and has been studied in a great variety of ways and contexts. In most situations a final measure of diagnostic quality can be defined only in the subjective sense, but there is a strong tendency to objective analysis of diagnostic elements. Spatial frequency analysis of "diagnostic" information can be performed by introduction of increasing unsharpness in radiographic images (Feddema). Copies of diagnostic films made with increasing distances from the original image decrease the modulation transfer fuction, and realize an equivalent filtration of higher frequencies. Our experimentation shows that gallbladder lithiasis, peptic ulcer or bone fracture are seen in radiographs with a poor modulation transfer function (below 10 cycles/cm), but also that most of the rhumatoid or metabolic bone changes, all breast radiography, almost all vascular opacifications need the better image quality. In these cases, it is frequent to diagnose a disease only by the perception of a very small detail (cortical erosion or striation, small irregularities of vascular walls, micro calcifications in a breast).

Table I gives some usual spatial frequencies determined by progressive low pass cutoff frequency analysis.

OBJECTS	SPATIAL FREQUENCY (cycles per cm.)
Gastric ulcer	0.5
Colonic polyp	1
Gallbladder lithiasis	2
Miliary tuberculosis	5
Small vessel occlusion	30
Cortical striation (bone)	40
Breast calcifications	20 - 40

From daily clinical experience, we could assume that 90 percent of diagnostic interpretations depend upon large modifications of shape, contour or structure. Only in a fraction of examinations the perception of small details or poorly contrasted images is involved. Image analysis shows that nonoptimal radiologic quality suffice in many cases when dose reduction is a primary condition.

It could be interesting, however, to determine the frequency spectrum of the X-ray diagnostic pattern. A knowledge of that frequency content permits to assess whether the spectrum can be transmitted by the radiodiagnostic chain, and with what quality (6, 16).

Moreover, it is of interest to know to what extent the spectral analysis of the diagnostic patterns of a pathologic x-ray image differ from a normal one. This approach could be a way to automated diagnosis by image analysis.

Our experimental work has the purpose to appreciate image quality and diagnostic differences by study of spectrum computation on radiologic digitalized images.

Image acquisition is obtained by digitalization with a vidicon special TV camera. From the resulting file, we take a 128 pixels square part used as the data file.

The two-dimensional Fourier transform is made by two successive one-dimensional transforms along lines and columns. This transform uses a 128 points FFT. The file is rearranged to have lower frequencies in the image center. The modulus the transform is then computed; to have a better visual perception, the final values are the logarithm of this modulus (contrast compression) after adding a constant to keep a finite amplitude for a zero value. The visualized values G are:

$$G = A \, \ell n(1 + ||F||^2)$$

Preliminary results show that spatial frequency spectrum could be a good and objective analysis of physical quality of image (7). But the interest of that analysis appears particularly in the displaying of differences between normal and pathological structures in some cases. Our experiments show that these differences are present in bone disease (Fig. 3) (Paget or vertebral osteoporosis), chest iseases (alveolar vs interstitial patterns) and vascular textures.

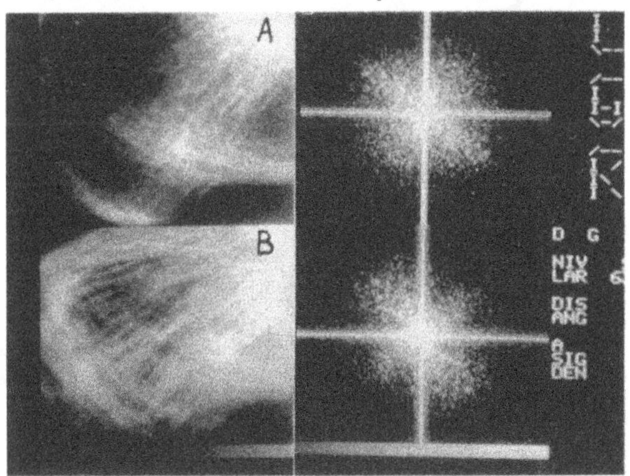

Figure 3. Fourier spectrum frequency analysis

A. Normal calcaneum
B. Paget's disease of calcaneum
Paget's spectrum contains more low frequencies due to spongy bone trabeculae enlargement.

It is important to note that the frequency content depends on the object and on the imaging system. If the image is magnified, the frequency spectrum will be shifted downward. The frequency content of the object is a very large field for new studies. From anatomical measurements of structures of diagnostic importance, one could define goals for the imaging machine and make a selection among the numerous radiographic techniques available (3).

Filtering image analysis is very close from the preceding method. Image filtering may change the ability of the eye-brain system to analyze the image and sometimes enhance the perception of diagnostic details. We had experimented different filters upon digital images from direct digital radiography or secondary digitalization (Figure 4).

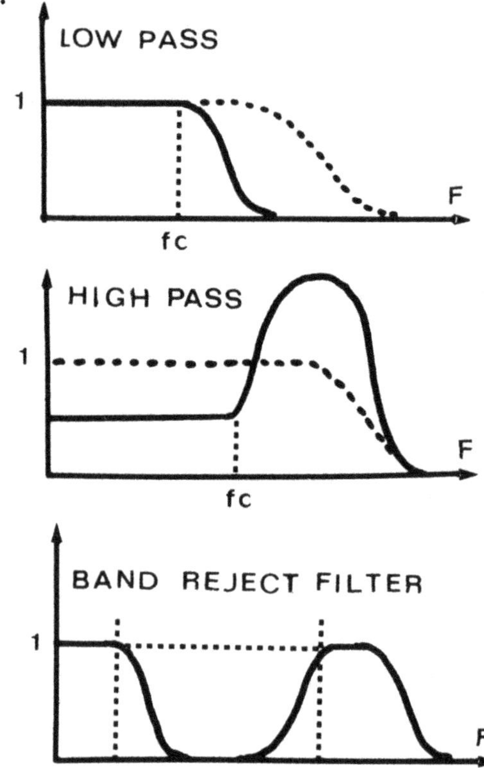

Figure 4.
Three frequency responses

The low pass filter. The first order low pass (passes the lower frequencies) could be used with the following difference equation:

$$y(n) = b_1 y\ (n-1) + a_o x(n) + a_1 x(n-1)$$

$$\text{with } b_1 = (1 - c) \ / \ (1 + c)$$

$$a_o = 1 \ / \ (1 + c)$$

$$a_1 = a_o$$

The low pass filter will smooth the image, and it is used primarily to remove "noise" from the image. It could give a better visual analysis of low-contrast small objects (ROSSMANN). In bone lesions where a small change of density is the pathologic image (Paget's disease, sclerosing metastases), the high frequency structures of spongy bone reduces the perceptibility (1). Low-pass filtering eliminate largely the disturbance by the fine structures of spongy bone, and improves the visibility of large and dense bone lesions.

The high pass filter. The first order high pass has the same form of difference equation, except with

$$a_o = c \ / \ (1 + c)$$

$$a_1 = -c\ (1 + c)$$

The high pass filter will sharpen the image, but will also lighten the image as the average gray shade level is reduced or lowered.

Image filtering may be a good initial stage in automatic analysis, such as organ measurements or recognition.

The High Emphasis filter. To keep from losing information, all frequencies are retained and the amplified higher frequencies are added back to the original signal. This is accomplished with a band reject filter where the low pass cutoff frequency is set much higher than the high pass cutoff frequency.

Another method of this kind of filtering is the analogic logetron. These filters will produce sharper edges, but will also have a tendency to produce artifacts and to darken the image in certain regions.

Conclusion

Image filtration could be very useful to lower the noise level. A reduction of noise in CT scanner imaging is possible by a factor of 4 to 8 with simple described low filters, but with some sacrifice in spatial resolution. Experimental measurements with a complex phantom indicate that filtering allows smaller lesion of low contrast to be detected. (Figure 5)

It is necessary to be very cautious with filtration analysis: filtering edge enhancement can generate a variety of treatment artefacts which can interfere with visual image analysis. Fine grained noise texture enhanced image yield subjective impression of higher acuity and contrast but, in fact, gives a lower signal/nose ratio, and a bad enhancement can induce reticulate pseudostructures, in chest X rays or mammographic image analysis.

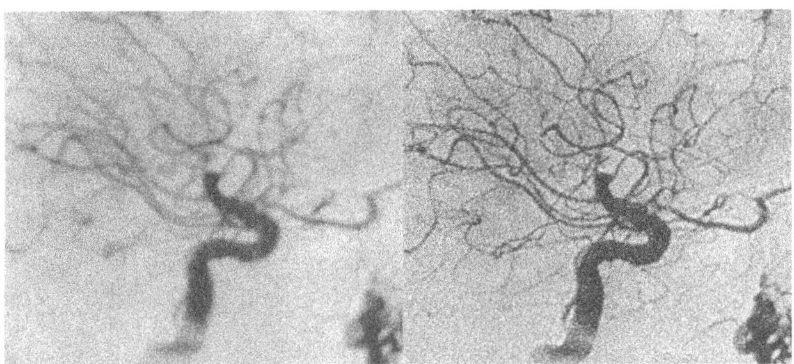

Figure 5. High pass filtration and contrast enhancement by computer processing of cerebral angiogram. Note the best visibility of smaller vessels.

Subtraction technique analysis is a photographic or electronic image analysis used to eliminate unwated images from a radiograph. (15). Strictly speaking, the method does not add any information, but it makes diagnostically important informations easier to see.

Subtraction eliminates the constant part of the image by superimposition of a negative and a positive film of the same region. If one of these films differ on only certain details, such as vascular opacification, subtraction gives a very high improvement of vessels' perceptibility. We have experimented association of high pass filtration and subtraction with very good results on visibility of smaller cerebral or pancreatic vessels.

Pseudo - color image processing and analysis.

Black and white images are limited to one parameter, brightness, whereas colored images have three parameters brightness, hue and saturation.

The additional parameters of color analysis permit more information to be conveyed, and theoretically a best perception of contrast. Color radiography can improve discrimination between areas of slightly different x-ray intensity, when these are displayed not only as changes of brightness but also as a change of hue.

On the assumption that there is more information on a radiograph that can be seen by the observer, a colored analysis and display could be done in a simple TV system (6).

The TV camera video signals are evaluated by electronic circuits which sort the information into three channels depending upon the density of the elements of the radiograph. The final display is a full-color conversion of the original black and white radiograph.

The question arises whether there is a need in radiography for this information analysis and recording. Color displays had not gained wide acceptance, probably because psychological habits and limitations are still unknown.

Densitometric analaysis is a very important way of image analysis, and perhaps the most useful. Many techniques permit image density determination: point by point measurements, density profiles, isodensity curves, histograms of densities. Application of image analysis to determination of bone mineral density is very interesting, but very difficult: Radiographic film analysis (13) gives many errors (nonlinear response, development, artifacts) and classical methods employing a densitometric scale polychromatic X ray and large beam are the causes of large measurement errors (5 to 10 percent).

Measure of the linear attenuation coefficient (or of the Hounsfield number H_n) is closely related to the mineral content of bone. For a certain X ray energy, H_n is a characteristic of normal or pathological bone, sufficient to detect a demineralization.

Substitution for imaging of films by linear counters used in CT scanners or DDR reduces errors to 3 percent. The theoretical possibilities of CT censitometry had been tested by an experimental work on vertebral columns of 14 patients who died after acute disease. The correlation between ashes weight - H_n was positive, but only moderate. Intravertebral fat remains an important cause of errors, and multiple energy imaging analysis could be an improvement. The efficiency of these techniques is under investigation in several centers.

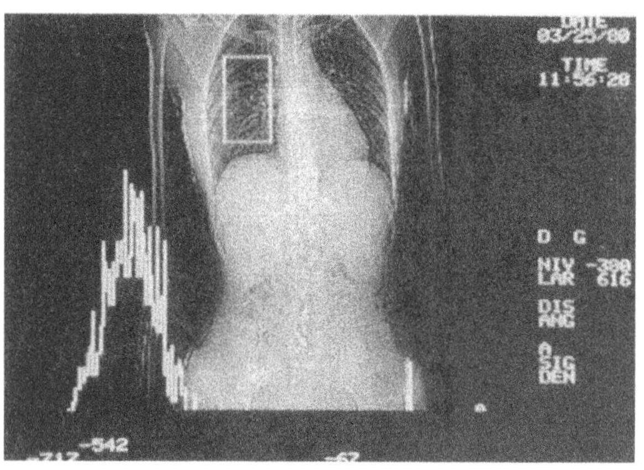

Figure 6. Histogram of pulmonary densiti from direct Digital Radiography.

Texture and boundary recognition are very important steps in image analysis. The most successful application of these methods are studies of arterial system of the brain or of the abdomen (5,19).

CLINICAL APPLICATIONS

In mammography one of the major initial areas of investigation is the process of evaluating and correlating the many visible structural patterns which are seen in the enhanced images and very difficult to see in non enhanced images, with a possible disease state of precancerous nature. A best visibility of radiating cancerous extensions constitute an interesting improvement in some cases of deep breast tumors (10).

From chest X-rays, the earlier approach was taken by Hall (8) with an evaluation of texture features in the inter-rib regions. Kruger used the digital texture analysis and feature extraction from optical Fourier transform. The study of Ledley (12) was based on histograms of the X-ray image. More recently, Savol and Hoy worked on the field of computerized recognition of individual small rounded opacities. The recognition accuracy of the best apparatus is around 80p The evaluation of early lesions of pneumoconiosis is one promising area.

A computer image processing technique has been developed by Jet Propulsion Laboratory (Selzer, et al.,) to automate the measurement of atherosclerosis in the femoral and coronary arteries (19).

In the long range the use of the computer to extract and display information may also, in some limited field of radiodiagnostic, lead to automatic screening.

These first clinical applications of image analysis in radiology are promising, but many of them have required sophisticated techniques and equipment that do not lend themselves to large routine applications.

From a medical point of view, the most important results of image analysis are: image quality determination, magnification, no-screen films, automatic or semi-qutomatic measurements, bone densitometry and subtraction. The usefulness of other results are uncertain: e.g., pseudo-color processing and analysis, enhancement of "regions of iconographic interest", spatial frequency spectrum, and automatic image analysis in medical routine practice.

CONCLUSION

Radiologists had generally been directing their attention in improving the quality of the fixed radiologic image. Less attention has been directed toward extracting more information from the image than what is readily apparent to the eye. The sole method of extraction employed widely has been subtraction of angiograms.

We now see that it is becoming possible to use electronical subtraction systems, high resolution television systems, and computerized image enhancements.

Many studies remain necessary to obtain precise indications for the numerous methods of image analysis actually available in radiology.

REFERENCES

1. CEDERLUND J. , HEMMINGSSON A., JUNG B., LUNDQUIST H., MOBERG H.O. "Image enhancement by digital - analog filtration." Acta. Radiol. Diagn. 1979 20 154 - 160.

2. CLEARE H.M. "Future prospects for screen film radiography." in Small vessel angiography Mosby Cy St. Louis 1973.

3. FEDDEMA J. , BOTDEN P.J.M. "Adequate diagnostic information" in Television in diagnostic radiology Aesculapius Publ. Comp. Birmingham (Alab.) 1969.

4. GENANT H.K. , BOYD D. Quantitative Bone Mineral Analysis Using Dual Energy Computed Tomography. Invest. Radiol. 1977 12 545 - 551.

5. GEORGES A., GOUTTE R., PROST R., AMIEL M.
"Amélioration des images radiologiques par traitement du signal."
J. Radiol. 1979 60 221 - 224.

6. GONZALEZ R.C., WINTZ P.
Digital Image Processing.
Addison - Wesley Publ. Comp. Reading. Mass. 1977.

7. GOODENOUGH D., DOI K., ROSSMANN K.
"Optical spatial filtering of Radiographic Images with Binary Filters."
Radiology 1974 111 433 - 438.

8. HALL E.L.
"Overall classification from Zonal classification."
Proc. of 3rd Intern. joint Conf. on Pattern Recognition 1976.

9. KATRAGADDA C.S., FOGEL S.R., COHEN G., WAGNER L.K., MORGAN C., HANDEL S.F., AMLEY S.R., LESTER R.G.
"Digital Radiography using a Computed Tomographic Instrument."
Radiology 1979 133 83 - 87.

10. KIRCH R.L.A., LARSEN G., THOMAS J.J.
"Digital computerized mammographic image enhancement : a preliminary report."
Biosigma. Paris Avril 1978 Vol. 2 251 - 257.

11. LAVAL-JEANTET M., LAVAL-JEANTET A.M., LAMARQUE J.L., DEMOULIN B.
"Evaluation de la minéralisation osseuse vertébrale par tomographie computérisée."
J. Radiol. 1979 60 87 - 93.

12. LEDLEY R.S., HUANG H.K., ROTOLO L.S.
"A texture analysis method in classification of Coal Worker's Pneumoconiosis."
Computers in Biol. Med. 1975 5 53 - 67.

13. MEEMA H.E., TAVES D.R., OREOPOULOS D.G.
"Comparisons between X - ray photodensitometric and gamma-ray Absorptiometric findings of Bone Mineral Measurements, and the Evidence of their Convertibility."
Invest. Radiol. 1976 11 550 - 555.

14. NEVATIA R.
"Locating object boundaries in textured environments in 'Digital Image Processing".
EHO 133 - 9
IEEE Trans. on Computers 1976.

15. ORT M.G., GREGG E.C., KAUFMAN B.
"Subtraction Radiography : Techniques and limitations."
Radiology 1977 124 65 - 72.

16. ROSSMANN K.
"An approach to Image Quality Evaluation Using Observer Performance Studies."
Radiology 1974 113 541 - 544.

17. SAVOL A.M., HOY R.J.
"Biomedical pattern recognition for early detection of pneumoconiosis from chest X - Rays."
Biosigma. Paris Avril 1978 Vol. 2 245 - 250.

18. SCHOTT O.
"The X-ray pattern and its properties as input parameters in X - ray television"
in Television in diagnostic radiology
Aesculapius Publ. Comp. Birmingham 1969.

19. SELZER R.H., BLANKENHORN D.H., CRAWFORD D.W., BROOKS S.H., BARNDT R.
"Computer measurement of arterial disease from angiograms."
Biosigma. Paris Avril 1978 Vol. 2 267 - 271.

20. TER-POGOSSIAN M., PHELPS M.E., HOFFMAN E.J., EICHLING J.O.
"The extraction of the yet unused wealth of information in diagnostic radiology."
Radiology 1974 113 515 - 520.

21. TULLY R.J., CONNERS R.W., HARLOW C.A., LODWICK G.S.
"Towards Computer Analysis of Pulmonary Infiltration."
Invest. Radiol. 1978 13 298 - 304.

22. TURNER A.F., KRUGER R.P., THOMPSON W.B.
"Automated Computed Screening of Chest Radiographs for Pneumoconiosis."
Invest. Radiol. 1976 11 258 - 266.

INTRAVENOUS ANGIOGRAPHY USING COMPUTERIZED FLUOROSCOPY APPARATUS†

Charles A. Mistretta, Ph.D., Robert A Kruger, Ph.D., David L. Ergun, M.S.
Chorng Gang Shaw, M.S., C.M. Strother, M.D., A.B. Crummy, M.D.
J. F. Sackett, M.D., D. Myerowitz, M.D., W. Turnipseed, M.D., M. Van Lysel, M.S.
W. Zarnstorff, Ph.D., R. Lieberman, M.D., and F.F. Ruzicka, M.D.

Department of Radiology
The University of Wisconsin
Madison, Wisconsin 53706
U.S.A.

ABSTRACT

Following several years of development and testing using animals, a digital image processor designed to perform generalized subtraction imaging tasks has been interfaced to an image-intensified television fluoroscopy apparatus in the University of Wisconsin Clinical Sciences Center. So far, 175 patients have been examined using three time-subtraction modes. In Mask-Mode-Radiography, images of opacified arteries are subtracted from a mask image obtained just prior to the arrival of iodine injected into an antecubital vein. Fully processed subtraction images are obtained at a rate of about one per second and stored on a video disc in real time. This mode is used for all arteries outside of the heart and may be ECG-gated for cardiac imaging. Left ventricular motion is well visualized in Mask Mode Fluoroscopy. In this mode the mask is taken prior to the injection of contrast. Then 60 subtraction images per second are stored on video tape. For wall motion studies this can be done at conventional fluoroscopic exposure levels. We have had limited success in seeing coronary bypass grafts and coronary arteries, but further improvements are needed. In Time Interval Difference Mode short term changes in iodine concentration are displayed. This mode is obtained from Mask Mode Fluoroscopy by reprocessing.

1. INTRODUCTION

We have believed for many years, that the greatest potential benefits from image processing will not come from processing of single images, but rather from formation of generalized subtraction images [1]. When the dependence of the x-ray transmission image on the variables x, y, z (spatial variables), energy and time is examined, it is seen that standard single projection radiography, whether done with a film or a modified computerized tomography scanner (Computed Radiography) consists of a zero order term plus derivative terms involving the spatial variables x and y in the detector plane. Processing of single projection images can proceed through the variables x and y or through grey scale operations but information associated with the energy, time or depth dependence of attenuation is no longer accessible.

The success of computed tomography was to a large extent due to the fact that, although by indirect means, it achieved complete isolation of the generalized subtraction image associated with the z (depth) variable. If one imagines an x-ray beam passing from head to foot, the CT image represents the differential attenuation occurring between depth z and $z + \Delta z$ where Δz is the slice thickness. Thus CT is equivalent to the isolation of the z derivative term in a Taylor series expansion of the x-ray transmission function about a point in (x,y,z,ε,t) space.

†The techniques described in this paper were developed under support from the National Science Foundation, Grants #APR 76-19076 and ENG 7824555.

During the last several years, we have studied a variety of generalized subtraction imaging techniques involving the z, ε and t variables, initially using analog storage tubes and more recently using digital techniques [2,3,4,5,6,7,8].

This paper reports on the use of computerized fluoroscopy, i.e. real time digital processing of video information from image-intensifier fluoroscopy systems, to obtain time subtraction angiograms following injection of iodinated contrast material into a peripheral vein in the antecubital region.

2. APPARATUS AND METHODS

The x-ray apparatus used for our initial studies of 175 patients consists of a conventional .6 mm (nominal) focal spot tube filtered by 4.6 mm of aluminum, and a 4.5"-6"-9" Cesium Iodide image intensifier tube. Although satisfactory images were obtained with a standard Plumbicon television camera, we are presently using a 26 mm frogs neck Plumbicon which has somewhat better dynamic range and spatial resolution.

Prior to digitization at a rate of eight bits per 100 nanoseconds, the video signal is logarithmically amplified to ensure that the iodine signal isolated by subtraction will be independent of the local grey shade in the unsubtracted image. This, along with convenience and the possibility of multiplication of the iodine signal, is a major advantage over film subtraction techniques.

Depending on the imaging mode the data may be integrated over several television fields in any of three 256 × 256 × 13 bit memories. Data is repeatedly cycled through memory to permit integration or continuous display. Image subtraction and other hardware based algorithms are performed on data passing from the various memories into a processing pipeline.

Processed data may be stored on video tape, video disc or, in modes which involve serial time-separated exposures, data may be transfered to conventional digital storage. For real time digital storage high speed tapes and discs are now available, but are quite expensive [9]. As pointed out by Brennecke [10], writing presubtracted and amplified data on analog storage media effectively increases the signal-to-noise ratio of images upon playback. We have found it convenient to redigitize data stored on tape or disc in order to eliminate patient motion artifacts. In some cases analog storage contributes a significant amount of noise to the final subtraction. However, such reprocessing usually produces better images than the originals when motion is involved. If motion artifacts are sufficiently well cancelled, the noise associated with analog storage can limit image quality. Digital storage is obviously preferable if available and economically feasible.

The x-ray factors used for intravenous angiography depend greatly on the type of information sought. For carotid angiography we typically use 60 kVp, tube currents of 200-300 mA, and integrate for 1/15 seconds. For observation of coronary bypass grafts, similar exposure rates may be employed continuously for three or four seconds following opacification of the left ventricle. The time of the latter may be observed using low dose fluoroscopic subtraction. For studies of left ventricular wall motion, fluoroscopic currents (a few mA) may also be used.

The signal-to-noise ratio of the television camera is on the order of 500 to 1 for a bandwidth of 5 MHz, which is sufficient to digitize 512 picture elements per horizontal line in real time. The lens aperture for the Plumbicon is chosen for each type of examination. When maximum detail is desired, such as in most arterial imaging, we have used an aperture which produces near maximal Plumbicon current for about 300 μR/video field at the image intensifier. This should permit visualization of a 1 mm vessel filled with contrast material diluted by a factor of twenty. In some cases this exposure, which is already a factor of 10-15 higher than used for cine fluoroscopy, is integrated over a few video fields, if motion permits.

2.1 Injection Procedure

Our injection procedure has been fairly well standardized after lengthy experimentation. A number 16 2" long Angiocath is inserted into an antecubital vein, preferably the basilic. A 5% dextrose solution (30-40 cc) is drawn into an inverted syringe. Then a similar amount of contrast material is drawn in and, due to its higher density, layers below the dextrose solution. This combination is injected at a rate of 12-14 cc/sec. The dextrose solution prevents the contrast material from pooling in the venous system. Reflux of contrast material into large veins, such as the jugular veins in the neck can sometimes interfere with the image if this persists during the taking of the mask image.

Depending on the particular examination, two or three views may be required. On our present apparatus this requires a separate injection for each view. A biplane apparatus would be useful in this regard. However a moveable source-detector arrangement might permit subtraction images at several angles if sufficient storage for multiple mask images is available.

2.2 Mask Mode Radiography

In this mode, which is used for serial imaging of arteries, an image is digitized immediately following the injection but before opacification of the arteries of interest. Then at a rate typically set a one image every 1-1.5 seconds, subtraction images are formed and stored on a video disc. In this mode a digital disc is preferable, especially if motion requires choosing an alternate mask. This can be done by choosing one of the early subtraction images as an alternate mask. Because all images have been formed by subtraction from the original mask, this mask cancels as a common element. If analog storage is used, the recording of such alternate masks as enhanced subtraction images is very important as discussed earlier.

2.3 Mask Mode Fluoroscopy

In this mode a preinjection mask is necessary. Since the injected iodine arrives quickly at the right side of the heart, failure to obtain a mask before injection could cause right heart structures to persist in the left heart images, although they would occupy the portion of the grey scale opposite from that of iodine. In our early studies we used masks which were integrated over a large fraction of the heartbeat, resulting in a blurry compromise mask which sufficed to suppress non-iodinated anatomy well enough to permit amplification of left heart structures by a factor of about 8-10. For obtaining optimal images of coronary bypass grafts or coronary arteries, phase-matched masks will be preferable but will require some post-processing. Again, if analog storage is to be used, a blurred mask can be used to permit subtraction and amplification of information before storage.

For imaging coronary vessels exposure rates as high as 500 mR/sec are presently used for time periods of about 4 seconds. So far we have had greater success in recognizing these vessels during continuous exposure because of the fact that this motion helps to separate them from simultaneously opacified but more stationary pulmonary structures. A display capable of repeating a brief sequence of high exposure rate fluoroscopy would be useful for helping the observer to become oriented to the image sequence.

2.4 Time Interval Difference (T.I.D.) Mode

This mode displays short term variations in iodine contrast. Typically four video fields are integrated and subtracted from a similar and usually immediately preceding image integral. The advantages of this mode include immunity to respiratory motion and, in the heart, display of dyskinetic regions as anomalous grey shades. This has been demonstrated in infarcted dog hearts [8] and will be illustrated in the patient examples below.

3. RESULTS

Examples of Mask Mode Radiography are shown in Figures 1 through 6. Figure 1a shows conventional left and right common carotid arteriograms. These are to be compared with Figure 1b which is an intravenous angiogram obtained with 40 cc of iodine injected at 14 cc/sec. The most notable feature is the ulcer at the origin of the right internal carotid artery. This is seen well in the intravenous examination.

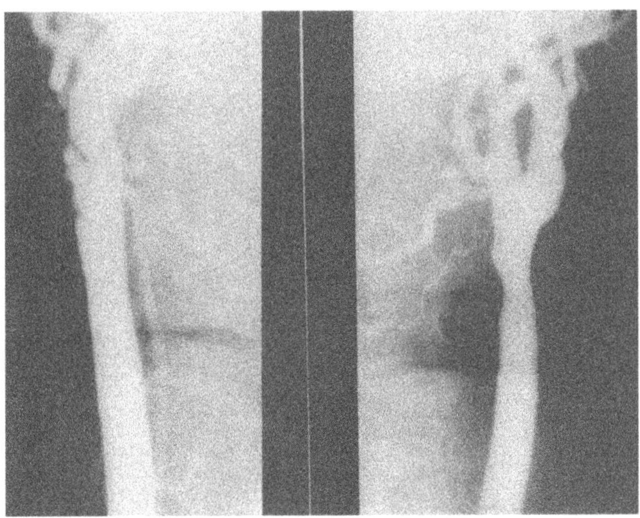

FIG. 1a. Left and right selective common carotid angiograms obtained with intra-arterial injection.

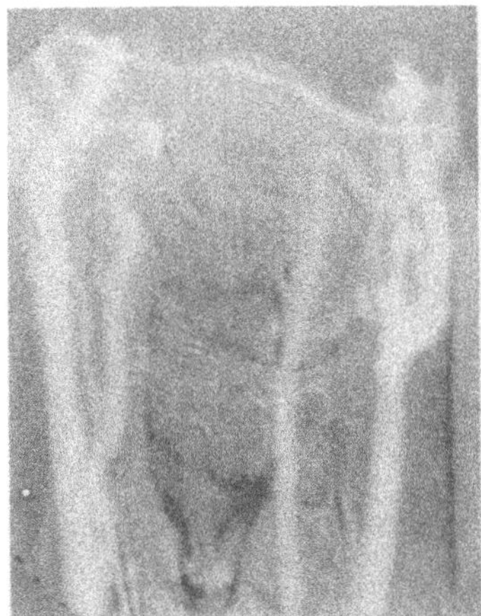

FIG. 1b. Intravenous angiogram of the same patient as in Figure 1a. 40 cc of contrast material were injected at 14 cc/sec.

Generally two or three projections are required to evaluate the carotid bifurcations as shown in Figure 2 in which the right internal carotid is observed to be occluded. A similar occlusion is seen in Figure 3 which compares conventional and intravenous results.

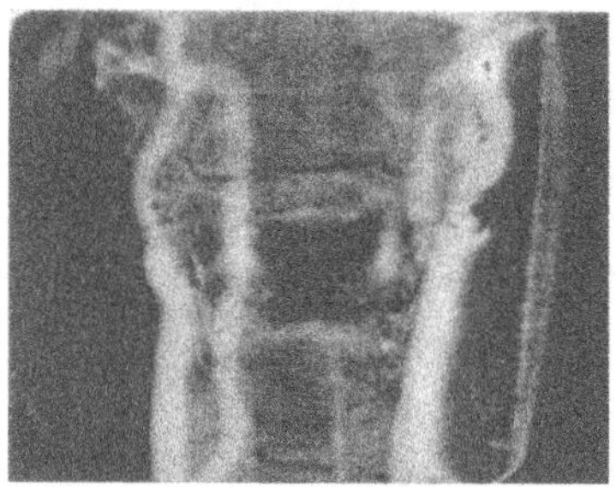

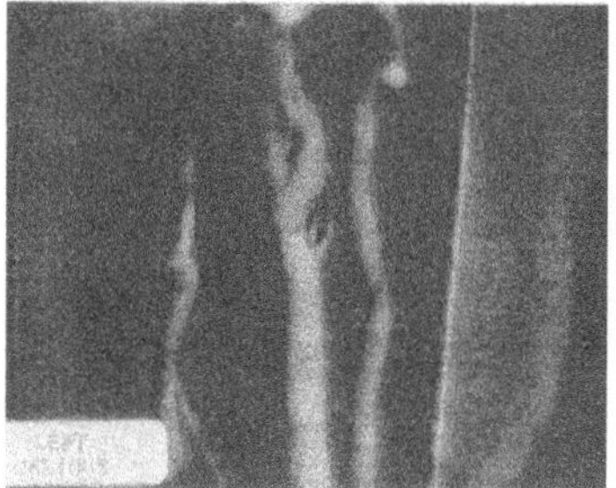

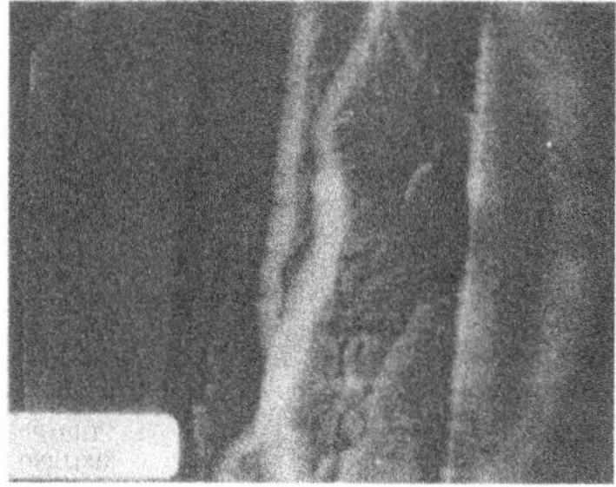

FIG. 2. Antero-posterior and oblique projections of the carotid arteries. Injection factors are in Figure 1. Typical exposure factors are 60 kVp, 250 ma, 1/5 sec.

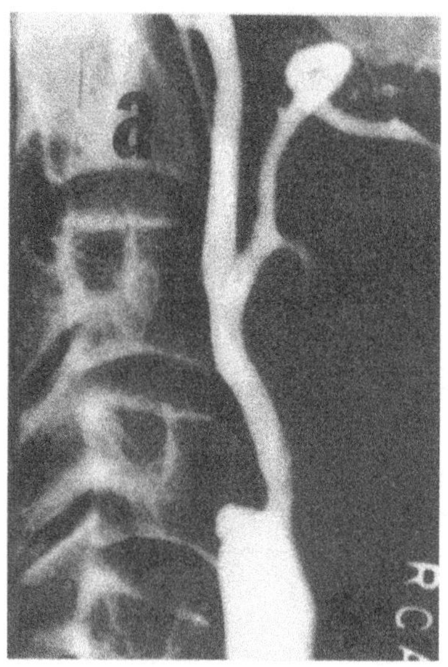

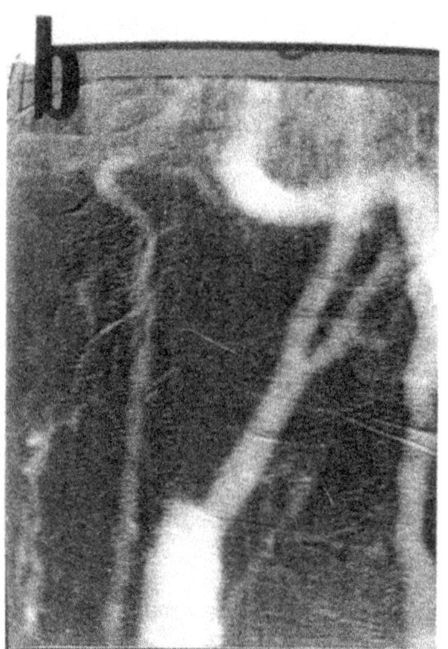

FIG. 3. Comparison of conventional (a) and intravenous (b) carotid angiograms showing occlusion of internal carotid artery.

For examination of the abdomen and leg vessels, we usually use a single 60 cc injection. Figure 4 shows an examination of the abdominal aorta in the region of the renal arteries. Bowel motion can be a problem in this type of examination. However some suppression of peristalsis can be achieved using glucagon.

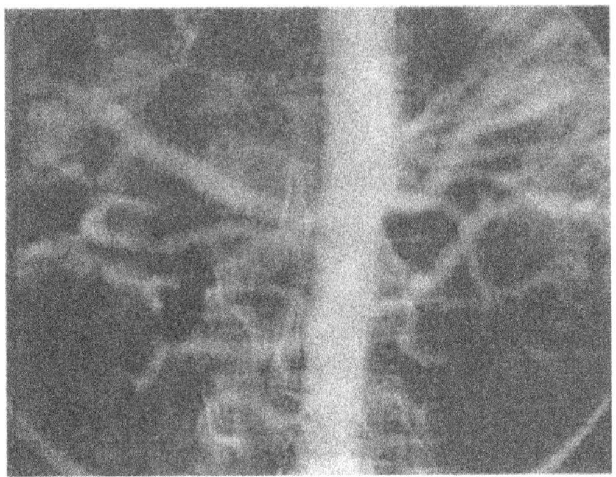

FIG. 4. Intravenous examination of the abdominal aorta following a 60 cc injection.

A particularly useful application involves follow-up studies of peripheral vein grafts such as those shown in Figures 5 and 6. These examinations are almost always successful because motion can be suppressed.

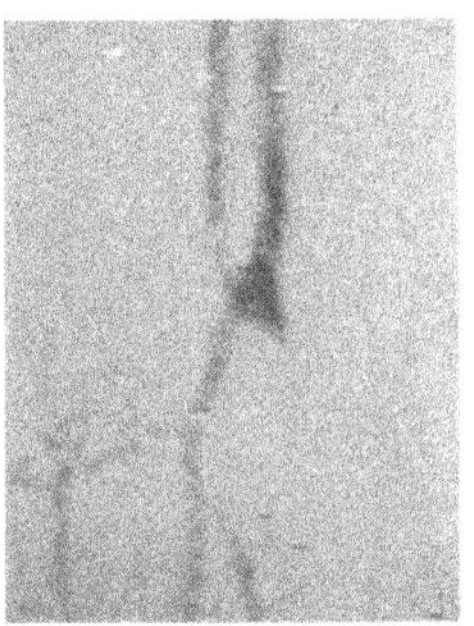

FIG. 6. Distal anastomosis of femoral-popliteal vein graft following a 60 cc injection.

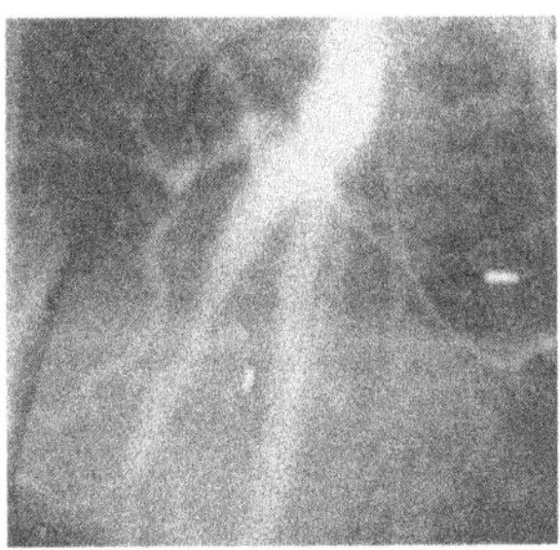

FIG. 5. Proximal portion of femoral artery vein graft following a 60 cc injection.

The use of Mask Mode Fluoroscopy is illustrated in Figure 7 which shows diastolic and systolic phases of the left ventricle in a patient having an akinetic portion of the inferior border. Evaluation of the ventricle can be done at conventional fluoroscopic exposure rates. However, evaluation of bypass grafts and coronary arteries requires a rather high exposure rate. Figure 8 shows a patent left anterior descending bypass graft. Better visualization is possible in the dynamic display from which this image was taken.

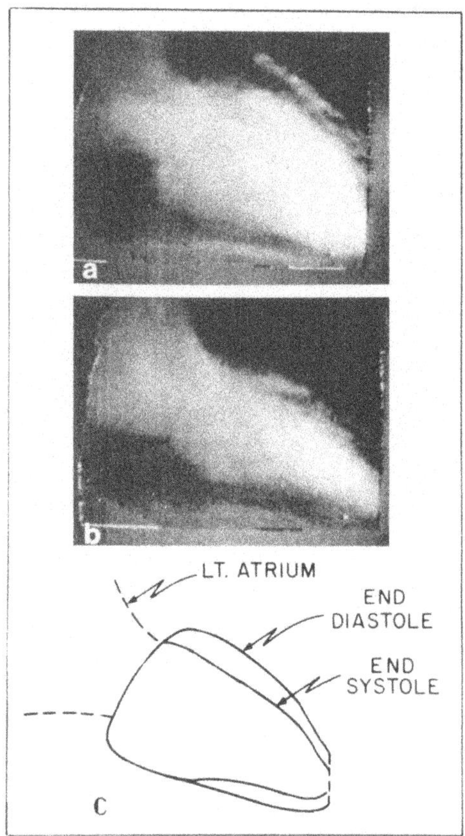

FIG. 7. Diastolic and Systolic phases of left ventricle following a 50 cc intravenous injection.

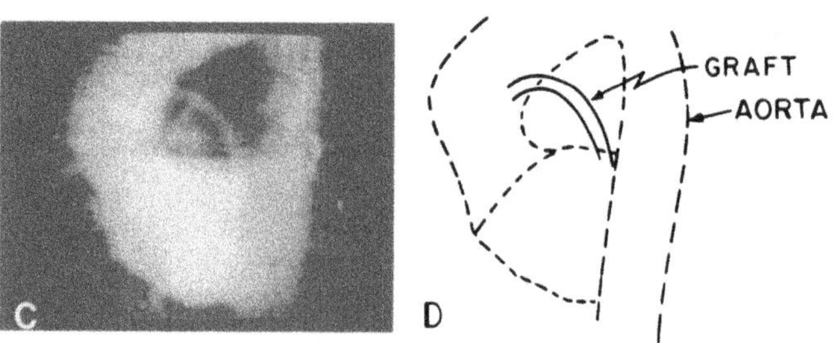

FIG. 8. Patent coronary artery bypass graft observed during high exposure rate (500 mR/sec) fluoroscopy of four seconds duration.

In Figure 9 the use of T.I.D. mode is illustrated. In this mode expansion of the ventricular border produces white signals. Contraction produces black signals. In Figure 9a and 9b a healthy heart is shown. The borders of the ventricle are uniform during contraction and expansion. In Figure 9c and 9d, the heart of Figure 7 is shown in T.I.D. mode. The absence of signals along the inferior border directly show the akinetic region. Figure 9 was generated by redigitization of Mask Mode Fluoroscopy data stored on video tape.

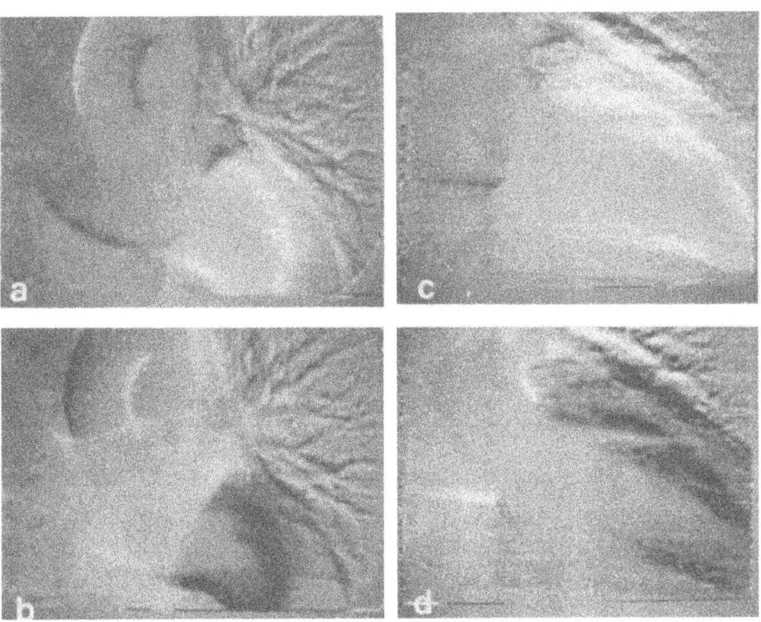

FIG. 9. T.I.D. images of normal (a and b) and diseased heart (c and d).

4. CONCLUSIONS

Digital time dependent subtraction imaging using computerized fluoroscopy apparatus shows great promise for evaluation of pathology in a number of anatomical sites. Because of the dilution of the contrast material which occurs in the intravenous technique, conventional arteriography will continue to provide superior results and may still be required to visualize subtle lesions, especially in the heart where coronary arteries will be especially difficult to separate from overlying iodine.

The evaluation of coronary bypass graft patency seems very promising, however we have only validated our results in a limited number of comparisons with conventional angiography. It should also be noted that the graft may fill during the course of several heartbeats and be visualized even if flow is severely limited by serious narrowing of distal vessels.

There are several areas in which image quality can be improved. Our present images are limited in spatial resolution by a nominal .6 mm focal spot which has been measured to be greater than 1.0 mm at the tube currents (> 200 ma) used for many of our examinations. In view of the 1.5-1.7 magnification factor of our present x-ray system, this focal spot is probably a greater limitation than our 512 picture element mode when the image intensifier is used in 6" or 9" mode.

Recording of data on analog storage devices adds noise, especially when reprocessing is required. Digital recording of real time fluoroscopy requires expensive devices. However, conventional digital discs may be used for serial radiographic examinations.

For imaging of coronary vessels the use of phase correlated masks in order to provide improved cancellation of anatomy may prove to be important. Regarding the advantages of radiographic versus continuous fluoroscopic visualization of coronary vessels, we are not sure which will ultimately be preferable.

We believe that the approach we have taken, using dedicated digital hardware, with perhaps microprocessor control, will prove to be the most advantageous approach toward dissemination of this technique. Images similar to ours have been obtained at the University of Arizona where a concurrent developmental effort has been underway using a much more extensive digital system, based on a VAX computer and intended for a wider variety of applications such as digital acquisition of chest radiographs [9].

REFERENCES

1. Mistretta CA: The use of a general description of the radiological transmission image for categorizing image enhancement procedures. Opt Eng 13:134-137, Mar-Apr 1974.

2. Mistretta CA, Kelcz F, Ort MG et al: Absorption-edge fluoroscopy using quasi-monoenergetic x-ray beams. Investig Radiol 8:402-412, 1973.

3. Kelcz F, Mistretta CA: Absorption edge fluoroscopy using a three-spectrum technique. Med Phys 3:159-168, May-June 1976.

4. Kruger RA, Mistretta CA, Crummy AB et al: Digital K-edge subtraction radiography. Radiology 125:243-245, October 1977.

5. Kruger RA, Mistretta CA, Lancaster J et al: A digital video image processor for real-time x-ray subtraction imaging. Opt Eng 17:652-657, Nov-Dec 1978.

6. Kruger RA, Mistretta CA, Houk TL et al: Computerized fluoroscopy in real time for noninvasive visualization of the cardiovascular system--preliminary studies. Radiology 130:49-57, Jan 1979.

7. Ergun DL, Mistretta CA, Kruger RA et al: A hybrid computerized fluoroscopy technique for noninvasive cardiovascular imaging. Radiology 132:739-742, Sept 1979.

8. Kruger RA, Mistretta CA, Crummy AB et al: Digital K-edge subtraction radiography. Radiology 125:243-245, October 1977.

9. Ovitt TW, Nudelman SN, Fisher D et al: Computer-assisted video subtraction for intravenous angiography. Presented at the Work in Progress: General Diagnosis Session of the RSNA, Chicago, Illinois, November 27-December 2 1977.

10. Brenneke R, Brown RK, Bursch J et al: Computerized video image processing with application to cardioangiographic roentgen image series. [In] Nagel HH, ed: Digital Image Processing. New York, Springer, 1977, p. 244.

INTRAVENOUS CEREBRAL ANGIOGRAPHY AND IMAGE PROCESSING

by

Jean-Pierre MARC-VERGNES, M.D.
LHEC - INSERM FRA 40
C.H.U. PURPAN
31059 TOULOUSE Cedex

ABSTRACT

Cerebral angiography (CA) is a current means of diagnosis. This paper describes: a) the classical intra-arterial method for CA, its drawbacks and risks, b) the physical non-invasive techniques developed to avoid these risks, c) the intravenous angiography with film subtraction technique, and d) digital analysis of raw angiographic images of extracranial cerebral arteries.

1. INTRODUCTION

CA meets an important medical need for both diagnosis and research. In routine practice, the morphological aspects of brain vessels are often required to choose the medical or surgical treatments, especially in cases of vascular malformations, atheromatous lesions and brain tumors. In clinical research, the lesions of the vascular walls are known to be instrumental in the outbreak and the evolution of cerebral vascular diseases. But to what extent is not defined. In particular, their relationships with other factors such as blood viscosity, platelets agregability, vessel wall elasticity and tissue metabolism are not clearly understood. If any significant headway is to be made in this field, it will involve carrying out prospective studies where physiological parameters would be compared to morphological aspects. The feasibility of these studies depends on non-traumatic and easily repeatable techniques for visualizing the entire arterial tree, including extra and intracranial vessels.

The intra-arterial classical method of CA provides very fine images; but this process is painful, expensive, and involves exceptional but real pathological risks.

Other diagnostic tests have been proposed to avoid these risks. They include non-invasive methods such as thermography, oculoplethysmography, carotid phono-angiography. Doppler Velocimetry, and visualization processes such as ultrasonic imagery. However, none of these supersede X-ray angiography which remains the best method of visualization of vascular abnormalities.

The intravenous injection of contrast medium is another means to avoid the risks of the intra-arterial injection. But the vessel contrast thus obtained is poor. Several processes can be used to improve the contrast and to extract the useful information. The film subtraction technique is a simple one which often gives excellent results. Image processing techniques are also suitable for this purpose. The objective of this paper is to show and compare some applications of these techniques.

2. INTRA-ARTERIAL CA

CA was first described by Egas Moniz (1) in 1927. Since then, it has been greatly improved. Now its technical modalities and results are fully described in numerous papers and handbooks (2,3).

The technique is based upon an intra-arterial injection of contrast medium. The arrangement and situation of the cerebral arteries allows detection on two different levels; and extracranial one, between the aortic arch and the skull, with only four large vessels, superficially located, at least for the carotid axises, but radiologically superimposed with the very complex image of the cervical spinal column, and an intracranial one, well protected by the skull, with numerous little arteris-- least 20 anastomic arches about 1 mm in diameter around each hemisphere -- the images of which overlaping each other. Thus, the injection is performed into aortic arch for visualizing the supra-aortic vessels (Fig.1) or into a selected artery for visuali-

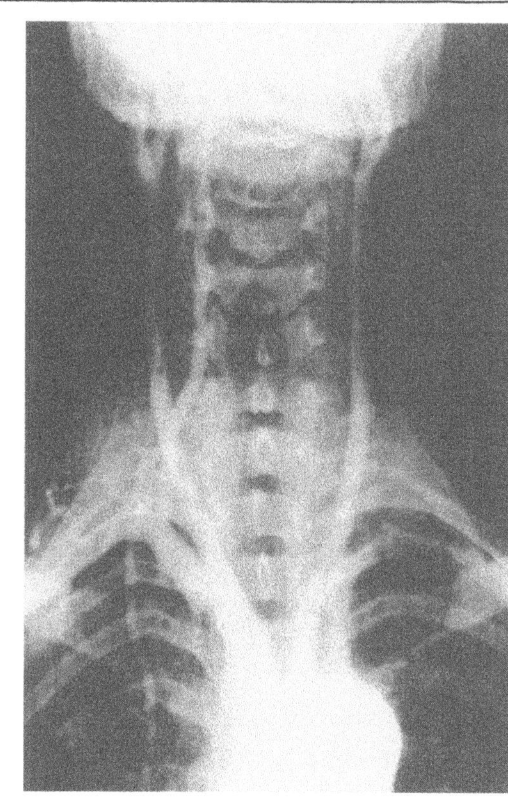

Fig.1.

Intraarterial angiography of supra-aortic arteries.

zing the intra-cranial vessels(Fig.2). Several techniques are used to catheterize or to directly puncture the arteries. But, in any case, they are highly technical, painful and expensive examinations which involve risks of embolism or hematoma. General anesthesia is sometimes required. A weak but non-negligible rate of permanent stroke, even of death, is reported in all the studies dealing with this topic (4,5,6,7). The visualization of both extra and intracranial arteries is required in cerebral vascular diseases.

3. NON-INVASIVE TECHNIQUES

The superficial situation of the carotid arteries offers the opportunity to apply several non-invasive physical methods for demonstrating their atherosclerotic lesions They are thermography, thermometry, oculodynamometry, oculoplethysmography, carotid phono-angiography, Doppler Velocimetry. The latter can also be applied to vertebral arteries. All these techniques only provide indirect functionnal informations which are in agreement with the angiographic morphological findings only in cases of occlusion or important stenosis on the extracranial arteries (8). On the whole, they are almost useful to decide to perform angiography or not.

Ultrasonic imagery (9,10) gives very encouraging results. But, at the present time, its resolution rate is not sufficient to make out small lesions and to follow their evolution. In addition, it can only visualize one part of the arterial cervical tree and seems to be unable to demonstrate intracranial arteries. Thus it does not supersede X-Ray angiography. However, it could be useful when there is some contra-indications to contrast medium or for surveying a ponctual lesion. For this, it deserves encouragements.

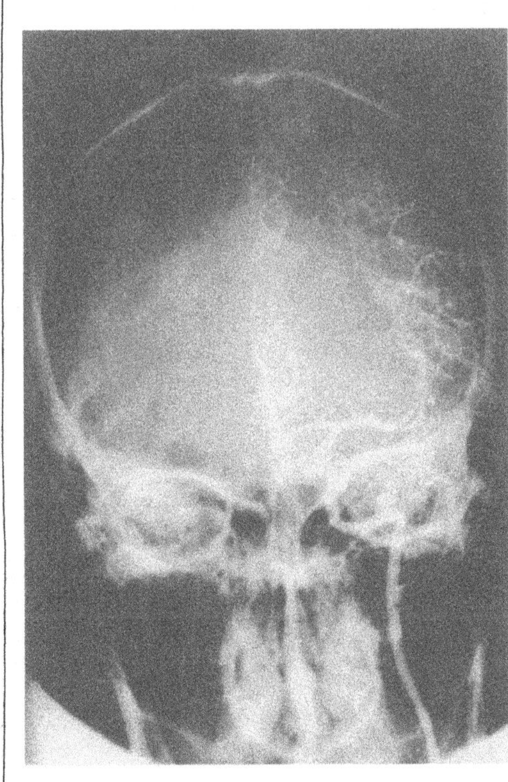

Fig.2.

Intraarterial angiography of intra-cranial arteries.

Computerized tomography (CT) brings valuable informations about cerebral lesions. It can also visualize the arteries after contrast product injection. But, it only shows slices of the vessels and its principle does not allow to follow the vessels on all their path-length. Moreover, its resolution is insufficient to visualize the intraluminal abnormalities. Therefore, CT is not a convenient method for studying the cerebral vessels.

4. INTRAVENOUS CA AND FILM SUBTRACTION TECHNIQUE

The idea of replacing intraarterial injection of contrast medium by an intravenous one for visualizing cerebral arteries is not new. In the 50ies and the early 60ies, some attempts were made to apply it, namely by VIALLET and al (11), by BANNISTER and MURRAY-LESLIE (14), by STEINBERG and EVANS (12), and by SCATLIFT and GREENPAN (13). But these techniques providing insufficient contrast at cerebral level were given up. Improvements in contrast media and systematic use of film subtraction technique have permitted to re-actualize and to modify this technique (15,16).

The investigation is carried out without local and general anesthesia or premedication. Patients must only be fasting. A teflon catheter (14 G Cathlon needle) is inserted into the basilic or the cephalic vein of the arm. After that the circulation time between arm and tongue is measured, two serial angiographies are carried out ; the first one in the anteroposterior (AP) projection and the second one in oblique projection, the patient's head being rotated to the right or left depending on the clinical situation. 1 ml/kg of sodium methyglycamine Ioxitalamate is injected in

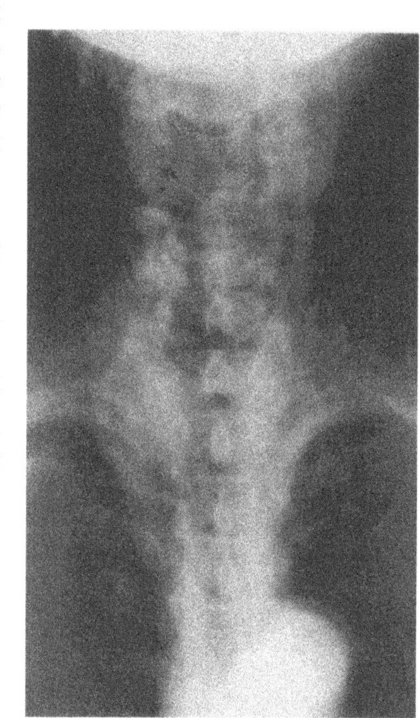

Fig.3a: Intravenous angiography. Raw image of supra-aortic arteries.

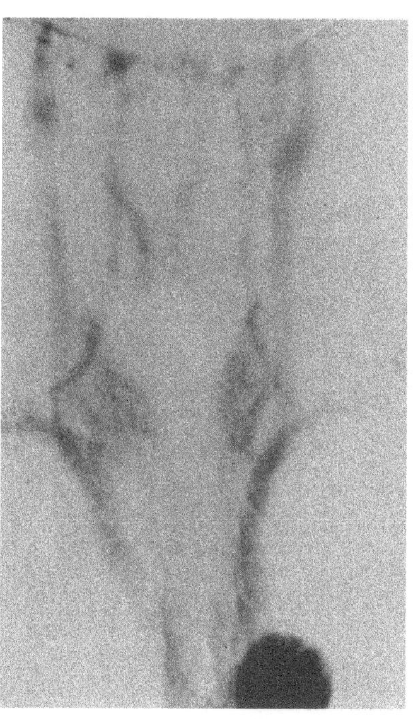

Fig.3b: Intravenous angiography. Image of supra-aortic arteries obtained by film subtraction technique.

four seconds for each series. An automatic pneumatic injector (Caillon, Model 602 V.D.) with two syringes is used, the first seringe is filled with cold (from 10°C to 15°C) contrast medium and the second with 50 ml of dextran solution, which is used to flush out the contrast agent. Ten films are exposed in each series ; the first one is used for subtraction and the other nine, beginning four seconds before circulation time, are exposed at a rate of one per second.

The technique allows to study the common carotids, carotid bifurcations, internal carotids up to the carotid siphons, and vertebral arteries simultaneously (Fig.3 a and 3 b). After more than one thousand cases, 81 % of the studies are good or excellent, providing the same informations than the intraarterial CA. 19 % are poor or ininterpretable. These bad results are due to reflux of contrast material into the jugular vein on the injected side, masking the origin of the vertebral artery, and/ or to changes in the patient's position between the reference film and the serial films.

At the intracranial level (Fig.4 a and 4 b); the contrast is poor and the practical results are often insufficient for clinical purpose.

Two other technical restrictions must be emphasized. The risks associated with the contrast medium lead to limit dosage to 2 doses of 1 ml/kg, so that no more than two projections are possible. Simultaneous biplane angiography can avoid this drawback.

The manual film subtraction technique is time consuming, expensive, and difficult to perform in all the radiological centers.

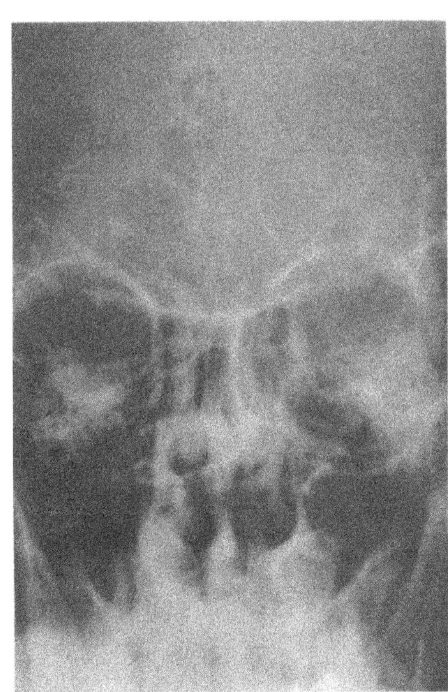

Fig.4a:Intravenous angiography. Raw image of intracranial arteries.

Fig.4b:Intravenous angiography. Image of supra-aortic arteries obtained by film subtraction technique.

5. DIGITAL ANALYSIS

The vessel images obtained after contrast medium injection are quickly moving images, and the informations needed for medical decision are very abundant. For instance, the size of an image of extracranial or intracranial vessels is about 20 cm^2 and that of pathological details could be less than 1 mm. Thus, the devices used for data collection, storage and digitization determine the possibilies of datal analysis of angiographic images. A compromise must be choosen between speed and accuracy.

Using X-Ray image intensifier and video camera, real time digital subtraction can be performed ((17,18,19). This process offers actual advantages in speed and versatility compared to film subtraction technique. But it calls for some comments. First, it shows the same impossibilities than the film subtraction technique when patients move or when the contrast medium flows back into the veins of the neck. Second, video cameras are not perfectly linear, and this defect is difficult to rectify because the video signal is unstable. Furthermore, the image resolution is that of the camera and cannot exceed 100 real gray levels and 300 micrometers as pixel size. These performances seem sufficient to correctly visualize the extracranial vessels. But, the images thus obtained must be compared with those provided by intraarterial angiography and by intravenous film subtraction technique to know if there is not a significant loss of information. At the intracranial level, this device is obviously inadequate.

Another approach is to digitize directly raw radiological films by means of a microdensitometer and to extract the useful information by means of image enhancement methods. For this purpose, we use the following devices : a) a SCANDIG rotating-drum microdensitometer, b) a MINITRIM terminal with a logic unit for pseudo-color treatment, an image memory (512 X 512 X 8 bits), an auxiliary graphic memory, a joystick and a TV monitor, and c) a SOLAR 16/40 minicomputer with a 64 K words of 16 bits core memory, a 2 X 5 MØ unit and the usual peripheral devices.

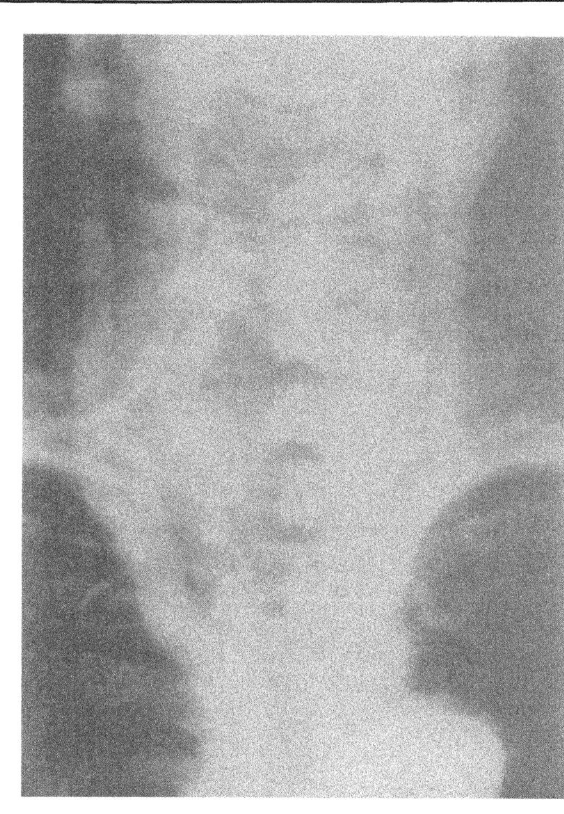

Fig.5

Digitized image of supra-aortic arteries. Same patient as in Fig.3a and 3b.

The data are digitized with a step of 100 micrometers and a gray scale of 256 levels. Figure 5 shows the digitized picture of the image shown in figures 3 a and 3 b. Its dynamic covers a range of almost 200 gray levels. The low density tissues take a part of almost 50 levels while the dynamic of the vessels covers a range from 0 to 130-140 gray levels. In a given area, the vessel density is quite similar to that of the bones.

An image enhancement algorithm using histogram hyperbolisation (20) improves the image quality (Fig.6). However, this result is not so good than that obtained with the film subtraction technique (see Fig. 3-b).

The edge enhancement algorithms can be easily applied to the aortic arch the density of which is very high and different from that of the others structures. But they do not provide good results at the level of carotid and vertebral arteries. Only visual results (Fig.7 d) are obtained. Automatic contour detection cannot be performed.

Of course, this procedure is not suitable for routine medical practice. It is too slow and requires high technical installations and competences. But it is useful to

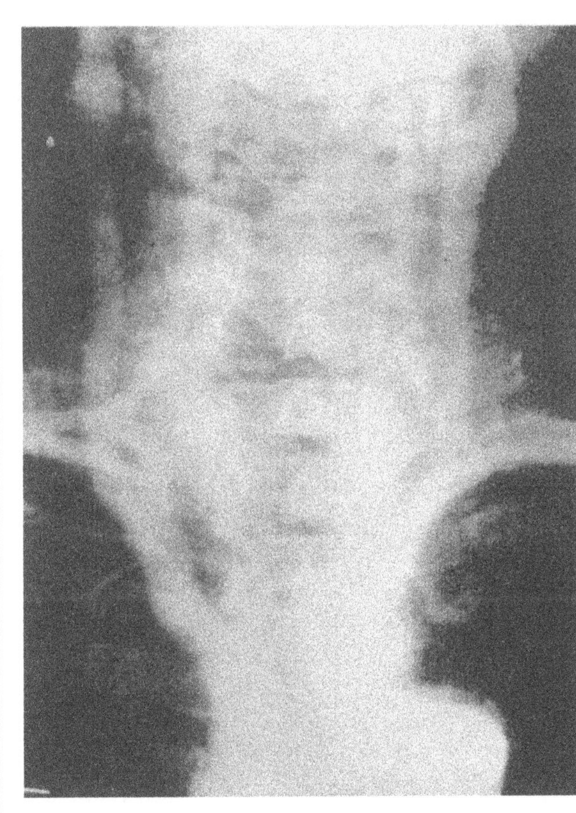

Fig.6

Contrast enhancement of the image presented in Fig 3, and 5.

salvage examinations to which the subtraction techniques cannot be applied. Moreover it will allow to define the real digitization needs and to design specialized processes intended for real time extraction of vessel images from raw film.

6. CONCLUDING REMARK

From a medical point of view, the main interest of image processing applied to CA arises from the feasibility of extracting useful informations from low-contrast images. This provides the opportunity to replace the intraarterial injection of contrast medium by an intravenous one. Subtraction techniques-film subtraction or real time digital subtraction- are the simplest ones to achieve this purpose. But they cannot be always applied and their results must be appreciated in comparison with those of the classical intraarterial CA . Enhancement methods seem to be able to palliate the insufficiencies of the subtraction techniques.

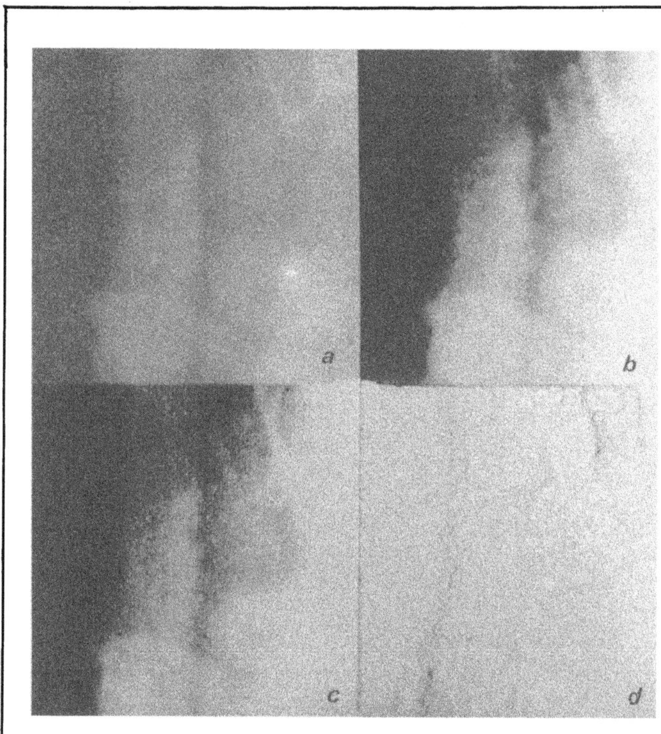

Fig.7

Contrast enhancements (b,c) and contour detection (d) applied to the carotid level.

ACKNOWLEDGMENTS

We are indebted to members of the "Laboratoire de Traitement d'images du LSI" (ERA n° 298-CNRS), in particular : A. BRUEL, M. ADELANTADO, R. JEANSOULIN, and Ph. MARTHON and to those of the "Laboratoire d'Hémodynamique et d'Energétique Cérébrales" (FRA n° 40-INSERM), in particular : P. CELSIS, M. DUCOS de LAHITTE, C. MANELFE, A. RASCOL, and G. SETIEN.

REFERENCES

1. MONIZ E. : Injections intracarotidiennes et substances injectables opaques aux rayons X. Presse méd. 35 : 969-971, 1927.

2. KRAYEN BUHL,H., and RICHTER,H. : Die Zerebrale Angiographie. Georg Thème, Verlag, Stuttgart, 1952.

3. BONNAL,J., and LEGRE,J. : L'angiographie cérébrale, Masson et Cie. Edit., Paris, 1958.

4. GUIRAUD B., MANELFE C., SALANDINI A.M., SANCIER A., TOUIBI S. & RASCOL A. : Etude rétrospective et prospective des risques de l'angiographie dans les accidents ischémiques cérébraux. Concours Médical. 1978,9, 106-111.

5. MANI R.L., EISENBERG R.L.,Mc DONALD E.J., et al. : Complications of catheter cerebral arteriography : Analysis of 5 000 procedures. I. Criteria and incidence. Amer J. Roentgen. 131 : 861-866, 1978.

6. MANI R.L., EISENBERG R.L. : Complications of catheter cerebral arteriography :

Analysis of 5 000 procedures. II. Relation of complication rates to clinical and arteriographic diagnoses. Amer.J.Roentgen. 131 : 867-870, 1978.

7. MANI R.L., EISENBERG R.L. : Complications of catheter cerebral arteriography : Analysis of 5 000 procedures. III. Assessment for arteries injected, contrast medium used, duration of procedure and age of patient. Amer.J.Roentgen. 131 : 871-874, 1978.

8. GROSS W.S., VERTAM J.Jr., VAN BELLEN B., et al. : Comparison of non-invasive diagnostic techniques in carotid artery occlusive disease. Surgery 82 : 271-278, 1977

9. REID J.M., SPENCER M.P. : Ultrasonic Doppler technique for imaging blood vessels Science, 176 : 1235-1236, 1972.

10. POURCELOT L., BESSE D., PEJOT C., et al. : Visualization du sang circulant par effet Doppler. Biosigma 78, April 24th-28th, 1978. Paris. (Secrétariat d'Etat à la Recherche Scientifique et Technique). Colloque International sur les signaux et les images en Médecine et en Biologie. Imp. EMF. 2ème trim. 78, pp. 407.

11. VIALLET P., SENDRA L., CHEVROT L., et al. : Angiocardiopneumographie élargie. Méthode d'opacification vasculaire générale par voie veineuse. Ed.Masson et Cie. Paris. 1959.

12. STEINBERG I., EVANS J.A. : Technique of intravenous carotid and vertebral arteriography. Amer.J.Roentgenal. 85 : 1138-1145, 1961.

13. SCATLIFT J.H., GREENSPAN R.H. : Radiographic evaluation of major arteries of the neck by intravenous aortography. Acta.Radiol. I : 404-416, 1963.

14. BANNISTER R.G., MURRAY-LESLIE R.M. : Venoangiography in the study of cerebro-vascular disease. Brain, 86 : 161-172, 1963.

15. MARC-VERGNES J.P., DUCOS de LAHITTE M., RASCOL A., et al. : Non-invasive assessment of atheromatous lesions of extracranial cerebral arteries by intravenous angiography. "Proc. of the 9th International Salzburg Conference on Cerebral Vascular disease, sep 1978", pp. 88-89 (Excerpta Medica, Amsterdam, 1979).

16. DUCOS de LAHITTE M., MARC-VERGNES J.P., RASCOL A. et al. : Intravenous angiography of extra-cranial arteries. accepted for publication by Radiology. 20 November 1979.

17. KRUGER R.A., MISTRETTA C.A., LANCASTER J; et al. : A digital video image processor for real-time X-Ray subtraction imaging. Optic. Eng. 17 : 652-657, 1978.

18. OVITT T.W., CAPP M.P., FISHER H.D. et al. : Computer-assisted video subtraction for intravenous angiography. Optic. Eng.17 : 645-651, 1978.

19. MISTRETTA C.A., KRUGER R.A., ERGUN D.L., et al : Intravenous angiography using computerized fluoroscopy apparatus - This Seminar.

20. FREI,W. : Image Enhancement by histogram hyperbolisation. J.Comput.Graphic Image Proc., 6, 293-301, 1977.

21. ASHKAR,G.P., and MODESTINO,J.W. : The contour extraction problem with biomedical applications. IEEE Transactions on Computers, Vol.C.26, N°3, Mars 1977, pp 216-224.

DIGITAL ANALYSIS OF X-RAY RADIOGRAPHS

by
Jack Sklansky, Eng.Sc.D.
School of Engineering
University of California
Irvine, California 92717

ABSTRACT

We describe several recent advances in computer algorithms for the analysis of x-ray radiographs, with attention to a) visual enhancement, b) detection of abnormalities, c) data compression of boundaries, d) measurement of distances and textures, e) visualization of three-dimensional structures from two projections, and f) interactive generation of quantitative and graphical reports.

1. INTRODUCTION

Routine diagnosis in hospitals, clinics and dentists' offices often involves the construction and interpretation of radiographic images of human tissue. In almost every instance the image of the tissue of interest is partially obscured by non-pertinent tissue or artifacts, distorted and blurred by the imaging system, and corrupted by human vision. The interpretation and reporting of these images is further limited by the technology of pictorial reproduction and by the human ability for verbal expression. These problems of acquiring, interpreting and reporting of radiographic images lead to substantial errors and inadequate reporting.

Advances in imaging techniques, digital electronics, image detectors and scanning devices, image processing software, and digital display devices over the past ten years have alleviated several of these problems, and have generated hope that further alleviation will be brought about by computer technology. The advances in computer hardware and algorithms for image analysis exploit a broad range of techniques often associated with the interdiscipline of automatic pattern recognition [1]. We discuss several of the advances in computer algorithms, with special attention to some of the research at the Pattern Recognition Project (PRP) of the University of California, Irvine, U.S.A. In that project we use the following major devices: a) an Optronics rotating-drum microdensitometer, b) a Perkin-Elmer 7/32 digital computer with 327,680 bytes of core memory, c) two Control Data Corporation 67-megabyte disc memories, d) a Genisco digital color graphic display system, with a capability of displaying a 512 × 640 × 8 digitized image with a color overlay, e) a Versatec printer/plotter, with a capability of printing half-tone digitized images, f) a Qume impact printer/terminal, g) two cathode-ray-tube/keyboard terminals, h) a Pertec magnetic tape drive, and i) a Diablo 10-megabyte disc memory.

2. PRINCIPAL TASKS OF THE COMPUTER

In radiographic image processing, the tasks of the computer may be placed in the following six categories:

Enhancement
Detection
Compression
Measurement
Visualization
Reporting

Below we describe recent technological advances in each of these categories.

3. ENHANCEMENT

Digital image filters, usually implemented on digital computers, have been instrumental in improving or "enhancing" the visual quality of radiographic images. In particular these filters can a) suppress the visual degradation produced by random noise (such as film grain, electronic noise, and Compton scatter) b) suppress blurring such as the geometric unsharpness produced by extended focal spots, c) suppress geometric distortions such as the barrel or pincushion effects in television cameras, d) transform the distribution of gray levels so as to match the perceptual characteristics of human vision, and e) change the relative sizes of the spatial harmonics so as to increase the visibility of small, low-contrast details.

The following are a few of the properties considered desirable for such filters:

1. The filter should consume only a small amount of digital memory.
2. The filter should be fast.
3. The filter should preserve the edges of objects in the image.

Because of the desirability of small memory consumption and high speed, and because the variations from one pixel to its neighbor are usually slow, filters that are recursive are usually desirable. Such filters modify only a small part of the filter's memory during each scan of the image by the filter.

The "Normalized Zonal Notch" (NZN) filter, recently developed at PRP, has many of these desirable properties. The purpose of the NZN is to enhance the edges and small details of an image, while suppressing the dynamic range. This filter is defined as follows:

$$q(\underline{x}) = \alpha \frac{p(x) - \bar{p}(x)}{\text{Max } (\sigma(\underline{x}), s)} \bar{\sigma} + \beta \, \bar{p}(\underline{x}).$$

where

$\underline{x}$ = position vector of a pixel
$p(\underline{x})$ = image (digital picture function) at input of filter
$q(\underline{x})$ = image at output of filter
$\bar{p}(x)$ = mean of $p(\underline{\xi})$ over all $\underline{\xi}$ in a zone $N(\underline{\xi},\underline{x})$ centered at $\underline{x}$
$\sigma(x)$ = standard deviation of $p(\underline{\xi})$ over all $\underline{\xi} \in N(\underline{\xi},\underline{x})$
$\bar{\sigma}$ = mean of $\sigma(\underline{x})$ over all $\underline{x}$ in the input image
s = minimum allowed divisor: prevents excessive amplification of noise

α,β are scaling factors
$N(\underline{\xi}, \underline{x})$ is defined as a subset of $W \times W$ square window centered at $\underline{x}$ such that

$$| \, p(\underline{x}) - p(\underline{\xi}) \, | \leq T.$$

Both W and T are determined empirically for any given class of images. For chest radiographs, $W \cong$ spacing between adjacent dorsal ribs, $T \cong 25\%$ of dynamic range of the unfiltered image.

This filter is a hybrid of the zonal notch [1] and the statistical differencer [2].

The effectiveness of the NZN filter is illustrated in Figure 1. The image at the left is a reproduction of an original chest radiograph; the image at the right is the result of applying our NZN filter to the digitization of the image at the left. Note that the trachea and the lower vertebrae were made visible by the NZN filter, even though they were virtually invisible in the original film.

4. DETECTION

The automatic detection of the boundaries of blood vessels, ribs, vertebrae, clavicle, and tumors can help the radiologist in both the quantitative and qualitative analysis of a radiograph. At the PRP we have found that an accurate detection of the boundary of the image of a candidate nodule helps to classify the candidate correctly as nodule or nonnodule.

4.1 Piecewise linear detection of boundaries of major blood vessels and skeleton

Using a 1200μm-wide pixel, we (at PRP) noted that the boundaries of major blood vessels and ribs are nearly straight within a 20 × 20- pixel window. We exploited this property in a piecewise linear detector of these boundaries.

For this detector we considered, and discarded, the well known Hough straight line detector [4,5]. The reason we discarded it is that the reliability and sensitivity of the Hough straight line detector is a spatially varying function when the noise in the image is significant [5]. Furthermore the tolerance of the Hough line detector for deviations from straightness is also spatially dependent. The technique we devised has neither of these disadvantages, while maintaining high sensitivity and reliability. Our technique evolved from the straight line detector described by Griffith [6].

Our straight line detector operates as follows. A thresholded digital gradient $\underline{g}(\underline{x})$ of the given image is computed, the threshold serving to suppress noise. Every nonzero pixel of $\underline{g}(\underline{x})$ has both magnitude and angle. Thus $\underline{g}(\underline{x})$ is a digital vector field. This vector field is covered by a set of n × n windows, with the edges of the windows aligned with the horizontal and vertical coordinate axes. Although n may be adjusted to any value between 4 and 32, usually we have set n = 20.

A horizontal (3 × n)-pixel rectangle R_H is formed. The number of horizontal $\pm$ 30° nonzero elements of $\underline{g}(\underline{x})$ in R_H is counted. Similarly a vertical rectangle R_V is formed and the number of vertical $\pm$ 30° nonzero elements of $\underline{g}(\underline{x})$ in R_V is counted. This is repeated for all possible (3 × n)-pixel horizontal and vertical rectangles in the window. The histogram of each of these counts (horizontal and vertical) is produced, and the peaks, if any, of the histograms are found.

All of the pixels at points $\{\underline{x}_i\}$ are then rotated by a small angle Θ (say Θ = 7 degrees), spatially quantized, and the peaks, if any, of the histograms computed again. The rotation is accomplished by the transformation

$$\underline{x}_i' = \underline{R}(\Theta)\ \underline{x}_i,$$

where

$$R(\Theta) = \begin{pmatrix} \cos\Theta & \sin\Theta \\ -\sin\Theta & \cos\Theta \end{pmatrix}.$$

When a peak of sufficiently large size is detected, an n-pixel-long line segment is generated as a representation of a detected line segment.

The capability of our straight edge finder is illustrated in Figure 2, which shows the result of applying our straight edge finder to a digitized chest radiograph. The superposition of the detected straight line segments forms parts of the boundaries of the ribs, heart, trachea, and major blood vessels.

4.2 Boundary following of nodules

To obtain a powerful suppressor of false positives we developed a heuristic follower of nodule boundaries that incorporates much of the gestalt of a nodule boundary, while limiting the search space so as to be relatively fast. Our boundary follower's incorporation of gestalt gives it a capability for jumping large gaps; its estimate of "heuristic cost" is an effective feature for classifying the candidate nodule as nodule or nonnodule.

The gestalt guidance is implemented by moving the search counter clockwise around the estimated center c within an annular region determined by the radius R. (The center c and the radius R are determined by our circle detector [7]. The space around c is divided into four quadrants. Within each quadrant the candidate paths for the boundary are grown as a tree in which the pixel at each node, except the root, has a unique predecessor corresponding to the current minimal-cost path through that pixel. The root of each tree in the first quadrant is an arbitrarily chosen pixel on the initial radial edge of that quadrant. Our cost function depends on the accumulated moduli of the edge elements from the nearest boundaries of the estimated annular region, and an estimate of the distance from the end point of the current path to the current goal. (The current goal is a segment of the second radial edge of the current quadrant.)

The end points of the paths accepted for each quadrant are the start points for the next quadrant, from which the paths for the next quadrant are grown. This process is repeated five times, once for each quadrant.

The "fifth" quadrant is a second search in the first quadrant, using the end points of the fourth quadrant as start points for the second search of the first quadrant. The second search in the first quadrant is needed, because the start points in the first search of the first quadrant were chosen arbitrarily. This technique incorporates what we believe are the best features of the earlier versions of heuristic search boundary followers [8,9]. We find that it is computationally more economical than those boundary followers, as a result of its use of an expected cost tree search.

The computed boundaries for a set of two nodules and two false positives (nonnodules falsely detected by our circle detector) are shown in Figure 3 to illustrate the performance of the search procedure.

In a preliminary data set of 15 nodules, we found that the ratio of the number of search nodes to the length of the computed boundary serves as a powerful discriminator of nodules from nonnodules. These and other preliminary results indicate that our computer procedure is a sensitive, robust technique for following boundaries containing large gaps [10].

5. COMPRESSION

For the construction of a description of a digitized image, it is often useful to represent the image as a set of boundaries, each closed boundary enclosing a region represented by an array of local statistics of the grey levels within the region. Descriptive features may then be extracted from the boundaries and from the parameters of a model of texture fitted to the local statistics of the region. The parameters of the texture model are a form of image compression, which helps in the extraction of textural features. A compact representation of the boundaries of candidate nodules also helps to obtain fast algorithms for the extraction of features for the classification of these candidate nodules.

For the efficient representation of boundaries, we constructed a fast scan-along minimal-perimeter polygonal (MPP) curve finder. We applied this MPP finder to the boundaries of ribs and lungs, yielding a reduction of the memory space occupied by these boundaries by factors of 15 or more, with a peak error of just one sampling cell [11].

This method of boundary data compression is derived from our earlier work on a theory of minimum-perimeter polygonal approximations of digital closed curves [12]. Since our approximations are polygonal curves whose vertices are a subset of the points in the given digitized curve, we refer to these approximations as rectified minimum-perimeter polygons (RMPP's).

Our method assigns the first point in the boundary sequence to a vertex of the RMPP. We call this first point a source. A circle of radius ε is centered at the next boundary point; and the angular orientations of the two tangent rays to this circle from the source are computed. We refer to one of these as the upper tangent ray and the other as the lower tangent ray. Another circle of radius ε is centered at the next boundary point, and the angular orientations of its two tangent rays from the source are computed. The two upper tangent rays are compared. Of these two, the lower one is retained, and the upper one discarded. This yields a downward ratcheting action of the upper tangent ray. In a similar manner, one constructs an upward ratcheting action of the lower tangent ray. In Figure 4, which illustrates this concept, ray t_3 is ratcheted downward or clockwise; ray b_3 is ratcheted upward or counterclockwise. In the simplest form of our RMPP finder, when the two ratcheting rays meet or cross, the most recent boundary data point examined before the meeting or crossing is chosen as a new source. This new source is the next vertex of the RMPP. The set of sources generated in this manner is the set of vertices of the RMPP.

We modified our RMPP algorithm to preserve points of high curvature. The geometric concept underlying this modification is illustrated in Figure 5. In this modification, the lengths of the recent candidate linear segments of the RMPP are compared, and the longest one retained. This results in a slight increase in the perimeter of the polygonal curve, but with significantly improved representation of the shape of the boundary.

In our tests of the RMPP, we use the interpixel distance as a unit of length; thus the interpixel distance is 1.

Figure 6 shows the result of applying our RMPP algorithm to the digitized contour of the image of a rib on a chest radiograph. Here the allowed peak error is $\varepsilon = 1$. The data compression ratio, defined as the number of points in the input data divided by the number vertices in the computed MPP, is 28.5. In this figure the original data points are so close to the polygonal approximation that they cannot be seen without magnification. A magnified view is shown in the insert.

Figure 7 illustrates the result of applying the RMPP finder to a digitized boundary of the image of a lung on a chest radiograph, with $\varepsilon = 1$. This achieved a data compression ratio of 15.6.

Our procedure for computing piecewise linear approximations of digitized curves has the following attractive properties.

1. The amount of computer memory required for the procedure is relatively small, and is independent of the number of points in the digitized curve.

2. The procedure can accept digitized curves whose points are nonuniformly spaced.

3. The size of the error can be restricted to any nonnegative number below a specified bound. (Greater values will result in an ill-conditioned situation.)

4. Our procedure is a "scan-along" technique, in the same sense that the sequence of points specifying the digitized curve can be approximately pipelined with the sequence of vertices of the computed polygonal approximation.

5. The set of vertices of the computed polygonal approximation is a subset of the points in the given digitized curve. This constraint contributes to the savings of space in the main computer memory and to the simplicity of the computer program of the RMPP finder.

6. MEASUREMENT

The clinical practice of modern radiography rarely extracts quantitative measurements from a radiograph for diagnostic purposes. The measurements that are extracted are almost always qualitative or rough approximations. These approximations lead to significant variations in diagnosis. We suggest that quantitative measurements, carried out with the aid of a computer, will reduce the errors and variability of these measurements, and hence will lead to a greater reliability in diagnosis.

An example of such measurements is the computation of the cardio-thoracic ratio and other physical dimensions associated with the diagnosis of cardiomegaly (enlarged heart). Figure 8 illustrates the line segments found by the computer program developed by R. Kruger, et al. for the detection of rheumatic heart disease [13].

Another example is our measurement of the extent of prominent ducting in mammograms. This measurement could be useful in evaluating the belief of some radiologists that if more than 25% of a woman's breasts contain prominent ducting, then her risk of developing breast cancer is significantly greater than that for women having less than 25% prominent ducting [14].

To obtain this measurement, each digitized mammogram was segmented into 64 square sections, each 1.25 cm wide. Twelve statistical featues were extracted from each section, and entered into a near-Bayes-optimum quadratic classifier. The classifier's error rate was 14.6%.

7. VISUALIZATION

Human beings vary considerably in their ability to visualize stationary or time-varying objects from cross sections or projections. Such an ability is particularly valuable in radiography, where two or more central projections of a single object are often required to determine the shape and location of a lesion.

Computed tomography has been of great help to radiologists in this task of visualization. Nevertheless, a set of tomographic slices is a far from ideal form for aiding visualization. Furthermore, tomography of the entire thorax requires many slices and projections -- leading to a very high dose if a full reconstruction of the thorax is desired.

Recently we investigated the feasibility of modeling the three-dimensional structure of the rib cage from just two nearly conventional posterior-anterior chest radiographs [16]. A major purpose of this model is to help the radiologist or surgeon visualize the rib cage from any viewpoint.

Toward this end we represented each rib by an estimate of the rib's medial axis. We estimated this axis from the medial axis of the image of each rib. A fast program that computes this medial axis directly on the boundary sequences of the boundaries of the rib images was devised at our project [15]. These estimated images of the medial axes provided the basic data for our modeling procedure.

Our modeling procedure is as follows: we determine the coordinates of two source positions; we find pairs of corresponding points in the two projections of the rib cage (from the source/object/film-plane geometry); and we use this information to estimate three-dimensional coordinates of points on the medial axis of the ribs. The geometry of this configuration of two sources, and the equations relating the two projections of a point to the coordinates of that point in 3-space is shown in Figure 9.

From a careful investigation of physical, mathematical, and computational constraints, we developed the following seven steps for implementing the above procedure.

Step 1. Obtain two PA chest radiographs from x-ray source positions on a line normal to the film plane through the spine, the center of the rib cage, and the center of the film. Measure the z-coordinate of each source location along an axis perpendicular to the film plane. Obtain the source coordinates x,y from Step 4.

Step 2. Find the rib images in both radiographs. A rib image is defined by two open boundaries, each of which is represented by a simply connected string of x,y coordinates (a string of two-element position vectors).

Step 3. Compute the medial axis of each rib image. (For this purpose we constructed a high-speed algorithm that computes the medial axis from the sequential data representing the rib boundaries.)

Step 4. Determine the location of the origin 0 of the cylindrical coordinate system needed for Step 5 and 6. Describe this location in terms of x,y and z. 0 is by definition the point at which the line joining the two source positions intersects the film plane. Because this line is perpendicular to the film plane, the x,y coordinates of 0 are also the x,y coordinates of both source positions. A small number of control points (located between the chest phantom and the two source positions) and a least-squared-error procedure are used to determine the location of 0.

Step 5. For each medial axis found in Step 3, find pairs of corresponding points in both projections. Because of our source/object/film plane geometry, each pair of corresponding points in the film plane lies on a radial line emanating from 0.

Step 6. For each pair of corresponding points, compute the three-dimensional position vector of a point on the medial axis of a rib.

Step 7. Compute views of the rib cage model using currently available software for computer graphics.

Application of this procedure to a chest phantom resulted in rib cage coordinates with substantial noise in the depth coordinate z, while x and y were well behaved [16]. To suppress the noise in our computation of z, we used Roberts' thorax model [17]. According to this model, which agrees quite well with measured data, the section of each rib from the costochondral junction to the "angle" a) lies in a plane perpendicular to the midsaggital plane and b) lies on a circular arc. Inclusion of these constraints in our modeling procedure resulted, in almost all instances, in a satisfactory model of the rib cage. Figure 10 shows three orthographic views of a resulting model of the rib cage.

8. REPORTING

The final product of a radiologist's task of image analysis is often a report describing the medical significance of various parts of the image. This is especially important in a clinical setting.

Computer-aided reporting of medical radiographs has been implemented in the United States at John Hopkins University and at the University of Vermont, exploiting cued question-answer displays.

At the PRP we have developed a new approach toward this type of reporting. Our system provides the radiologist a means to interact directly with the radiograph via a digital cathode-ray-tube display. Virtually no training of the radiologist in the use of the computer system is needed. Via the cathode-ray-tube display, our computer program asks the radiologist to use an ultrasonic graphic pen to encircle regions of the image to be enlarged and visually enhanced. The radiologist encircles the region of interest, and in response the cathode-ray tube displays an enhanced high resolution enlargement of this region. Each such region is labeled and keyed to the digitized image of the full radiograph.

The radiologist orally records his or her analysis of each of these regions into a tape recorder. This taped material is subsequently transcribed into the computer's memory. The report is then issued by the computer on a dot-matrix printer-plotter, which uses our software for digital half-tone printing of the radiographic images.

9. CONCLUDING REMARK

In digital radiographic image analysis -- as throughout the technology of digital computers -- the allocation of tasks between the computer and the human user is both important and difficult. Among the six tasks of radiographic image analysis described in this paper, our experience indicates that measurement and visualization are maong the most difficult for the unaided human. On the other hand, measurement is a relatively easy task for the digital computer.

Thus measurement techniques should receive special attention in current short-range research on computer-aided radiography.

ACKNOWLEDGMENTS

We are indebted to many members of the UCI Pattern Recognition Project for the research reported here, in particular: D. H. Ballard, V. Gonzalez, M. Katz, C. Kimme-Smith, E. J. Pisa, W. Root, P. V. Sankar, F. Towfiq, G. Wassel, and H. Wechsler.

This research was supported by the National Institute of General Medical Sciences of the U.S. Public Health Service under Grant No. GM-17632 and by the National Science Foundation under Grant No. ENG77-17081.

REFERENCES

1. J. Sklansky (ed.), Pattern Recognition -- Introduction and Foundations, Dowden, Hutchinson and Ross, Inc., Stroudsburg, Pennsylvania, 1973.

2. A. A. Schwartz, J. M. Soha, "Variable threshold zonal filtering," Applied Optics, Vol. 16, No. 7, July 1977, pp. 1779-1781.

3. W. K. Pratt, Digital Image Processing, Wiley & Sons, New York, 1978.

4. R. O. Duda, P. E. Hart, "Use of Hough transformation to detect lines and curves in pictures," Communications of the Association of Computing Machinery, Vol. 15, Jan. 1972, pp. 11-15.

5. J. Sklansky, "On the Hough technique for curve detection," IEEE Transactions on Computers, Vol. C-27, No. 10, Oct. 1978, pp. 923-926.

6. S. K. Griffith, "Edge detection in simple scenes using a priori information," IEEE Transactions on Computers, Vol. C-22, No. 4, April 1973, pp. 371-381.

7. C. Kimme, D. H. Ballard, J. Sklansky, "Finding circles by an array of accumulators," Communications of the Association of Computing Machinery, Vol. 18, No. 2, Feb. 1975, pp. 120-122.

8. A. P. Ashkar, J. W. Modestino, "The contour extraction problem with biomedical applications," Computer Graphics and Image Processing, Vol. 7, No. 3, June 1978, pp. 331-355.

9. D. H. Ballard, J. Sklansky, "A ladder-structured decision tree for recognizing tumors in chest radiographs," IEEE Transactions on Computers, Vol. C-25, No. 5, May 1976, pp. 503-513.

10. J. Sklansky, P. V. Sankar, et al., "Computed detection of nodules in chest radiographs," Proceedings of IEEE Computer Society Conference on Computer-Aided Analysis of Radiological Images, Newport Beach, California, June 1979.

11. J. Sklansky, V. Gonzalez, "Fast polygonal approximation of digitized curves," Pattern Recognition, 1980.

12. J. Sklansky, "Measuring concavity on a rectangular mosaic," IEEE Transactions on Computers, Vol. C-21, pp. 1355-1364.

13. R. P. Kruger, J. R. Townes, D. L. Hall, S. J. Dwyer III, G. S. Lodwick, "Automated radiographic diagnosis via feature extraction and classification of cardiac size and shape descriptors," IEEE Transactions on Biomedical Engineering, Vol. BME-19, No. 3, May 1972, pp. 174-186.

14. J. N. Wolfe, "Breast pattern as an index of risk for developing breast cancer," Am. J. Roentgenol, Vol. 126, June 1976, pp. 1130-1139.

15. B. Shapiro, E. J. Pisa, J. Sklansky, "Skeletons from sequential boundary data," Proceedings of the 1979 IEEE Computer Society Conference on Pattern Recognition and Image Processing, Chicago, August 1979, pp. 265-270.

16. E. J. Pisa, "Computing the geometry of the rib cage from two chest radiographs," Technical Report TP-79-8, Pattern Recognition Project, School of Engineering, University of California, Irvine, California 92717, U.S.A., August 1979.

17. S. B. Roberts, Journal of Bioengineering, Vol. 1, No. 4, Oct. 1977.

FIGURES

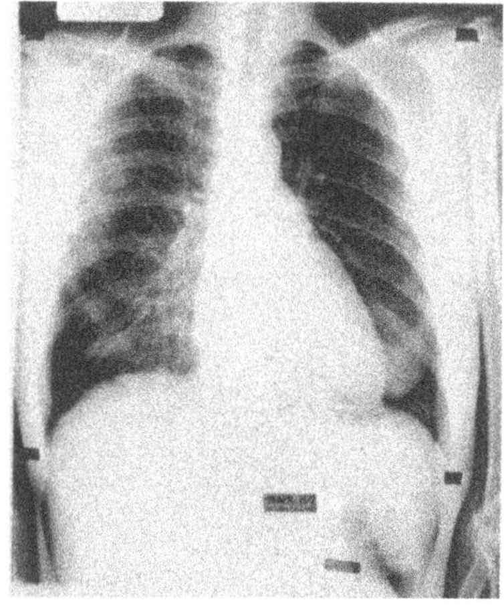

a. original chest radiograph

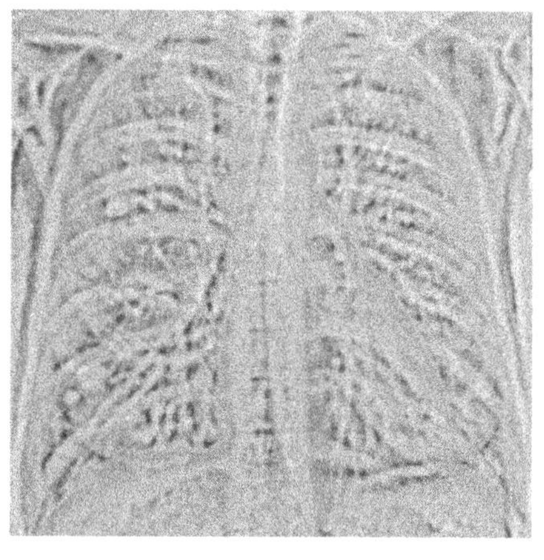

b. normalized-zonal-notch filtration of chest radiograph.

Figure 1.

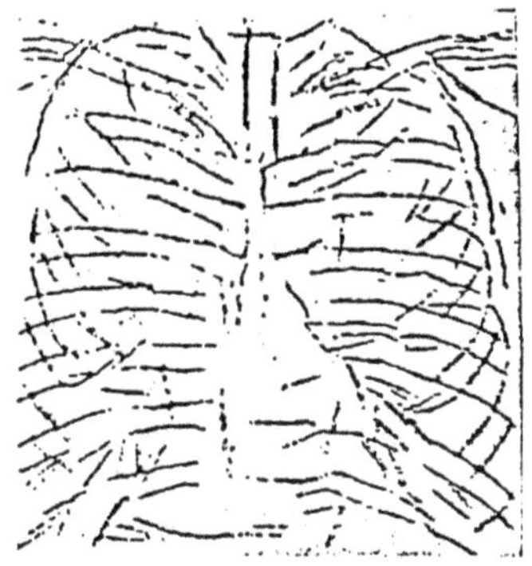

Figure 2. Application of straight edge finder to a chest radiograph.

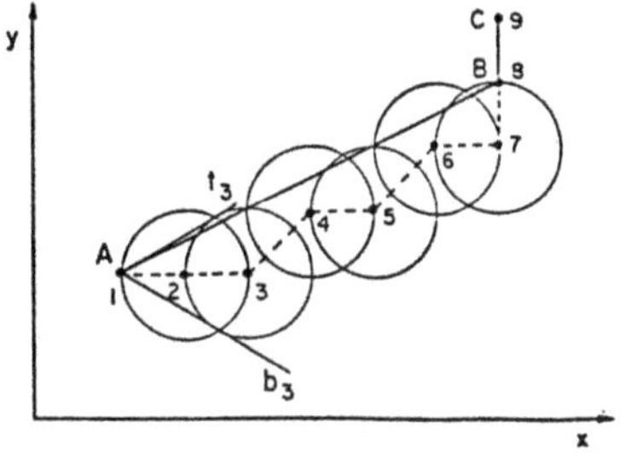

Figure 4. Tangent rays for finding the RMPP.

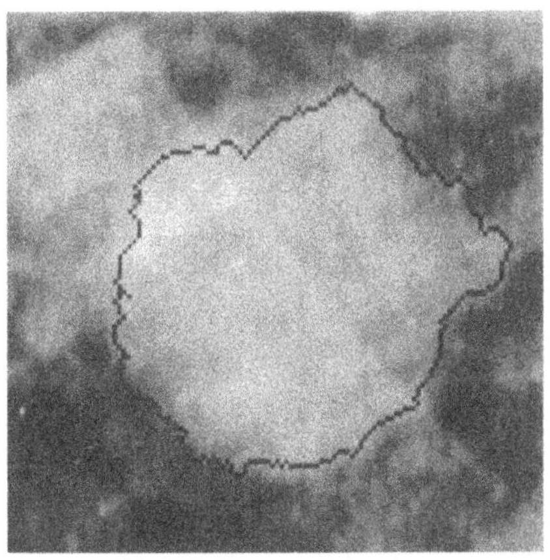

Fig. 3(a) nodule

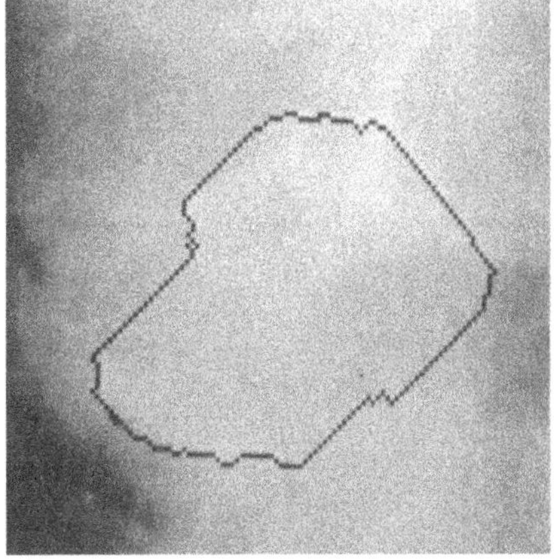

Fig. 3(c) nonnodule

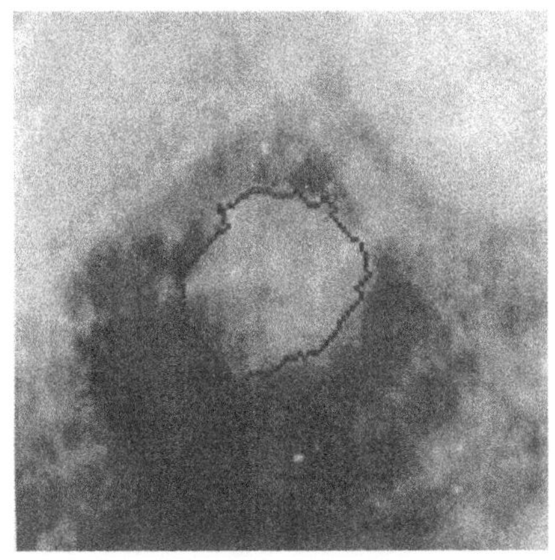

Fig. 3(b) nodule

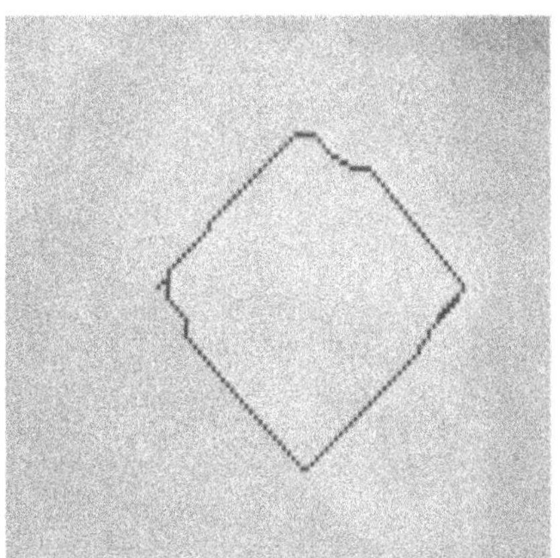

Fig. 3(d) nonnodule

Figure 3. Boundaries of nodules and nonnodules.

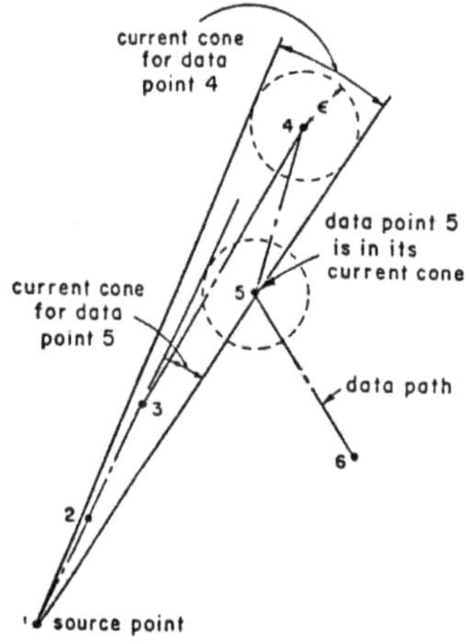

Figure 5. Peak detection for the RMPP.

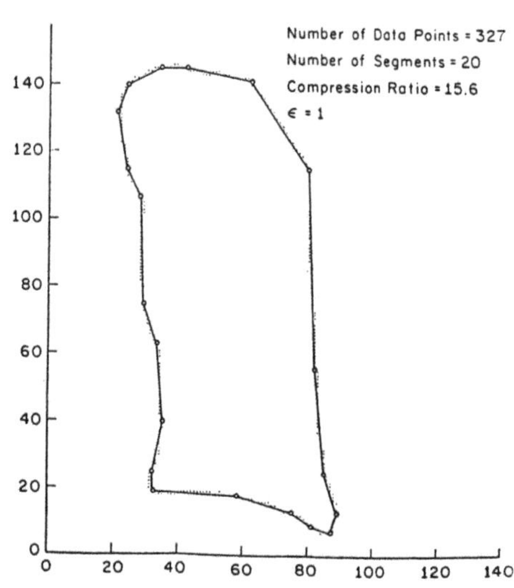

Figure 7. RMPP approximation of boundary of lung.

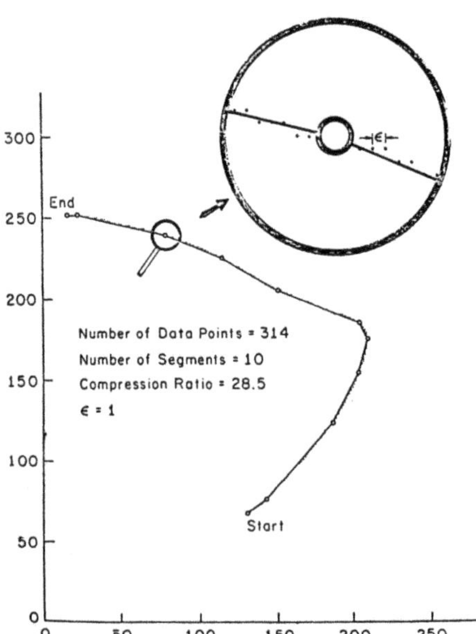

Figure 6. RMPP approximation of the contour of a rib.

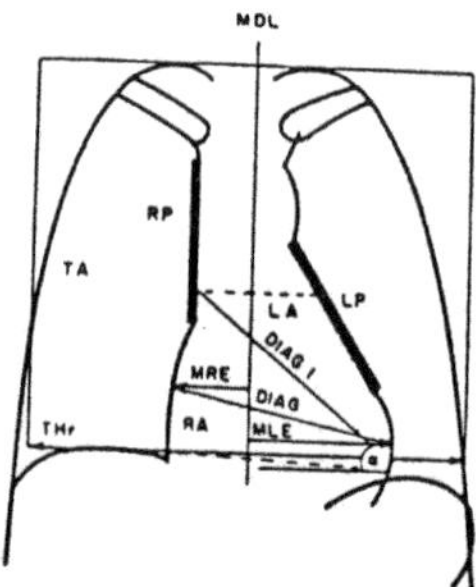

Figure 8. Line segments in a chest radiograph, for detecting rheumatic heart disease.

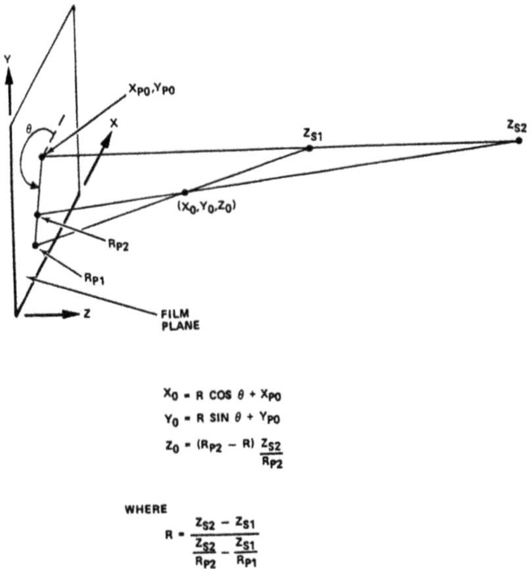

Figure 9. Reconstruction geometry.

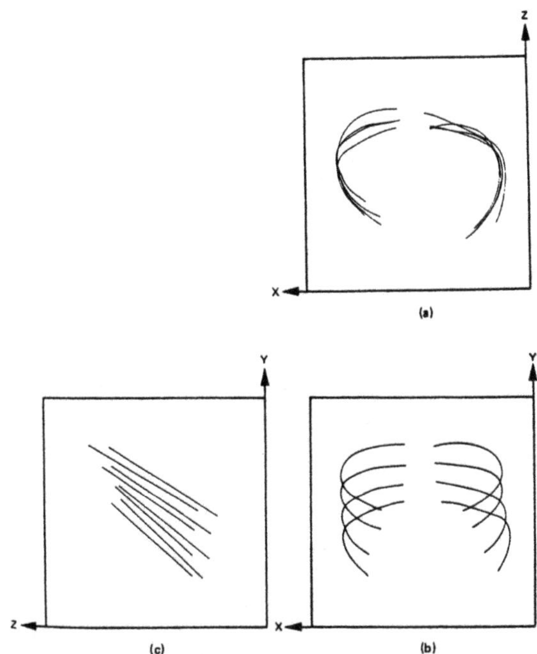

Figure 10. Three orthographic views of the reconstructed rib cage obtained from the model-driven algorithm. a) top view b) front view c) side view

ULTRASOUND SIGNAL PROCESSING FOR IMAGING AND DIAGNOSIS

by
Robert C. Waag
Department of Electrical Engineering and Radiology
University of Rochester
Rochester, New York 14627

ABSTRACT

The advantages of ultrasonic imaging in medicine have led to its widespread use as a diagnostic tool as well as numerous efforts to extend its clinical usefulness. Current research employing computer-based techniques exploits the utility of existing and emerging digital technology to analyze the distributions of amplitude in an image, perform frequency analysis of backscatter, determine angular dependence of backscatter, and assess structure dimensions, area and volume. The distribution of amplitudes in an entire image or a selected field may be described by histograms which yield statistics and can also be used for amplitude mapping to enhance features. Amplitude distributions may also be described by two-dimensional Fourier transforms which yield information in terms of spatial frequency amplitudes. Frequency analysis of backscattered signals provides data about the spacing of scatterers and also the attenuation properties of the propagation path. Angular-dependent backscatter has been used to describe volume scattering from tissue and also to characterize surface roughness. Assessment of structure size has been accomplished to assist in the evaluation of cardiac function as well as provide information about fetal development. Research results now available show the feasibility of extracting more information than reflector position and strength from acoustic signals. Opportunities for important contributions by digital processing appear to exist in three-dimensional imaging, analysis of frequency- and angular-dependent scattering, quantification of structure geometry, and multiple parameter analysis or combinations of techniques. Three-dimensional imaging requires new beam steering techniques, data storage, and time gating which may be conveniently accomplished using digital technology. Angular- and frequency-dependent scattering techniques now under development promise to yield detailed information about the mechanical properties such as compressibility and density as they vary throughout tissue. Quantitative analysis of structure geometry should be enhanced by edge-finding algorithms that operate on three-dimensional data and introduce automation into the calculation of parameters. Pattern recognition systems offer the potential of yielding new diagnostic parameters from weighted combinations of image features and tissue characteristics. Significant progress toward the development of an ultimate ultrasonic system for medical imaging can be expected as research continues.

1. INTRODUCTION

Ultrasound has been developed into an important tool in medical diagnosis, primarily because of its unique capability to image soft-tissues without exposure to ionizing radiation or the use of contrast agents [1,2]. Recent advances in instrumentation have included gray scale presentation from analog and digital scan conversion systems which have improved the visualization of detail within organs [3]. The availability of this tissue detail for analysis offers the possibility of computer processing to extend the diagnostic capabilities of ultrasound through determinations of amplitude distributions and spatial frequencies for emphasis and better evaluation of tissue detail as well as for quantification of ultrasonic data to improve differential diagnosis.

It is known among scientists and clinicians working in medical ultrasound that more information than time-of-arrival is contained in the ultrasonic echoes produced by tissue. This has led to a variety of investigations [4-8] with the common objective of extracting additional information to characterize tissue completely from its ultrasonic properties. Among the most promising of the various studies are those which involve complex computational procedures to obtain sound speed, absorption, and scattering characteristics. Digital technology can also be expected to become more important in the control of instrumentation and computer-based display systems will be utilized more and more to permit interactive viewing, analysis, and production of optimal archival images.

The objective of this paper is to describe selected digital processing techniques that are being studied to extend the diagnostic utility of ultrasound and then to identify additional developments that are expected to result in an ultimate system utilizing all the capabilities of ultrasound to provide diagnostic information. The current status of the field is shown in this paper through analysis of amplitude distributions in terms of histograms and various indicators of texture, determinations of backscatter as a function of frequency and angle, and assessment of structure geometry. Discussion of prospective developments is directed at selected topics in three-dimensional imaging, angular- and frequency-dependent scattering, quantification of structure geometry, and combinations of techniques.

2. CURRENT STATUS OF THE FIELD

2.1. Amplitude Analysis via Histograms

Amplitude analysis for the characterization of tissue can be carried out by the creation of histograms which show the relative frequency of occurrences of amplitudes in an entire image or a selected part of an image. Construction of histograms has demonstrated differences in amplitude distribution between normal abdominal organs and abdominal organs modified by disease (Fig. 1) [9]. These differences may be quantitatively expressed in terms of amplitude statistics. Histograms also provide convenient guidelines for flexible mapping of the available amplitude distribution for improved gray scale display that emphasizes small but significant differences in signal level. For example, a histogram of the entire field can be used as a guide to select amplitude bands for separating regions of differing backscatter amplitude. Employing this analysis in an in vitro study of dog hearts containing myocardial infarcts, low amplitude echoes from normal heart muscle and high amplitudes from regions of damage by reduced blood supply have been identified for the interactive production of trilevel images in which the abnormal areas were represented by white and readily differentiated from normal muscle, imaged as gray (Fig. 2) [10].

2.2. Texture Analysis

There are a variety of ways that texture, i.e. the spatial distribution of amplitudes, in an ultrasonic image can be characterized. Well known for its wide spread application in other fields is the technique of decomposition into spatial frequencies via a two-dimensional Fourier transform. This provides a description of reflector size, shape, and spacing in terms that can be useful because the information is presented in an entirely different form than in the original image.

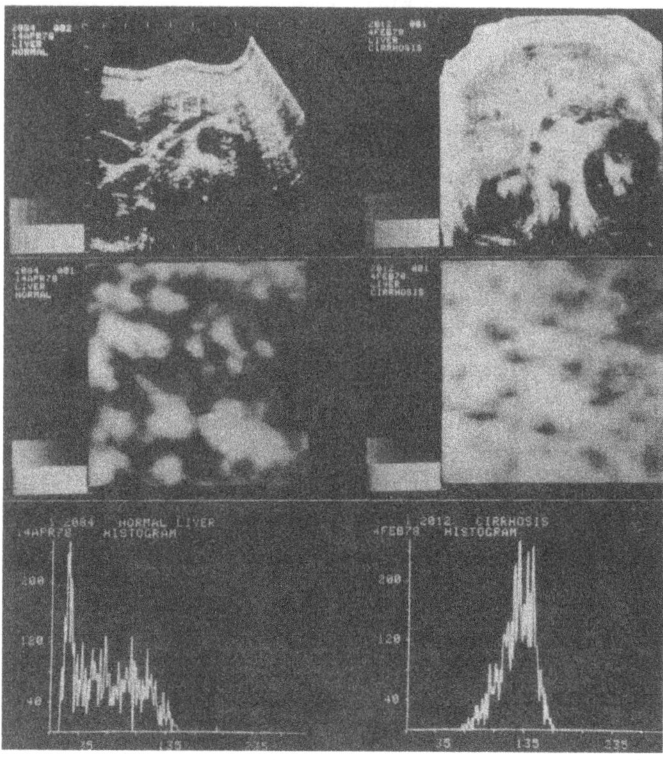

Figure 1. Tissue characterization by histogram analysis. Transverse upper abdominal scans contain windows identifying a portion of liver in a normal subject (left) and one with cirrhosis. The magnified images (8X) show the cirrhotic liver to contain densely packed echoes. The histogram analyses demonstrate a shift of echo amplitude in the cirrhotic liver toward the high range with relatively fewer low amplitude values. From Waag et al. [9].

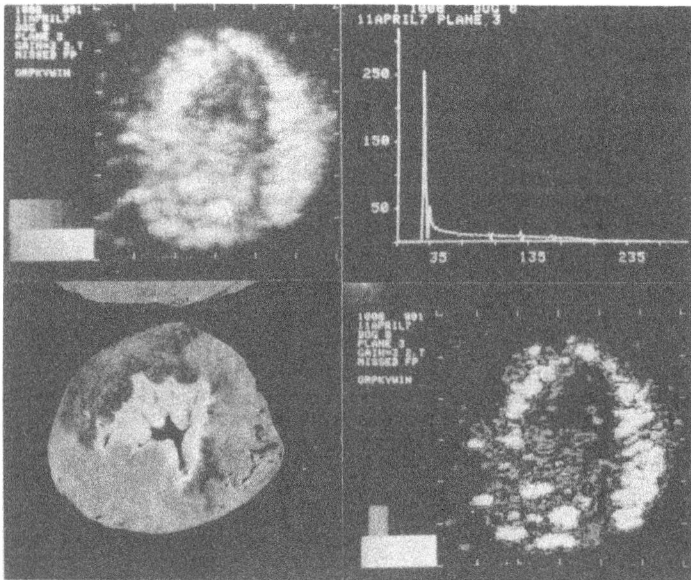

Figure 2. Amplitude processing of myocardial infarction. An original ultrasound image (upper left) of a dog heart cross-section, a histogram of its signal amplitudes, and a corresponding anatomic section are shown with a tristable image derived by amplitude processing. Dark areas in the anatomic cross-section represent regions of reduced blood flow. Other biologic studies demonstrated muscle damage in close agreement with the processed image in which the high amplitude echoes from abnormal tissue are shown as white. From Gramiak et al. [10].

Experience with texture analysis has indicated that in tissue such as liver containing relatively small, widely spaced and uniformly distributed reflectors, the two-dimensional distribution for frequencies has a tendency toward circular symmetry and higher mean radial frequencies than in disease processes which increase the size of individual reflectors or render them confluent (Fig. 3) [9]. Means obtained from averages in sectors oriented in the image at 90° to each other may be used to reveal spectral anistropy induced by differences in axial and lateral architecture. Frequency-based image filtration for emphasis of regions in which echo amplitude changes rapidly can be performed for enhancement of reflector boundaries). For example, the addition of a Laplacian-filtered version of an image to the original, unprocessed data produces an image in which reflected boundaries appear sharpened and echoes of small amplitudes are easier to recognize (Fig. 4) [9].

Color may be used to show the spatial frequency content of an image by dividing the available frequencies into three equal bands and then recombining them with color coding into an additive color image. The resultant image renders spatial frequency content of structures within the image in various hues which offer the possibility of demonstrating and quantifying tissue texture.

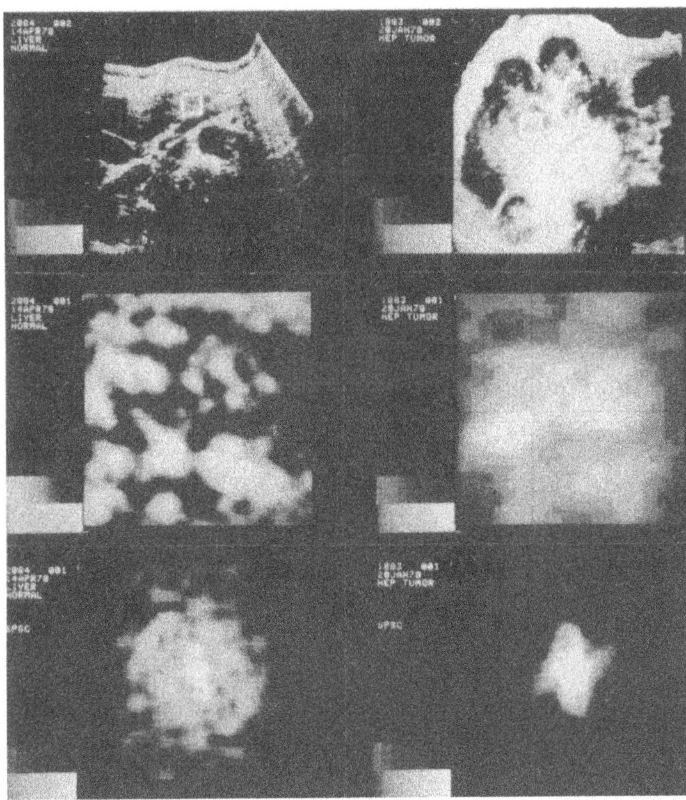

Figure 3. Spatial frequency description of tissue texture. Transverse upper abdominal scans in a normal subject (left) and one with primary liver tumors have been windowed for texture analysis. Magnified images (8X) and their spatial frequency distributions show the tumor to be composed of large, adjacent reflectors which fewer high frequency elements than normal liver. From Waag et al. [9].

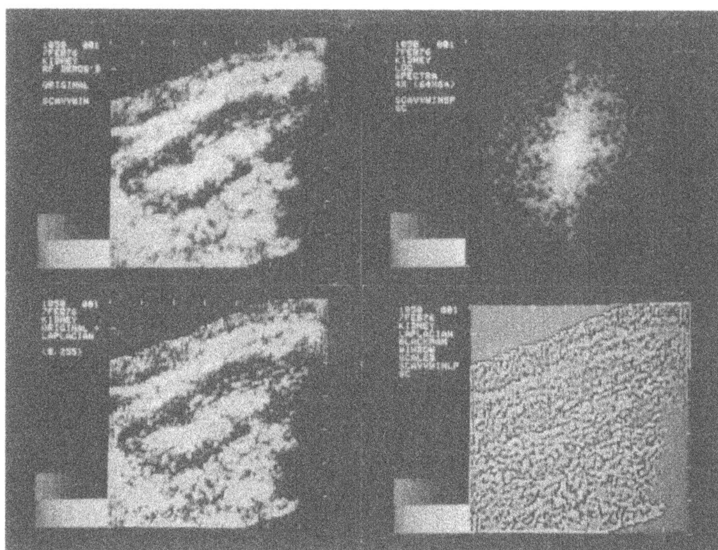

Figure 4. Edge enhancement. An original kidney image and its two dimensional Fourier transform are shown in the upper panels. The addition of a Laplacian-filtered version to original data results in sharper reflector margins with clearer delineation of low amplitude echoes. From Waag et al. [9].

2.3. Backscatter Frequency Analysis

Backscattered acoustic signals contain path length and scatterer spacing information that can be extracted by digital processing of RF wave forms treated as deterministic signals or as sample functions of a random process. Examples of frequency-dependent backscatter measurements of biological media are found in the work of investigators who have studied the eye and also in the work of investigators who have studied blood. In vivo data [11] obtained from an eye containing a detached retina shows backscatter peaks and nulls resulting from front and back surface echoes that interfere (Fig. 5). Spacing of peaks implies a retinal thickness of 190 microns. The eye, because of its relatively simple structure and uniformity among individuals is one of the few organs where useful in vivo scattering measurements have been made.

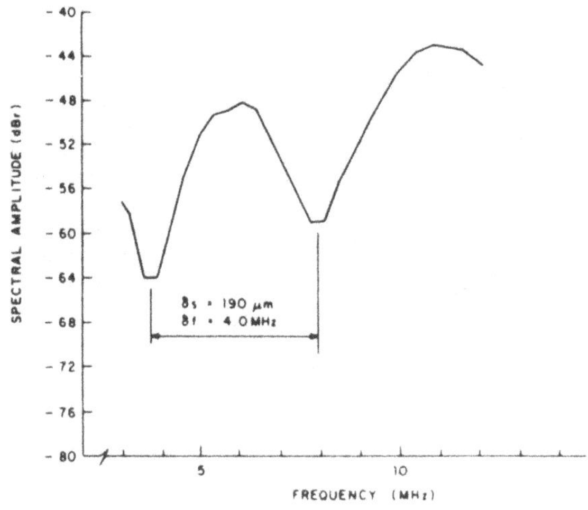

Figure 5. Spectrum of detached retina. The scalloping is the result of interference between the front and back surfaces of the thin retinal membrane. From Lizzi et al. [11].

Blood is a randomly organized medium that backscatter measurements [12] indicate a fourth-power Rayleigh scattering dependence at low red cell concentrations. Other measurements [13] of scattering by blood have been obtained and an analysis of data has indicated that the scattering phenomenon can be predicted analytically although a complicated model must be employed [14].

Fourier analysis of RF signals backscattered from normal and hypertrophic human hearts has been carried out at times when the hearts were contracted and relaxed [9]. In the normal, muscular contraction was associated with a narrowing of the spectrum as compared to the early phase of contraction and relaxation. In the presence of left ventricular hypertrophy, a similar cyclic narrowing was observed and was associated with an overall narrowing of the backscattered spectrum relative to the normal. These findings may be related to the change in muscle fiber diameter observed during contraction and in hypertrophy.

The volume scattering characteristics of a dog heart muscle damaged by coronary artery occlusion were also studied by recording the RF wave form of the backscattered signal and calculating the Fourier spectra. The damaged muscle exhibited more high frequency energy than normal muscle, probably as the result of changes in reflection in the presence of damage caused by poor perfusion [9].

2.4. Angular-Dependent Backscatter

Backscatter measurement as a function of angle have been made for liver, brain and spleen [15], and for arterial tissue [16]. The results indicate differences between scattering from different tissues. In addition, data from liver containing metastatic disease shows differences from data produced by normal livers (Fig. 6) [17]. Although the liver data is from a single determination of amplitude recorded as the specimen was rotated in front of the transducer in a water tank, it is a result from a medium usually considered random. Angular dependent backscatter has also been used in studies of surfaces [18].

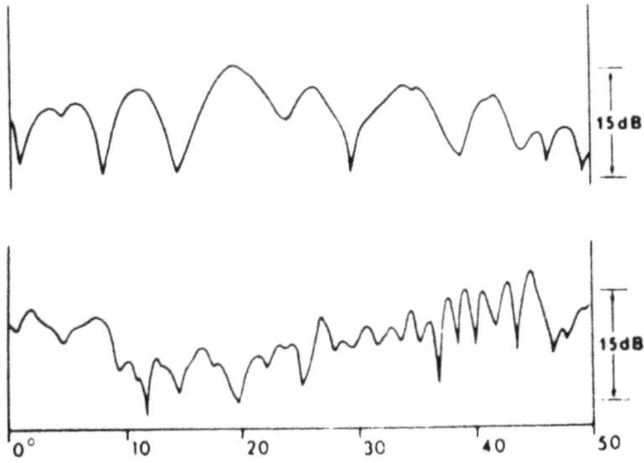

Figure 6. Observed backscattered Bragg diffraction patterns, taken at 1 MHz from normal liver parenchyma (upper) and secondary liver tumor (lower). The backscatter from the cancerous liver shows a higher rate of change with angle. From Hill et al. [17].

2.5. Assessments of Structured Geometry

Structure geometry can be assessed by available microprocessor-based instrumentation which allows determinations of dimensions, areas, and volumes as well as the rate of change of position. Current real-time systems and static B-scan imaging instruments have the capability to measure distance between two cursors which are positioned by controls on the panels of the instruments. Areas can also be calculated from boundaries identified by an operator. Determinations of cross-sectional area can be coupled with assumptions about symmetry in a third dimension to obtain estimations of volume that can be useful in characterizing things as diverse as left ventricular function and fetal development.

3. PROSPECTIVE DEVELOPMENTS

Predicting the future in diagnostic ultrasound is dangerous and challenging since the field is progressing so rapidly. However, information available from research now underway and knowledge of results obtained in other fields using computer methods to process and display signals suggest that research in a number of directions will make important contributions to extending the clinical utility of ultrasonic imaging. Outstanding among the areas with high promise for contributions to be made by digital processing are three-dimensional imaging, angle- and frequency-dependent scattering, quantitative determination of structure geometry, and multi-parameter display techniques.

3.1. Three-Dimensional Imaging

Extension of cross-sectional imaging to three dimensions requires data storage and time-gating in the presence of motion which can be conveniently accomplished using digital techniques. The need for data storage arises because the speed of sound limits the number of lines of acoustic information that can be obtained in a given interval of time. Current real-time cross-sectional imaging instruments are approaching the limits now.

Several approaches to develop three-dimensional images exist. Some of these have used various multi-jointed arms for determination of beam position within a volume [19]. Others have employed a random scanner in which position is determined from time-of-arrival of audible sound generated by spark gap [20].

New beam steering systems are also necessary to image structures ideally. An important improvement can be achieved by adding the capability to focus beams dynamically in the vertical direction and, thus, reduce the thickness of the scan plane not currently controlled electronically. This requires the incorporation of additional elements into the array to increase the aperture in the direction perpendicular to the scanning plane. Creation of a two-dimensional array would allow this type of narrowing of the scanning plane. It would also provide the capability to sweep the plane of scan electronically so that data may be collected from a three-dimensional region (Fig. 7) [21]. If a periodic dynamic process is to be imaged, data acquisition may be extended over over a number of periods (i.e. heart or respiratory cycles) and a gating technique used to develop images that correspond to specific phases of the cyclic process.

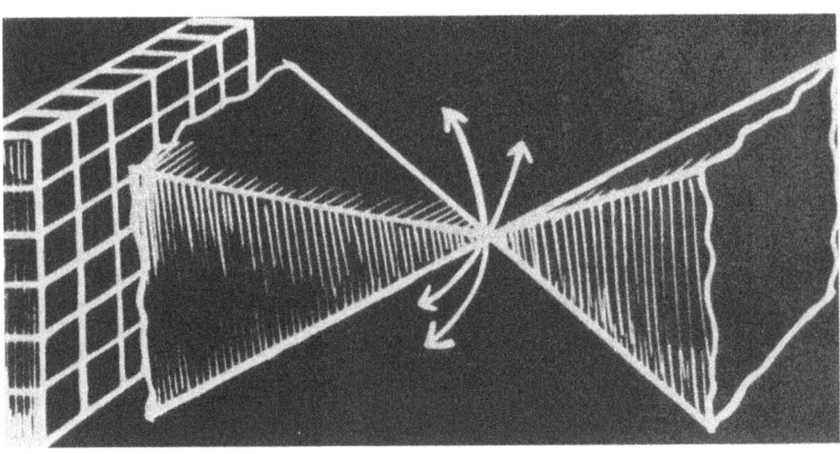

Figure 7. Two-dimensional phased array concept. The addition of elements in the vertical dimension allows two-dimensional focusing and beam sweeping through out a volume. The ideal of equal resolution in all three dimensions can be approached in this way. From Waag et al. [21].

Adaptive electronic control of instrument parameters offers the possibility of more rapid and efficient patient examination. Reasonable concepts for investigation are those already employed for automated control of spacecraft and compensation of communication channels. These concepts require periodic sampling of operational data, comparison with references, and on-line alterations to achieve specified system performance. Digital technology is ideally suited to carry out the computations required in the process of adaptation.

An ultrasonic system could adaptively determine amplifier gain as the ideal gain required for structure demonstration varies with range or beam angulation. This would require an estimation of the attenuation produced by reflection and absorption. In the heart, where limited acoustic impedance changes are encountered and absorption is produced primarily by myocardium and chest wall, the estimation of energy loss is simplified. Beam attenuation due to reflection may be derived from known tissue-fluid impedance differences or measured data. Absorptive losses can be derived from on-line measurement of absorber thickness when bondaries have been demonstrated by reflections.

3.2. Angular- and Frequency-Dependent Scattering

Extension of digital processing techniques now under development promises to yield detailed information about mechanical properties such as compressibility and density as they vary throughout tissues and, ultimately, to provide a non-invasive biopsy. Model studies demonstrate that reflector spacing can be inferred from scattering measurements when the structure is arranged regularly [22] as well as when structure is randomly distributed [23]. Randomly organized scatterers, however, require multiple determinations from which the average nature of structure or an estimation of structure variations can be obtained.

Results obtained at 6 MHz from collections of closely packed small spheres show more omni-directional scattering for an average particle radius of 83 microns than for an average radius of 93 microns (Fig. 8). Similar results have been obtained (Fig. 9) for particles having an average radius of 128 micrometers when the frequency was reduced on 6.0 MHz to 3.8 MHz.

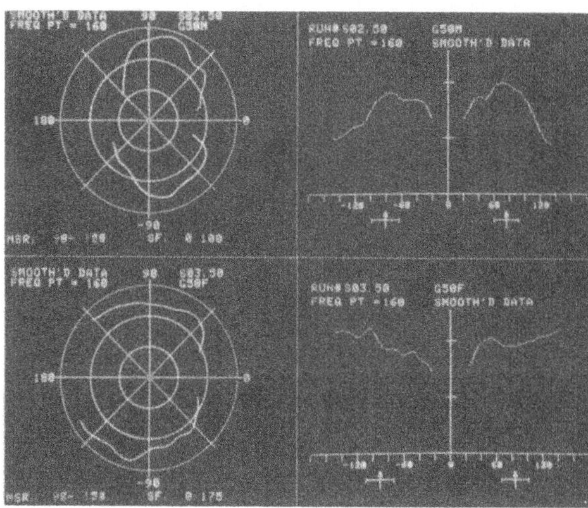

Figure 8. Size-dependent angular scattering by a random medium model. The polar plots and corresponding Cartesian plots show average intensity on a linear scale at 5.9 MHz for distributions of scattering with an average particle radius of 93 μm (top) and with an average radius of 84 μm (bottom). The increase in omnidirectional scattering for smaller scatterers is evident in both plots and also demonstrated by the mean scattering angle defined by arrows crossing standard eviation bars below the Cartesian plots. From Waag et al. [23].

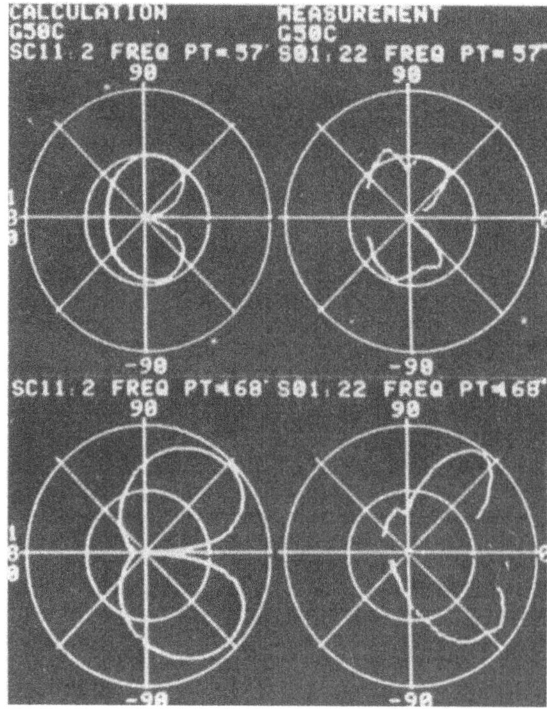

Figure 9. Frequency-dependent angular scattering by a random medium model. Measurements of average intensity are shown (left) on a logarithmic scane for a frequency of 3.8 MHz (top) and 6.0 MHz (bottom). The measured data obtained from a suspension of particles demonstrates more forward scattering as frequency increases and compares well with computations of scattering from a cloud in which the average particle radius is 128 micrometers. From Waag et al. [23].

The angular distribution of scattering from cirrhotic human liver has been observed to be considerably different from that of pig liver (Fig. 10) [24]. This is thought to be the result of the different distribution of collagenous structures which are known to produce scattering.

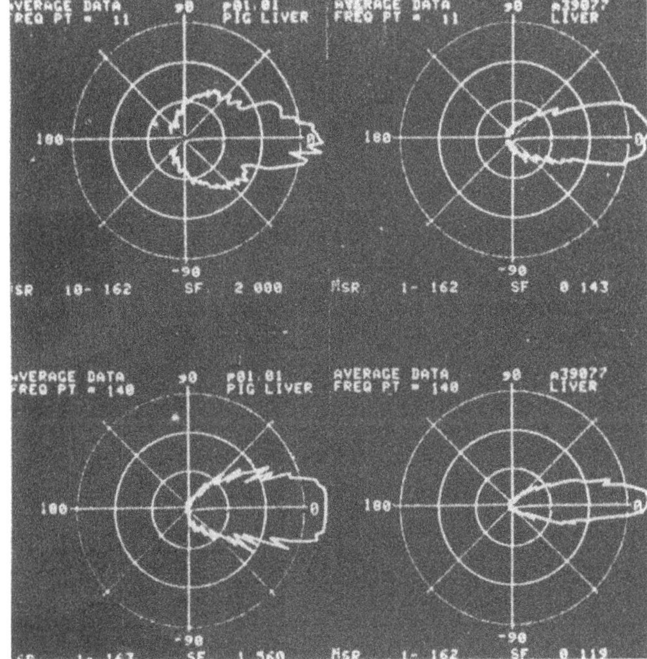

Figure 10. Comparison of average angular scattered intensity from normal pig liver and cirrhotic human liver. Specimens studied at 3 MHz (upper panels) show that the normal pig liver scatters more omnidirectionally than cirrhotic human liver and that, as frequency is increased to 6 MHz, the forward scattering component increases in both cases. This is consistent with scattering from collagen which is arranged in a smaller, more uniform matrix in the pig liver than in the cirrhotic human liver. From Waag et al. [24].

3.3. Quantitative Determination of Structure Geometry and Movement

Three-dimensional imaging systems allow quantitative determinations of structure dimensions, areas, and volumes without the need of special assumptions about symmetry as mandated by one- or two-dimensional imaging systems. However, the representation of three-dimensional information in analytically manageable ways is difficult.

One way that the three-dimensional data may be simplified is by means of modeling. For example, a number of spherical harmonics might be used to fit in a minimum-mean-squared-error sense the endocardial surface of the left ventricle at a given time. Then, similar fits at other instances of time can be used to study left ventricular function and wall dynamics.

3.4. Combinations of Techniques

Pattern recognition systems offer the potential of yielding new diagnostic parameters from weighted combinations of image features and tissue characteristics. Proceedings from a regularly held symposium describe new concepts and advances in the field [25,26]. Initial applications in medical ultrasound have been reported by investigators who were able to differentiate pyelonephrotic kidneys from normals and also by others who seek to characterize breast lesions through the use of new imaging parameters [27,28].

An ultimate ultrasonic system can be envisioned as a combination of the best methods for electronic beam sweeping and dynamic focusing, automation of data acquisition, data processing, and display of information. Displays will probably employ computer graphics and will likely utilize color representations to display in addition to signal amplitude, information describing tissue characteristics such as absorption as well as reflector spacings and compositions. The volume of data to be processed in such a multi-parameter system necessarily require a computer for control of peripherals during data acquisition as well as for signal processing and image reconstruction (Fig. 11).

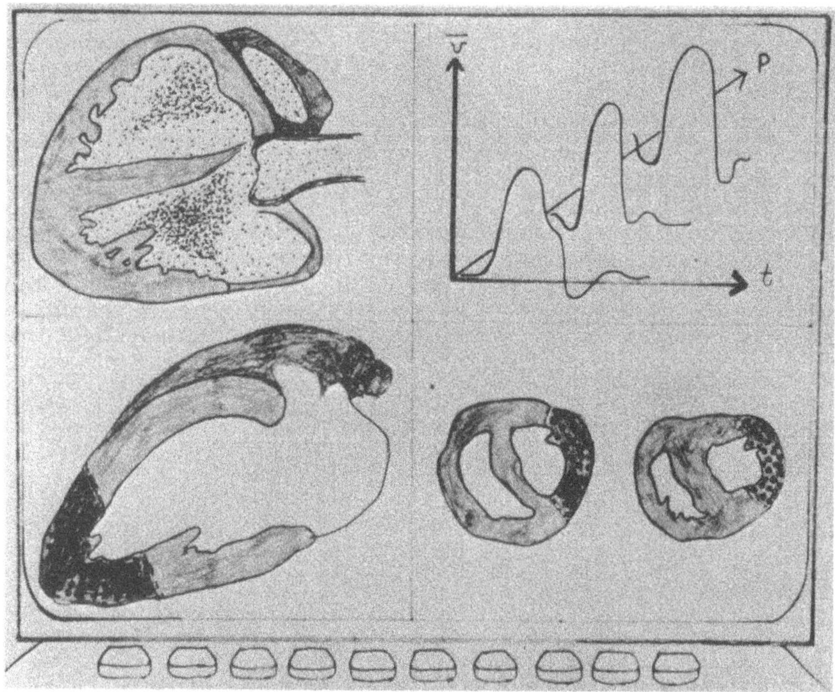

Fig. 11. Multiparameter display of simulated cardiac examination data. Solid structure and blood flow (strippled) imaging is depicted in the upper left next to a time (t) and position (P) display of the mean velocity (V) in a sample volume. An infarcted area (dotted) is shown below in a long axis plane (left) and two short axis planes (right). Viewing these images sequentially would provide motion information characterizing cardiac function. Computer graphics can also be used to introduce three-dimensional shading, interactive image rotation, and dynamic display of selected planes. From Waag et al. [21].

4. CONCLUSIONS

Although ultrasonic imaging has become widely used as a diagnostic tool in medicine today, existing research results show the feasibility of extending its clinical usefulness. A number of new techniques already proven in other fields and advancing digital technology which is providing more complex capability at reasonable cost offer great promise for applications in medical imaging. However, additional resarch is necessary to achieve an ultimate system and identify the range of clinical conditions in which ultrasonic imaging and tissue characterization can be used for patient diagnosis and management.

ACKNOWLEDGEMENTS

This report contains ideas developed as a result of long discussions with Dr. Raymond Gramiak whose contributions are gratefully acknowledged. The efforts of a dedicated staff as well as those of numerous graduate students are also contributed to the material in this report. This is also gratefully acknowledged.
Portions of this work have been supported by the National Institute of Health under Grants #HL15016 and HL16260 and the National Science Foundation under Grants #APR14890 and #DAR78-17840.

REFERENCES

1. R. Gramiak, and R. C. Waag, (editors), Cardiac Ultrasound, C. V. Mosby Co., St. Louis, 1975.

2. R. Gramiak, and S. A. Borg, "Ultrasound in the Diagnosis of Abdominal Disease", in C. Rob, (editor), J. Hardy, G. Jordan, W. P. Longmire, Jr., L. Maclean, T. Shires, and C. Welch, (associate editors), Advances in Surgery, Vol. II, Year Book Medical Publishers, Chicago, 1977, pp. 227-263.

3. D. White, and R. E. Brown, (editors), Ultrasound in Medicine, Vol. 3B, Engineering Aspects, Plenum Press, New York, 1977.

4. M. Linzer, (editor), Proc. Ultrasonic Tissue Characterization, National Bureau of Standards, Gaithersburg, Md., May 28-30, 1975, Spec. Publ. 453 (U.S. Govt. Printing Office, Washington, D.C.).

5. M. Linzer, (editor), Proc. Ultrasonic Tissue Characterization II, National Bureau of Standards, Gaithersburg, Md., June 13-15, 1977, Spec. Publ. 525 (U.S. Govt. Printing Office, Washington, D.C.).

6. S. A. Goss, R. L. Johnston, and F. Dunn, "Comprehensive Compilation of Empirical Ultrasonic Properties of Mammalian Tissues", J. Acoust. Soc. Am., 1978, 64, pp. 423-457.

7. R. C. Chivers and R. J. Parry, "Ultrasonic Velocity and Attenuation in Mammalian Tissues", J. Acoust. Soc. Am., 1978, 1, pp. 369-376.

8. P. N. T. Wells, "Absorption and Dispersion of Ultrasound in Biological Tissue", Ultrasound in Med. and Biol., 1975, 63, pp. 940-953.

9. R. C. Waag, P. P. K. Lee, and R. Gramiak, "Digital Processing to Enhance Features of Ultrasound Images", Proc. IEEE Computer Soc. Conf. on Pattern Recognition and Image Processing, May 31-June 2, 1978, Chicago, Illinois, IEEE Cat. No. 78 CH1318-5C.

10. R. Gramiak, R. C. Waag, E. A. Schenk, et. al., "Ultrasonic Detection of Myocardial Infarction by Amplitude Analysis", Radiology, March 1979, 130(3)., pp. 713-720.

11. F. L. Lizzi and M. A. Laviola, "Tissue Signature Characterization Utilizing Frequency Domain Analysis", in J. deKlerk and B. McAvoy, (editors), Proc. Ultrasonics Symposium, 29 Sept-1 Oct 1976, Annapolis, Md., IEEE Cat. No. 76 CH1120-5SU, p. 714.

12. K. K. Shung, R. A. Siegelmann, and J. M. Reid, "The Scattering of Ultrasound by Blood", IEEE Trans. on Biomedical Engineering, BME-23, 1976, 6, p. 460.

13. K. K. Shung, R. A. Siegelmann, and J. M. Reid, "Angular Dependence of Scattering of Ultrasound from Blood", IEEE Trans. on Biomedical Engineering, BME-24, 1977, 4, p. 325.

14. A. S. Ahuja, "Effects of Particle Viscosity on Propagation of Sound in Suspensions and Emulsions", J. Acoust. Soc. Am., 1972, 51, p. 182.

15. C. R. Hill, "Interactions of Ultrasound with Tissues", in M. de Vlieger, et. al., (editors), Ultrasonics in Medicine, Excerpta Medica, Amsterdam, 1974, p. 14.

16. F. E. Barber, III, "Ultrasonic Microprobe: For Modeling and Measuring the Angle Distribution of Echoes from Diseased Arterial Tissues", University of Washington, Ph.D. Thesis, 1976, Xerox University Microfilms, Ann Arbor, Michigan 48106.

17. C. R. Hill, R. C. Chivers, R. W. Huggins, and D. Nicholas, "Scattering of Ultrasound by Human Tissue", in F. J. Fry, (editor), Ultrasound: Its Applications in Medicine and Biology, Elsevier, 1979, Chapter 9.

18. M. de Billy and G. Quentin, "Ultrasonic Signal Analysis Methods Applied to Biological Tissues", in J. deKlerk & B. R. McAvoy (eds.), Proc. IEEE Ultrasonic Symposium, September 25-27, 1978, Cherry Hill, New Jersey, IEEE Cat. No. 78 CH1344-1SU, pp. 320-325.

19. D. L. Dekker, R. L. Piziali, and E. Dong, "A System for Ultrasonically Imaging the Human Heart in Three Dimensions, Comput. Biomed. Res., 1974, 7, p. 544.

20. D. L. King, S. J. Al-Banna, and D. R. Larach, "A New Three-Dimensional Random Scanner for Ultrasonic/Computer Graphic Imaging of the Heart", in D. White and R. Barnes, (editors), Ultrasound in Medicine, Vol. 2, Proceedings of the 20th Annual Meeting of the American Institute of Ultrasound in Medicine, Plenum Press, New York, 1976.

21. R. C. Waag and R. Gramiak, "Horizons in Ultrasound Technology", Proc. Conf. on Computerized Tomography in Radiology, April 25-26, 1976, St. Louis, Missouri, in American College of Radiology, 1976, pp. 309-311.

22. P. P. K. Lee, R. C. Waag, and L. P. Hunter, "Swept-Frequency Diffraction of Ultrasound by Cylinders and Arrays", J. Acoust. Soc. Am., 1978, 63, pp. 600-606.

23. R. C. Waag, P. P. K. Lee, R. M. Lerner, L. P. Hunter, R. Gramiak, and E. A. Schenk, "Angle Scan and Frequency-Swept Ultrasonic Scattering Characterization of Tissue", in M. Linzer, (editor), Proc. Ultrasonic Tissue Characterization II, National Bureau of Standards, Gaithersburg, Md., June 13-15, 1977, Spec. Publ. 525 (U.S. Govt. Printing Office, Washington, D.C.).

24. R. C. Waag, P. P. K. Lee, R. M. Lerner, L. P. Hunter, R. Gramiak, and E. A. Schenk, "Angle Scan and Frequency-Swept Ultrasonic Scattering Characterization of Tissue", in M. Linzer (ed.) Ultrasonic Tissue Characterization II, National Bureau of Standards, Gaithersburg, Med., June 13-15, 1977, Spec. Publ. 525 (U.S. Govt. Printing Office, Washington, D.C.), pp. 143-152.

25. Proc. of the IEEE Computer Soc. Conference on Pattern Recognition and Image Processing, May 31-June 2, 1978, Chicago, Illinois, IEEE Cat. No. 78 CH1318-5C.

26. Proc. of the Symposium on Computer-Aided Medical Images, Nov. 11, 1976, IEEE Cat. No. 76 CH1170-0C.

27. M. G. Czerwinski and K. Preston, Jr., "A Pattern Recognition Approach to Ultrasonic Tissue Characterization", Proc. IEEE Computer Soc. Conf. on Pattern Recognition and Image Processing, May 31-June 2, 1978, Chicago, Illinois, IEEE Cat. No. 78 CH1318-5C, pp. 21-24.

28. J. F. Greenleaf, R. C. Bahn, S. K. Kenue, and B. Rajagopalan, "Characterization of Palpable Lesions in Breasts Using Ultrasonic Transmission Tomography", presented at First International Congress on the Ultrasonic Examination of the Breast, October 8-9, 1979, Philadelphia, Pa., Conference Program, p. 53.

IMAGE RESTORATION IN CARDIAC RADIOLOGY

by
M. AMIEL, R. GOUTTE, R. PROST and P. VETTA
- Institut National des Sciences Appliquées de Lyon
Laboratoire de Traitement du Signal et Ultrasons
69621 VILLEURBANNE CEDEX
- Université Claude Bernard
Laboratoire de Radiologie Expérimentale
28, Avenue du Doyen Lepine 69500 BRON

ABSTRACT

The improvement of resolution in cardiac radiology may allow a best analysis of vascular structures and a more accurate measurement of stenoses. The resolution is limited by focal spot dimensions, detector imperfections and nearly periodical displacements of cardiac muscle. Having defined the main caracteristics of these different causes of degradation, we propose a digital method of restoration using a constrained deconvolution process.

In a pilot study the motion blur parameter identification is obtained from space invariant models. Other possible approaches of restoration (Wiener filtering, "gating tomography") are also considered.

1. INTRODUCTION

Improved resolution in cardiac radiology will lead to a more precise analysis of vascular structures and to a better quantitative analysis of stenoses.
With conventional radiology equipment the main factor for the present limits of this resolution are due to the finite dimensions of the focal spot, scattered radiation, imperfections in the detectors and to the complex movements of the cardiac muscle.

Optimal experimental conditions generally necessitate imperatives which may be contradictory. Thus, for example, reduction of motion blur by using short exposure times calls for a large focal spot. In the compromise which is generally used, the respective influences of geometric blur and of motion blur are equally important. Therefore efficient image restoration should permit the simultaneous reduction of the influence of these two causes of degradation.

In the specific case where instrumental characteristics are well known, and where simplifying hypotheses for linearity and invariance may be made, it is possible to develop a restoration process by deconvolution [1][2].

2. HYPOTHESES AND METHODS

The linearity hypothesis is generally well complied with by using a radiology system (Fig. 1)(bearing in mind a possible correction of the non-linear characteristics of certain detectors, the photographic film, for example).

On the other hand, the shift invariance hypothesis, even in the absence of motion blur, is only complied with around the immediate vicinity of the beam's central zone, since the point spread function depends on the coordinates x and y of the point considered in the plane.

Finally, so that this function is not dependant on the z coordinate of the point considered, the thickness of the object must be slight in front of the distance focal spot-detector.

Under these conditions it is possible to link the spatial distribution i(x,y) of optical density in the degraded radiography to distribution O(x,y) to density in the ideal radiography by the convolution operation

$$i(x,y) = O(x,y) * h(x,y)$$

with $h(x,y) = h_0(x,y) * h_d(x,y)$

$h_0(x,y)$ = point spread function

$h_d(x,y)$ = detector impulse response

$h(x,y)$ = impulse response of total system.

Thus in obtaining an "ideal" restored photograph O(x,y) remains a problem of deconvolution, since :

$$O(x,y) = i(x,y) * h(x,y)$$

whose solution in Fourier domain brings about a simple spectrum division

$$O(u,v) = \frac{I(u,v)}{H(u,v)}$$

Any resulting difficulties come from various factors : imprecise knowledge of H(u,v)(instrumental transfer function), noise and limits of band pass on the detector system. In fact, if output information is only accessible in the domain

$-u_c < u < +u_c$; $-v_c < v < +v_c$, only an estimate O(x,y) (principal values) of the

ideal solution O(x,y) may be obtained. If the signal/noise ratio decreases, cut off frequencies u_c and v_c become closer to the origin (u = 0, v = 0) and the quality of the estimate O(x,y) also decreases.

We were thus obliged to develop a super resolution algorithm (Fig. 2) in order to obtain a new estimate that corresponds to a wider spectral domain than that of the principal value. This constraint deconvolution algorithm uses the positivity properties of the signal to be restored, or, more generally, it uses the existence of amplitude bounds. This derives from the linear methods proposed by VILLE [3] and PROST [4] for the restoration of signals localised in space ; a simulated restoration example of an amplitude bounded signal is given Fig. 3.

This algorithm may be used in a two-dimensional form for the case of an image. In this application, bound α (amplitude threshold) is set to zero, to take into account the posivity of optical densities.

3. GEOMETRIC BLUR

Linear dispersion functions of the focal spot $h_0(x)$ and of the detector $h_d(x)$ (including amplifier, camera and film) are determined from the image from a suitably positioned 40 µm slit. The product of their Fourier transform gives the transfer function of the radiology system in the direction perpendicular to the slit. Figure 4 illustrates the results obtained for two perpendicular directions and shows a fairly good isotropy in the domain of low spatial frequencies. We admit then, as a first approximation, that the global transfer function H(u,v) presents a revolution symmetry. Figure 5b illustrates the results of deconvolution (solution with spectral extension) obtained from the original image 5a. (Kidney radiography with geometric blur, but without motion blur).

4. MOTION BLUR

We will now consider the problem of the restoration of images degraded by motion blur . [5][6].

In the particular case of cardiac x-rays, the principal difficulties are:

- The necessity of knowing, for each point of the object, considered as deformable, the time évolution of the speed vector. This is the problem of motion identification.

- The absence of simple properties of symmetry in the movement of the heart. Even if the study is limited to a thin cross-section of the object, perpendicular to the direction of the beam, projections of speed vectors are neither parallel to a given direction, nor of the same length. In addidion, the evolution as a function of time is governed by a complex law.

Thus, the system is globally variable, and it becomes necessary, in order to make certain symplifying hypotheses, to limit the study to specific cases.

We therefore suppose that in a limited zone of the cross-section of the object, projections of speed vectors are all oriented in the direction and have a common value a. The system then becomes locally non-variable, and the use of a restoration process by deconvolution is once again possible.

Physically, such simplifying hypotheses are justified if the study is limited to the blur in the immediate vicinity of a stenosis, for example, for X-ray radiographies obtained with relatively short pose time.

Our study was carried out using a model (ideal image) undergoing a flat motion where the parameters a and ψ are known. The resulting blurred image is used in an identification method to recalculate motion parameters. Lastly, a deconvolution process permits an estimate of the original ideal image (See Figure 6).

We use the complex cepstrum method for identification (7).

$$i(x,y) = O(x,y) * h(x,y)$$

Therefore $$I(u,v) = O(u,v) \cdot H(u,v)$$

With $$|H(u,v)| = \left|\frac{\sin\{\pi a(u\cos\psi + v\sin\psi)\}}{\pi a\,(u\cos\psi + v\sin\psi)}\right|$$

Following the axes u and v, modulus projections of H(u,v) present the respective periodicities :

$$\frac{1}{a\cos\psi} \quad \text{and} \quad \frac{1}{a\sin\psi}$$

But $$\ln I(u,v) = \ln |H(u,v)| + j\phi_{H(u,v)} + \ln |O(u,v)| + j\phi_{O(u,v)}$$

If we consider line i

$$\hat{\tilde{I}}(x,y_i) = \text{Modulus}\ F^{-1}\left[\ln |I(u,v_i)| + j\phi_I(u,v_i)\right]$$

and lastly, carrying out the summations :

$$\hat{\tilde{I}}(x) = \sum_{i=1}^{i=N} \hat{\tilde{I}}(x,y_i)$$

and similarly :

$$\hat{\tilde{I}}(y) = \sum_{j=1}^{j=N} \hat{\tilde{I}}(x_j,y)$$

The periodicity of $I(x)$ is $a\cos\psi$ and that of $I(y)$ is $a\sin\psi$ (Fig. 7).

Deconvolution of the blurred image is then possible by inverse filtering (Fig. 8).

In a real problem, the transfer function is not generally well known. This imprecision on $H(u,v)$ brings about supplementary difficulties during deconvolution by inverse filtering. It is note worthy that only exact deconvolution will allow the negative component of the restored signal, (without any physical significance) to be completely cancelled. This property may be profitably used to adjust the parameters of $h(x,y)$, whilst seeking to minimize the negativity of signals obtained after deconvolution of a line or colum.

4. CONCLUSION

The limitations of the restoration method of images degraded by motion blur are clear : invariance hypotheses are too imprecise, identification is limited to the case of flat motion and uniform speeds, and furthermore, noise has been neglected.

Interesting possibilities for future progress may be explored by using Wiener filtering which necessitates knowledge of the power spectral density of the ideal image, (which can be estimated from the spectral density of the blurred image) and also the PSF density of the noise, in isolation.

Lastly, another possible approach would consist of using the periodicity of cardiac movements in a "gating" technique. The aim here would be either to improve signal/noise ratio by processing a set of instantaneous images obtained in a particular state of the cardiac cycle, or to select projections to be used in tomographic reconstruction.

REFERENCES

1. A. Georges, "Restauration d'images par déconvolution numérique", Thèse de Docteur Ingénieur INSA de Lyon, France, 1978.

2. P. Marthon, "Contribution à l'étude de la restauration digitale d'images dégradées par des systèmes linéaires", Thèse de Docteur Ingénieur, Université Paul Sabatier de Toulouse, France, 1978.

3. J.A. Ville, "Sur le prolongement des signaux à spectre borné", Cablés Trans 1956, 1, 44.

4. R. Prost, R. Goutte, "Déconvolution when the convolution kernel has no inverse", IEEE ASSP 1977, 6, 542.

5. A. Omar Aboutalib, M. Murphy, L.M. Silverman, "Digital restoration of Images degraded by general motion blurs", IEEE Transactions on automatic control, Vol AC-22 n° 3, june 1977, pp. 294-302.

6. H.J. Trussell and B.R. Hunt, "Image Restoration of Space-variant Blurs by sectioned methods" IEEE Transactions on Acoustics, Speech and Signal Processing Vol 26, n°6, Déc 1978, pp. 608-609.

7. H.C. Andrews and B.R. Hunt, "Digital image restoration", Prentice Hall Inc, New Jersey 1977.

FIGURES

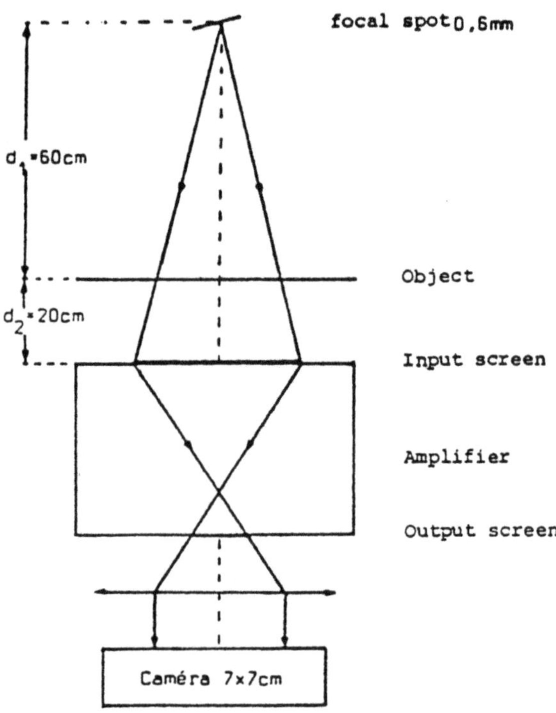

Figure 1. Schema of our radiological system

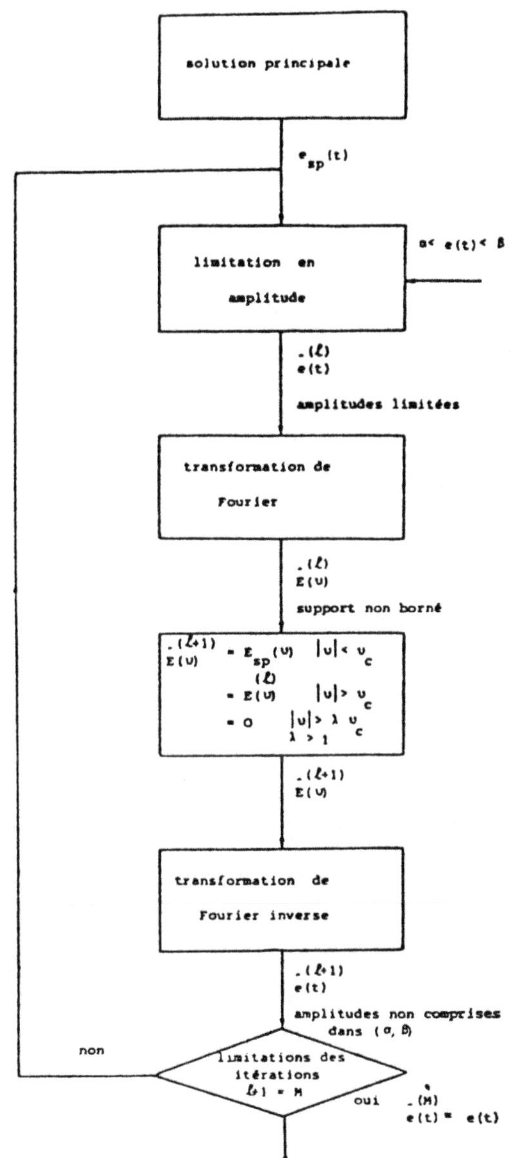

A restoration algorithm with spectral extrapolation for a signal with known (or approximately known) amplitude bounds.

FIGURE 2

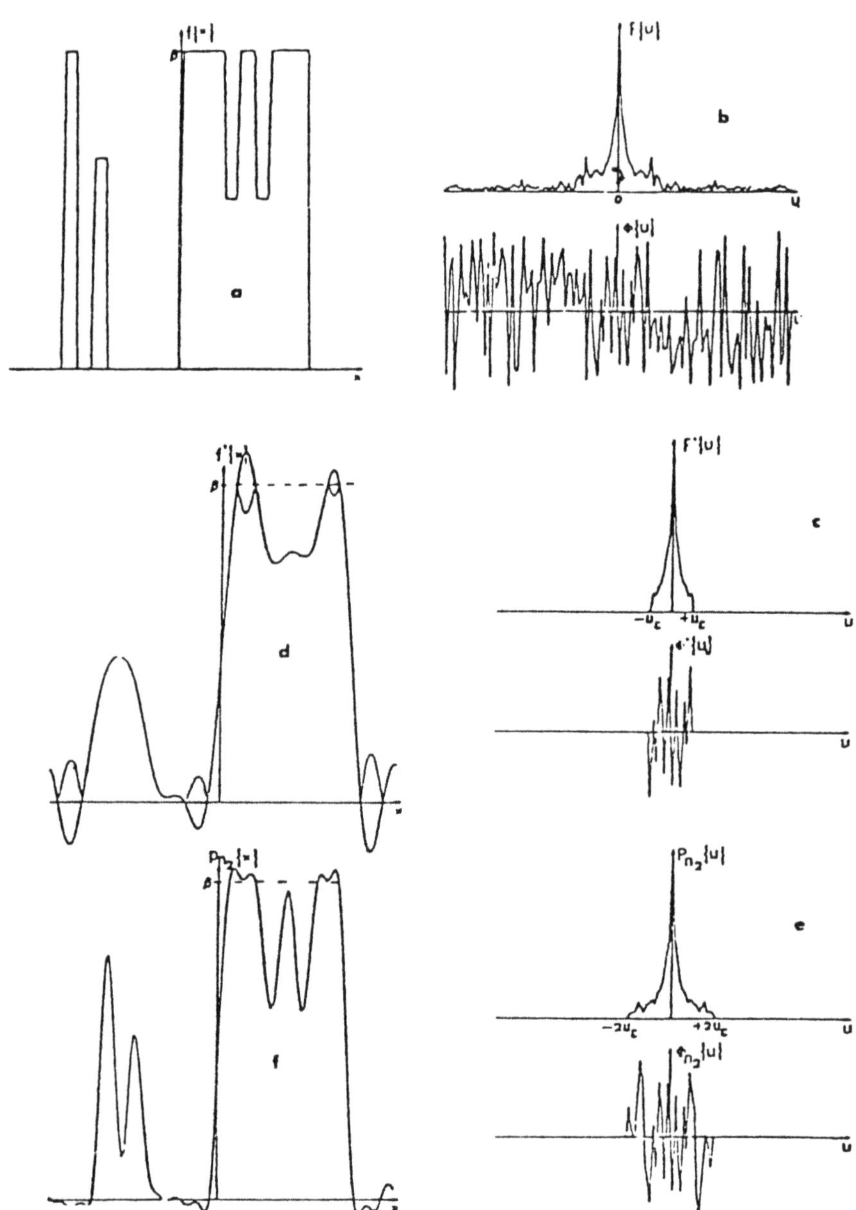

A simulated restoration example of an amplitude bounded signal ($\alpha = 0, \beta$).

a) The signal before deconvolution. *b*) The spectrum of the signal. *c*) The truncated spectrum, it is the spectrum of the principal value solution. *d*) The principal value solution. *e*) Extrapolation of the spectrum up to 2 ν_c. *f*) The result obtained by deconvolution with spectrum extrapolation.

FIGURE 3

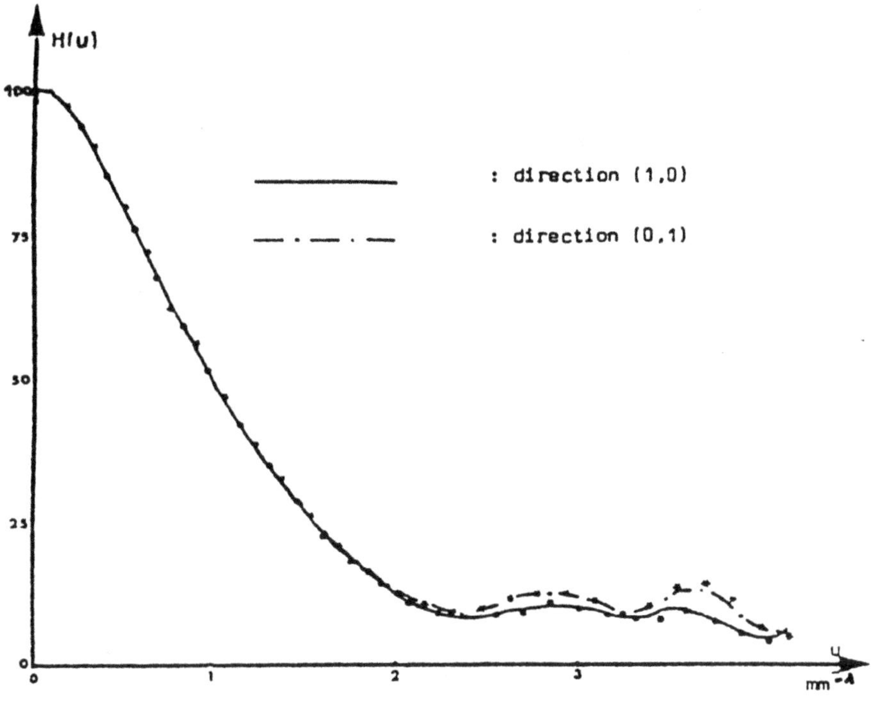

Figure 4. Transfer function of our radiological system in two perpendicular directions.

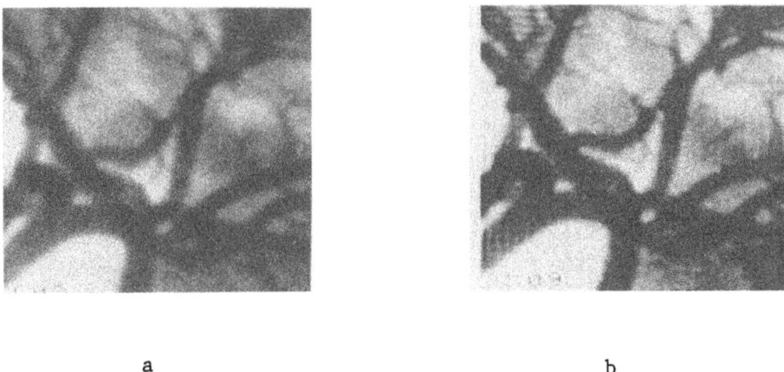

a b

Figure 5. Restoration of a kidney radiography.

a) The radiography before processing (positive image).

b) The restored radiography before the use of the algorithm for amplitude bounded signal (extrapolation of the spatial frequencies from $1.9mm^{-1}$ to $2,3\ mm^{-1}$).

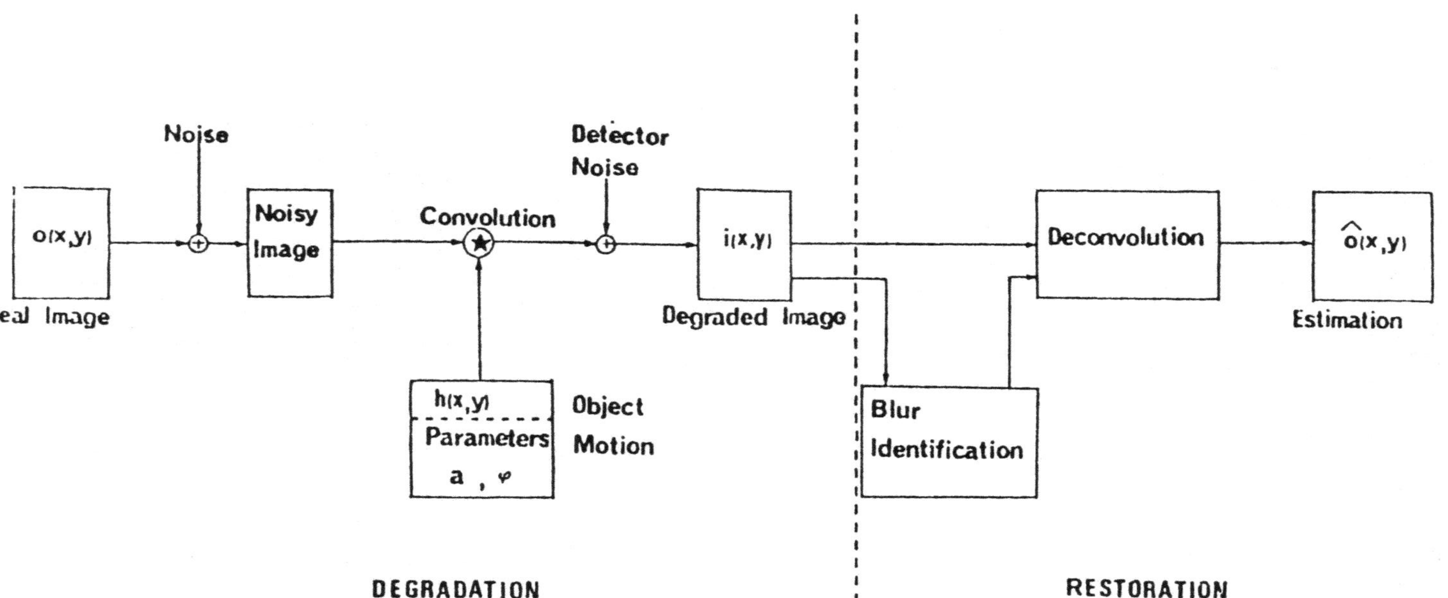

Figure 6. BLoc diagram of principle of Image Restoration after degradation by motion blur.

Figure 7. Complex Cepstrum of lines I(x) and colomns I(y).

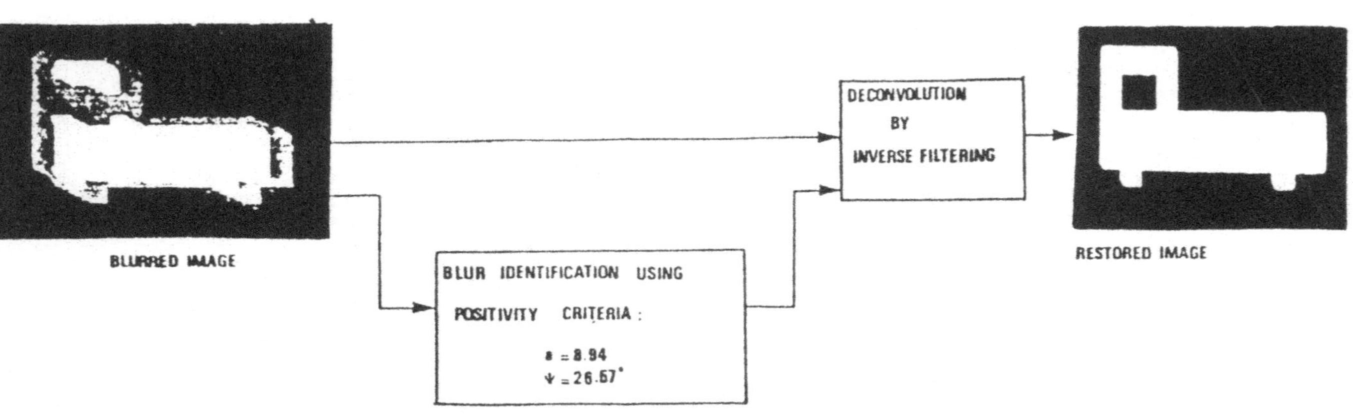

Figure 8. Results of indentification and deconvolution.

ULTRASONIC MULTITRANSDUCER INPUT SIGNAL ANALYSIS. M. BERSON, A. RONCIN, D. BESSE, Cl. PEJOT, L. POURCELOT. Service de Médecine Nucléaire et Ultrasons, C.H.R. Bretonneau, 37044 - TOURS CEDEX, France.

The increasing interest shown in rapid imaging by electronic commutation of multitransducers is linked to the inherent qualities of such equipment : immediate visualization of cross-sections, can be applied to most organs, straightforward use with instruments that are easily movable, no image distortion, etc... However with the early models developed, the quality of the image was poor compared to those obtained by manual scanning. This is due to the fact that in the multitransducer arrays, mechanical focusing cannot be made in the direction of the scanning.

After having developed a multitransducer model in 1972 our aim at the Laboratory of Biophysique of the Faculté de Médecine of TOURS, has been to further research on this type of apparatus in three directions :

- electronic focusing of ultrasonic beams at the transmission of the wave front as well as at the reception of echoes,
- electronic steering of beams in order to obtain images under incidences chosen by the operator, or in order to steer a Doppler line in the image,
- rapid visualization of circulating blood by means of high speed Doppler tomography.

I - FOCUSING OF THE ULTRASONIC BEAM.

I.1. Technique used :

Linear electronic scanning on a linear array consists in a step by step electronic translation of a group n of elements at transmission, and of the same group n, or a different group n', at reception. In order to focus each beam generated by the groups of transducers, a lens needs to be electronically reconstituted for each respective group.

Figure 1 shows that for transmission with a group of 12 transducers, focusing at F of the propagation axis requires a phasing of waves emitted by each transducer and therefore their excitation by pulses in some degree delayed. Delays T_1, T_2,... T_6 correspond to the different track times ($T_1 = 0$ for outside transducers, T_6 the maximum for central transducers) ; there is symmetry in relation to the axis of the group. Thus, during transmission one single focal area can be obtained.

For the reception the problem is the same (figure 2). The introduction of reflected signals at point F' in analog delay lines with suitable delays T'_1, T'_2, ... T_6' manages to get them back in phase, and their summation gives the echo resulting from their reflection in F', the focal point. Furthermore, a focusing in another point F" of the axis requires different delays. Thus an electronic variation in delays related to time enables one to obtain continuous focusing over the whole of the area interrogated : that is what is known as dynamic focusing. If the focal zone matches at any time the placing of the ultrasonic wave front transmitted, one obtains thereby much improved lateral resolution compared to classical echography.

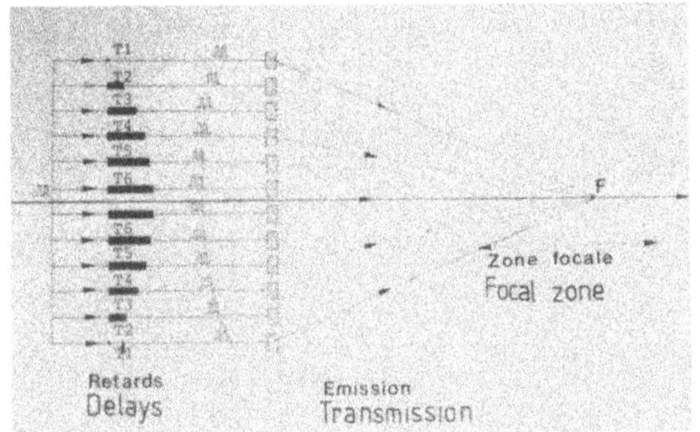

Figure 1 : Principle of electronic focusing of the transmitted ultrasonic wave using delay lines and an array of transducers.

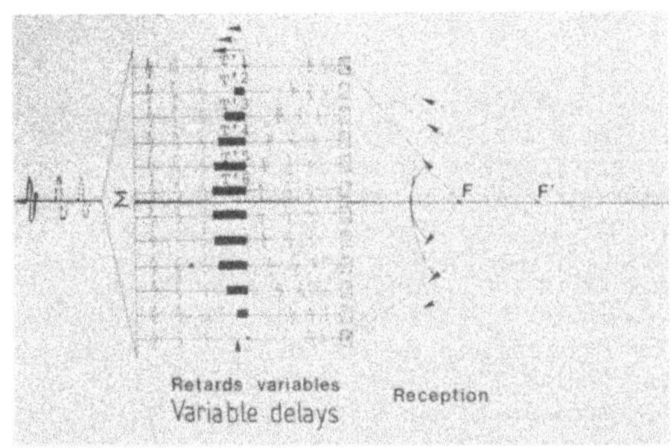

Figure 2 : Dynamic electronic focusing of the reflected waves. The focal area of the electronic lens follows the ultrasonic wave front.

For a given combination of delays one gets an area of focal zone whose length depends on the focal distance, the ultrasonic wavelength and the aperture (the number of transducers). Good dynamic focusing can then be obtained with only a few areas : it cuts out the continuous variation of delays which cannot easily be achieved in practice.

I.2. Theoretical and experimental research :

100 elements of 1 x 10 mm^2 with resonance frequencies of 2 and 3 MHz make up the array used.

Figure 3 shows the diagramm at 6 decibels and 3 MHz, of the resulting beam with focusing on transmission at 7 cm and dynamic focusing on reception. These results are obtained by using as a reflector a small steel ball bearing, of approximatively 3 mm in diameter, and by moving it laterally within the beam on each side of the axial maximum. There are two things we would like to point out :

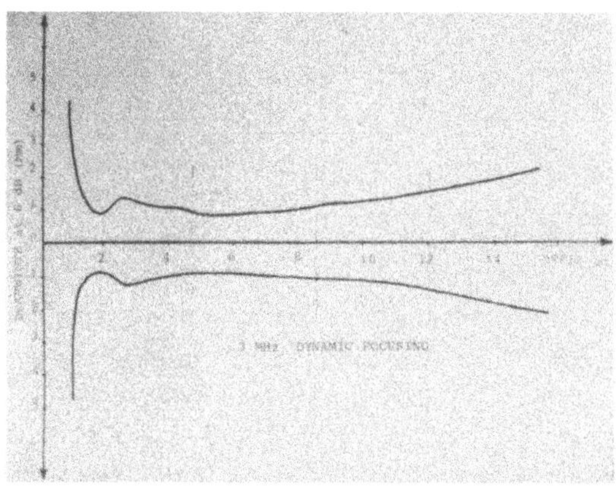

Figure 3 : Lateral resolution at 6 dB of a 3 MHz probe : dynamic focusing with 16 transducers, 1 x 10 mm^2 each.

1° The width of the resultant beam at 6 dB is between 1.75 and 2 mm, for depths between 2 and 10 cm ; on the other hand comparison with the results obtained without focusing, shows a more than half reduction in width over the whole depth of exploration. Hence a considerable advantage for lateral resolution on top of which there is a substantial increase in sensitivity.

2° We tried to use a minimum of focal areas in order to simplify electronic problems. Indeed the selection of areas requires electronic commutation : it is accompanied by transient noise which may take the form of continuous stripes in the image. They are very difficult to get rid of and 4 focal areas have proved to be sufficient

The final model will consist of a basic group of 24 transducers. On reception, a gradual increase in the number of transducers from the nearest focal area (3,5 cm - 12 items) to the furthest (14 cm - 24 items) makes it possible to work with a constant aperture. On transmission, the choice between several points of focusing : close up (4 cm), middle distance (7 cm) and far off (14 cm) is one way of optimising lateral resolution in relation to the chosen area in the image, or the dimensions of the organ being investigated.

I.3. Realisation and applications :

The step by step electronic translation of the group of 16 transducers on the array requires a multiplexing of delays and informations since each transducer, operating in 16 different positions in 16 successive groups, must be given 16 specific delays during each scan.

In each transmission network, the exciting impulses are suitable delayed and switched towards the pre-selected transmission groups, the transmitters being linked to the transducers. The same thing applies on reception : after selecting the reception groups, information is channelled by 16 analogous multiplexers towards 8 preamplifiers and 8 analog precision delay lines with intermediate outputs. After summation and amplification, focusing areas are selected by means of commutation. In order to avoid the stripes resulting from transient noise we chose to carry out these commutations almost at the end of the amplification network.

I.4. Clinical results :

The results obtained in vivo are noteworthy and the use over the last 3 years of this model (USABEL) in hospital has shown how efficient this method is in diagnosis. Probes of 3 to 5 MHz are used to visualize in real-time all organs that can be reached by ultrasounds.

II - COMPOUND SCANNING FROM ELECTRONICALLY STEERED BEAMS.

II.1. Aims of the research :

The goal of our research was, above all, to improve the quality of results by increasing the definition and quantity of informations appearing in the image and also to combine B echography with Doppler or T.M. modes.

II.2. Theoritical and practical aspects of the research :

Our aim was to realize a group of 3 images under 3 different incidences (figure 4). The first picture is obtained with normal scanning, the second one with an incidence of + θ and the third with a symmetrical incidence of - θ. Those 3 images are shown successively on the screen and superimposition is achieved optically. This method requires therefore the electronic steering of the beams under angles + θ and - θ, while maintaining the above mentioned focusing.

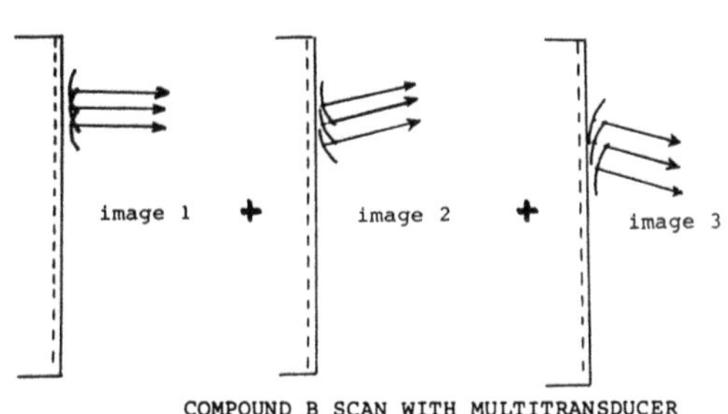

Figure 4 : In compound scanning with an array of transducers several images obtained under different angles are optically superimposed. Steering and focusing of the beams are performed electronically.

Figure 5 is a diagram of the realization principle of three successive images based on a group of 8 elements translated step by step along the array. The process described applies to reception (but it is identical in the case of transmission with a single focusing zone) : in image 1, signals are directed towards the focusing delay lines with delays T_1 to T_4, whose appropriate variation generates the dynamic focusing. In image 2, the adjunction of delays T'_1 to T'_8 results in the steering of the beam (their focusing is done by delays T_1 to T_4). For image 3, delays T'_1 to T'_8 are connected symmetrically to give deflection - θ.

We have adapted this technique to the arrays described above (100 transducers of 1 mm width) while keeping a basic group of 16 transducers. We have compared the width of the beam at 6 dB on transmission/reception for 16 elements of 3,5 MHz, at normal incidence and with an angle of about 12 degrees. One can observe that the beam is slightly larger in deflection. This result is linked to the limited number of transducers and the fact that they are somewhat too wide.

It is also essential to optimize delay and amplitude of the signals given by each transducer.

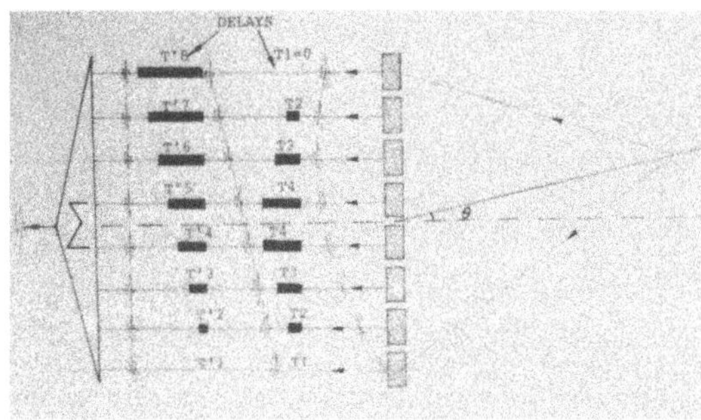

Figure 5 : In compound scanning, two sets of delay lines are used for focusing (T_1 to T_4) and steering (T'_1 to T'_8). Multiplexers are needed for translating these delays lines along the array of transducers.

These working conditions are likewise responsible for the presence of a grating lobe and lateral lobes that are larger on the deflected beams. A width of 1 mm results in giving each transducer an high directivity which is increased by the fact that the separation of elements is presently made by only cutting the electrodes. We might hope for a noticeable improvement of the size of the main beam and for a reduction of lobes by using a smaller width of the transducers (about one wavelength), i.e. a larger number of basic elements, and a total cutting of the transducers.

II.3. Developments :

This is a rather complex system. In addition to the multiplexing of electronic signals, commutation must be carried out so as to introduce the delays for steering and to produce symmetry for images 2 and 3. Further more, given the position of the transducers in the group, it is important to electronically balance each of the 16 lines.

Line and image sweep voltages for the visualization screen are obtained by superimposing, during images 2 and 3, the normal time bases with their cosine and sine, in suitable proportions. The final setting of the display is best obtained by using small targets placed in water. A diagrammatic synopsis of the apparatus is given in figure 6.

II.4. Results :

Experiments carried out at 3,5 MHz on targets placed in water have shown that excellent results and superimposition of the images over the whole area interrogated can be obtained. In figure 7, one can see the image of 3cotton threads echographed under 3 distinct incidences: after reconstituting the slanted scans, the echoes of each thread have coalesced perfectly.

Applications in vivo have made it possible to obtain the first images of the liver, the kidney (figure 8), the aorta and the heart. One can observe here yet again an excellent visualization of the different structures being studied.

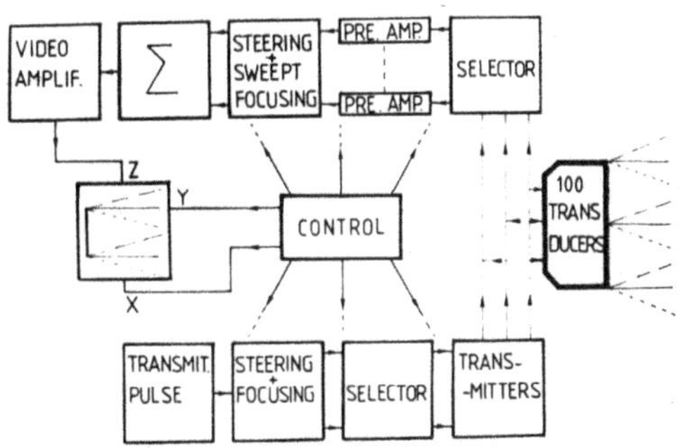

Figure 6 : Schematic diagramm of the real-time compound scanning system.

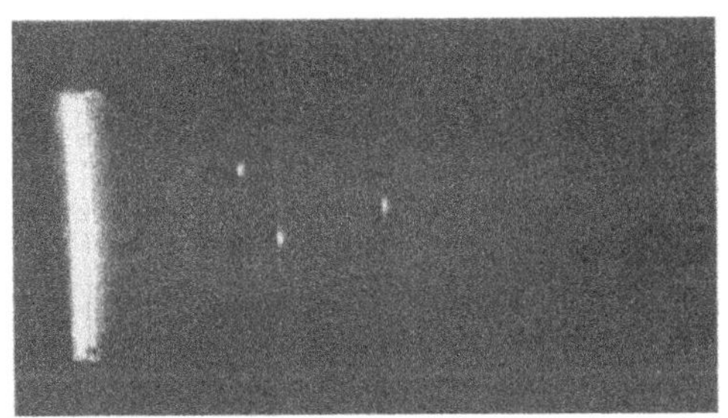

Figure 7 : Views of three cotton threads seen in water under incidences of 0°, + 12° and - 12°.

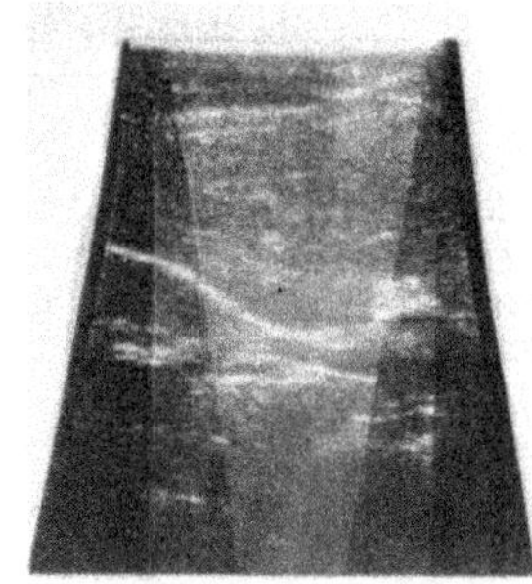

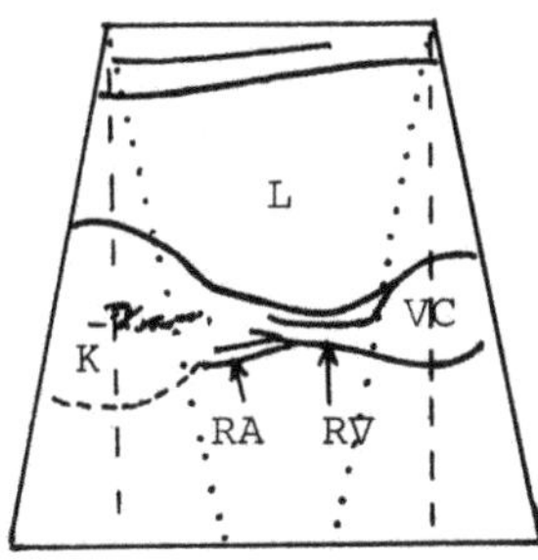

Figure 8 : Compound scanning in a normal subject. The horizontal cross-section shows liver (L), right kidney (K), renal artery (R.A.) renal vein (R.V.), vena cava (VC).

II.5. Discussion :

These are very encouraging results which show that with probes even better designed for the steering of the beams, it will be possible to obtain cross-sections under oblique incidences which are as good as classical views. Furthermore it is quite conceivable that this apparatus could be used in several ways :

a) classical electronic linear scanning,
b) images under oblique incidences at an angle chosen by the operator whilst continuing to use parallel explorating beams,
c) sectorial electronic scanning from a selected area of the array,
d) compound scanning using several superimposed incidences,
e) steering of the beams limited to one or a few lines, for T.M. or Doppler detection , associated with imaging.

The excellent localization of the volume of measure (a few mm^3) will doubtless make possible more accurate studies of parameters leading to the characterisation of tissues (diffraction, absorption, speed of sound). Three dimensions visualization which require a fairly homogenous resolution in all axes can be envisaged with such instruments. One should take into account how is important the combination of B and Doppler echographies : the use of this duplex system becomes relatively easy alongside multitransducer probes allowing the simultaneous visualization of the blood and other structures, or for the investigation of circulation in vessels that cannot be reached without supporting imaging (mesenteric, renal, coeliac arteries, portal vein). Finally a rapid visualization of excellent quality of organs such as the eye, the thyroïd gland, the breast or surface vessels, is quite likely thanks to the use of high frequency transducers.

III - REAL-TIME VISUALIZATION OF CIRCULATING BLOOD BY DOPPLER ECHOGRAPHY.

III.1. Principles :

The aim of Doppler imaging is to visualize moving structures, particularly the blood circulating in the vessels, by a transcutaneous and non-invasive method. This Doppler angiography is obtained by using a continuous or a pulsed Doppler system. The position of the probe and its orientation in the plane are detected by an electronic system which monitors the whole visualization (usually a remanence oscilloscope).

With a continuous wave apparatus the depth at which the Doppler signal is generated is not known. Consequently one can only get the projection of vascular axes as in angiography. The probe is moved in a way parallel to itself and sweeps accross the whole cutaneous area on the vessels being interrogated. Each time a Doppler signal is detected, the corresponding point on the visualization screen is lit up.

With a pulsed Doppler apparatus, cross-sections can be made as in echotomography, and those areas where a blood flow is detected can be visualized in depth. To this end, the probe is translated following a line on the surface of the skin. For each position of the probe, the shifting of the sample gate makes it possible to explore the depth in search of a Doppler signal.

It takes several minutes before a Doppler image can be obtained, which poses numerous problems for a routine check up or with fidgety patients. That is the reason why we have tried to develop real-time Doppler imaging so as to obtain a cross-section view of the circulatory blood in a fraction of a second. This is a tricky problem since there exist numerous limits in the rhythm at which informations are obtained.

III.2. Use of a multi-transducer system :

It was necessary to detect the Doppler signals at several points accross the vessel. Our first aim was therefore to design a multi-gated

Doppler apparatus (10 gates, 1,5 mm apart) working at a frequency of 4 MHz. With this apparatus one may trace the velocity curves at different depths inside the vessel or plot the real-time velocity profiles.

The rapid translation of the probe poses serious problems as it generates an interference Doppler signal caused by the displacement of the whole transmitter-receptor with regards to the reflecting structures. So the mechanical movement needed to be eliminated because of the continuous presence of a Doppler signal and we choose electronic commutation along an array. Consequently, the Doppler translation signal only appears during commutation : then the detector is fixed and can correctly detect the ultrasonic Doppler signal. The length of interrogation of each line is approximatively 1/200 of second, the probe being composed of 10 piézo-électric transducers. Image rate is approximatively 20/sec. In fact, owing to such factors as the amount of information, the reduction of commutation noise, etc... the present peak rate of the image, on the prototype that we have designed, is 15 per second.

The dimensions of the investigated area are 1,5 x 2 cm^2 and the overall image is made up of 100 dots. The image rate may be reduced at any time, or the scanning may be stopped in order to show the velocity curves and velocity profiles.

A diagram of the apparatus is shown in figure 9. An oscillator working at a frequency of 4 MHz monitors the basic electronic unit. Each of the ten transmitters is linked to a transducer of the probe ; the electric signals supplied by each receptor are selected by 10 gates and are sent through the amplifiers and attenuators. The velocity and direction of blood flow are detected for each depth ; the corresponding signals are then used to modulate the Wehnelt of the oscilloscope or to deliver the velocity curves and velocity profiles. The apparatus is sensitive to the direction of the blood flow and can therefore be used :

- either on its own as a multigated Doppler,
- or in junction with a real-time imaging system for a Doppler exploration following a line superimposed on the B scan,
- or else as a Doppler tomography system.

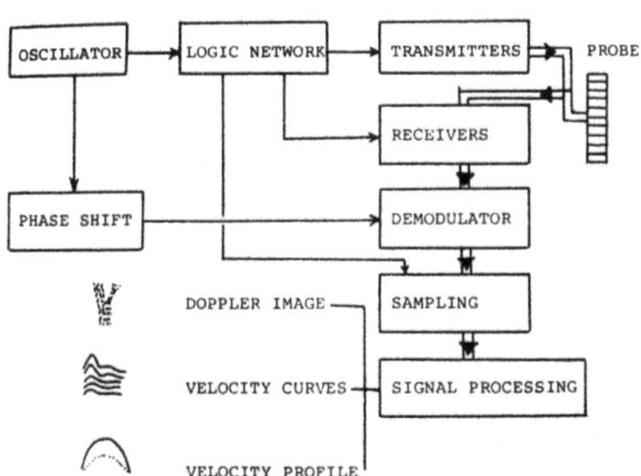

Figure 9 : Schematic diagramm of the multigated multitransducer Doppler system used for real-time blood flow imaging.

III.3. Results :

The possible application of this multitransducer multigated Doppler unit have been tested in vitro and in vivo. These experiments have shown that a fluid or a moving thread could be visualized fairly accurately with a grey scale in proportion to the speed. The display can only retain the positive Doppler informations (moving towards the captor) or the negative information (moving away) if necessary. This is useful in vivo for distinguishing arterial from venous circulation.

In vivo results were obtained with normal subjects (figure 10). Longitudinal and transversal cross-sections of the carotid arteries are obtained fairly easily. At each systole the image is lit up because of the increase in speed. During diastole, the external part of the common and internal carotids tends to disappear owing to the slow blood flow at this level. The external carotid disappears completely at the end of diastole since the flow is nil in this vessel at this time of the cardiac cycle. The jugular vein is eliminated by means of direction sensing presentation of the flow. A two-colour visualization system will make it possible to distinguish easily the two sets of information shown in the same image.

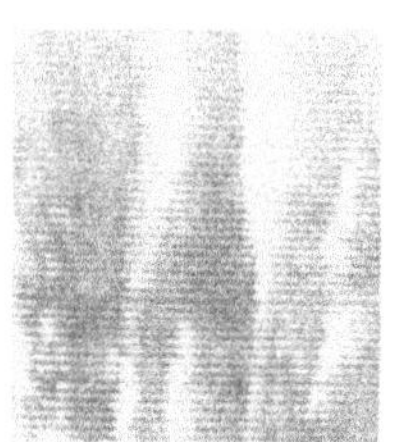

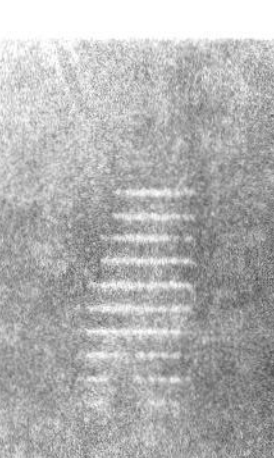

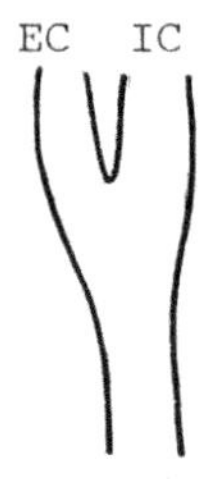

Figure 10 : Real-time cross sections of the carotid arteries : structures on the left (B mode echotomography, 5 MHz), blood on the right (multigated multitransducer system).These pictures are complementary and could be superimposed in the future.

The combined imaging of the anatomical structures and of the circulating blood, means for the future a powerful method of analysis of the vascular system and the heart. The realization of rapid imaging by B echography has already made it possible to obtain remarkable results. The visualization of the blood is much more complex but we can in the near future look forward to obtaining the superimposition of a small size Doppler image on a real-time echographic cross-section.

IV - CONCLUSION.

Rapid multitransducer echotomography systems have remarkable potentialities because of the numerous opportunities they make available in practice. Dynamic focusing, the steering of the beams, the visualization of the circulatory blood are examples of possible developments but one can expect a still greater evolution towards volume visualization and tissue identification, for instance. The quality of echotomographic images has become outstanding thanks to the real-time processing of ultrasonic signal which considerably alleviates the practical problems encountered by the operator. We can then look forward to an intensive use of this type of apparatus in a near future.

This work was supported by I.N.S.E.R.M. (ATP 35.76.67) and D.G.R.S.T. (contrat 76.7.1468) grants.

BIBLIOGRAPHIE.

1 - P. ALAIS, M. FINK, J. PERRIN : Acoustic imaging with an electronically focused and scanned array.
Ultrasonics in Medicine, Münich, may 75-80, 1975.

2 - D.W. BAKER, D.E. STRANDNESS Jr, S.L. JOHNSON : Pulsed Doppler techniques : some examples from the University of Washington.
Ultrasound Med., Biol., Vol. 2, pp. 251-262, 1976.

3 - J-P BOURNAT, P. PERONNEAU, A. HERMENT : Yes-no ultrasonic Doppler method of detection for vascular imaging.
Ultrasound Med., Biol., vol. 3, pp. 105-115, 1977.

4 - M. BRANDESTINI : Signalverarbeitung in perkutanen Ultraschall Doppler Blutfluss Messgeräten.
Dissertation I.B.T., Zürich, 1976.

5 - D. CARPENTER, M. DADD and G. KOSSOF : Multiple Mode, scanning linear array.
2nd meeting of the World Federation for Ultrasound in Medicine and Biology. July 22-27 1979, Miyazaki, Japan.

6 - P.H. DEFRANOULD and SOUQUET : Ultrasonic array design and performance.
Echocardiology, C.T. Lancée Ed.,published by Martinus Nijhoff, The Hague 1979, pp. 395-412.

7 - R.W. GILL : Pulsed Doppler with B-mode imaging for quantitative blood flow measurement.
Ultrasound in Medicine and Biology, vol. 5, pp. 223-235.

8 - C.M. LIGVOET, J. RIDDER, C.T. LANCEE : A dynamically focused multiscan system.
Echocardiology, N. Bom Ed., published by Martinus Nijhoff, The Hague, 1977, pp. 313-332.

9 - L. POURCELOT, J-M POTTIER, M. BERSON, Th. PLANIOL : A fast ultrasonic imaging system : USABEL.
Ultrasonics in Medicine, Münich, may, pp. 54-58, 1975.

10 - L. POURCELOT : Echo-Doppler systems. Applications for the detection of cardiovascular disorders. In : Echocardiology, N. Bom Ed., published by Martinus Nijhoff, The Hague, pp. 245-256, 1977.

11 - L. POURCELOT, M. BERSON, A. RONCIN : Real-time compound B-scans with multitransducers.
2nd Meeting of the World Federation of Ultrasound in Medicine and Biology. Miyazaki, Japan, july 22-29 1979.

12 - L. POURCELOT : Real-time blood flow imaging. In : Echocardiology, pp. 421-429, 1979, C.T. Lancée Ed., Martinus Nijhoff Publ., The Hague/Boston/London.

13 - L. POURCELOT, M. BERSON : L'imagerie à ultrasons. Possibilités et évolution.
R.B.M. revue européenne de Biotechnique Médicale, vol. 1, n° 5, septembre-octobre 1979, pp. 327-333.

14 - M.P. SPENCER, J.M. REID, P.S. PAULSON : Diagnosis of carotid artery disease and cerebral vascular insufficiency with Doppler angiography and ophthalmic artery sonography.
Cardiovascular applications of ultrasound. Ch. 21, R.S. Reneman,

Ed., Amsterdam, 1974, North Holland Publ. Co.

15 - D.E. STRANDNESS Jr., D.S. SUMMER : A new approach to arterial visualization. Ch. 19 in Cardiovascular application of ultrasound. R.S. Reneman Ed., Amsterdam, North Holland Publ. Co., 1974.

16 - F.L. THURSTONE, OT VON RAMM : Electronic beam scanning for imaging. Ultrasonics in Medicine, Rotterdam, june 1973, pp. 43-48.

HIGH SPEED CARDIAC X-RAY COMPUTERIZED TOMOGRAPHY

by

C. ROUX
E. TOURNIER

CENTRE D'ETUDES NUCLEAIRES
Laboratoire d'Electronique et de
Technologie de l'Informatique
85 X - 38041 Crenoble Cedex
France

ABSTRACT

The first part reviews the various studies of high speed X-ray computerized tomographic systems.

The second part deals with a new high speed multislice X-ray tomographic system which has been studied for cardiac imaging : a method for producing a sequence of very intense X-ray sources has been tested in using flash X-ray tubes. An annular array of about 150 tubes is technologically feasible on a 2 meter diameter ring. The main advantage of that solution is to obtain very intense pulsed beams.

A stationary solid state circular multidetector is needed. Cadmium-telluride detectors seem very well suited for pulsed X-ray beam detection.

The main expected characteristics are given and the initial test results illustrating the effectiveness of this technique are discussed.

1. INTRODUCTION

Currently available computerized tomographic systems (CT scanners) are able to produce high quality images of one section through the human body. But images of the beating human heart suffer degradation because of cardiac motion during the scan time.

We have undertaken studies to explore the feasibility of a high speed multislice CT system which allows the production of 4 images of 7 mm thick adjacent transverse section within a 20 ms scan time.

2. CARDIAC IMAGING : THE VARIOUS PROJECTS AND TECHNIQUES IN C.A.T.

2.1. Electrocardiograph (E.C.G.) gated computerized tomography

Principle

Several attempts have been made to use conventional CT scanners in cardiac imaging |1|, |2| : a gated image is formed from data collected during a selected phase of the cardiac cycle from series of consecutive heart beats. Presently there are two different approaches for obtainning data for the reconstruction :

1. Prospectively by synchronizing data acquisition with the cardiac cycle via E.C.G. control. Prior to performing the CT scan one decides which part of the R-R interval is to be examined. Then data acquisition occurs only during a specified time period keyed to an E.C.G. signal. If one wishes to examine another part of the cardiac cycle one must perform another CT scan with the data acquisition keyed to a different interval of the ECG cycle.
2. Retrospectively by selecting appropriate angular projection data and correlating them to corresponding segments of the E.C.G. (see fig. 1) without repeating the CT scan.

Results

The second technique is most often used because it is the most flexible : images of a heart during various phases of the cycle are produced. Contrast media are injected during the scan which is achieved with minor hardware and software modifications that permit longer scan time. The results shows that gating improves time resolution despite the loss of spatial resolution caused by the method itself.

The gated computerized tomography is limited by the relatively long data acquisition time which implies :

- That no respiratory motion nor cardiac aperiodicities may occur.
- That the whole activity from cycle to cycle and the injected contrast media must be stationary.

It seems in fact |7| that all these assumptions do not hold. Consequently, the reconstruction of the heart images requires development of high speed systems. Some of the most promising will now be briefly described.

2.2. High speed three dimensional CT system -

System design

A dynamic spatial reconstruction (DSR) system is under investigation in the biodynamics research unit of the Mayo Clinic-Rochester - USA |3|. The DSR scanner consists of 28 X-ray tubes equally spaced in a semicircle and 28 sets of image intensifiers and video cameras arranged in the opposing semicircle behind a curved fluorescent screen (Fig. 2).

Main characteristics

This system allows the production of 240 images of 1 mm thick adjacent transverse sections. One complete scan is performed within 10 ms by pulsing each of the 28 X-ray tubes in succession during 0.34 ms each. The entire system can rotate continuously around the patient to provide up to 240 equispaced wiews around 360° within 2 seconds (see table 1). A high speed computer interface will provide high-speed digitization (14 MHz), high speed storage and retrieval of the data. The computation time will be about 10 ms per cross section and about 2,4 seconds for each volume of 240 cross sections. A 3-D dynamic display will be developed in order to dynamically visualize both sections and volumes.

This DSR scanner seems very well suited for the production of three dimensionnal viewing of organ volume and the heart vascular system.

2.3. High speed multislice CT systems -

The main feature of these systems consists in the X-ray source : the classical Coolidge tube is not used but rather an X-ray source with circular anode and azimuthally swept pulsed electron beam or a multiple flash X-ray tube array.

2.3.1. Systems with swept electron beam X-ray source -

Design

The essential component of such systems is the X-ray generator : the rotational movement is achieved by an electronically controled electron beam and no mechanical motion is required (Fig. 3). Iinuma et al. |4| were the first to propose such a scanner whereas a similar system was constructed by Haimson |6|. The machine designed by Boyd et al |5| differs slightly since it uses a 180° geometry.

Specific aspects

The choice of this technique leads to difficulties that have to be resolved :

- The long drift distance and the high electron currents cause space charge defocussing which can enlarge the focal source size.

- The deflection, inflection and focussing coils introduce high order aberrations at the target plane.

- Small variations in electron energy leads to focal source movement.

Main characteristics

The most important characteristic of these systems is that they generate measurements of a large number of views (more than 200) within a very short time (from 10 to 50 ms). A generator power of about 150 kV with current of 200 mA is sufficient to develop tomographic images of 2 mm resolving power and of a few per cent density resolution (see table 1), However they do not allow a real 3-D reconstruction but rather multislice reconstruction.

2.3.2. High speed multiple flash X-ray tube system -

Such a system is under investigation in the CENG-LETI laboratories - Grenoble, France. The various features of this project will now be discussed.

3 - THE LETI PROJECT

3.1. Introduction

We propose to achieve a high speed multislice machine producing image qualities that can be compared to the ones produced by existing whole body CT scanners by means of technologies under development in our laboratories. The spatial and density resolution, the low scan time and the ability to produce sequential slice images will allow static and dynamic cardiac investigation.

Technological choices

The most important component of a high-speed scanner is the X-ray source which must have two qualities in order to obtain a good density resolution :

- It must be powerful enough to minimize the photon noise on the reconstructed image.

- It must permit the acquisition of a great number of view data to minimize artefacts caused by the high contrast structures surrounding the heart.

Because of its high power and its low study cost we have chosen a multitube flash circular X-ray source. The relatively limited number of views can be increased by machine rotation.

The second important component is the detection system. With regard to the very short pulse duration of the emitted X-rays, cadmium-telluride detectors seem very well suited for detection. Furthermore, their low cost will allow us to achieve high diameter detector rings with a great number of cells and subsequently a good spatial resolution multislice scanner.

Design (see figures 4,5,6)

The 360° circular X-ray source will permit 121 fan beam to be emitted within 20 ms. 2 or 4 1500 detectors rings will be assembled symetrically on each side of the X-ray source ring. Each fan beam will provide 310 data per view. The slow system rotation will allow a 60 ms scan and increase the X photons number three fold and the number of views up to 363 (see table 2).

Machine operation

- Static images (morphology - myocardium study - cardiac volumes) : one or two 60 ms scans can be produced to obtain images at various phases of the cardiac cycle. These acquisitions can be repeated during several cardiac cycles after a 30 mm patient shift.

- Dynamic investigation (wall motion) : 20 ms scans can be repeated during a whole cardiac cycle at a rate of 25, 16.7, 10 per second.

Furthermore, a high spatial and density resolution 120 ms scan mode is possible.

3.2. Image quality

The quality of the reconstructed image is specifically related to the choice of the X-ray source and of the detector. However two important aspects should be discussed : the number of views required and the reconstruction algorithm.

We have made some experiments with a thoracic phantom and tried to reconstruct images with various numbers of projections. The results (figures 7,8) clearly show the necessity of generating more than 100 views around an angle of 360°. A quantitative analysis of the relative standard deviation of three 169 points square zones (the image size was 362 x 362 points) has been made (fig. 9). The results depend on the surrounding density and shows the noise increases as the number of views decreases. However beyond 400 views their is no further image improvement.

The second important choice concerns the algorithm. Even with high speed systems, the number of views will not be great enough to make a data ordering into parallel geometry. Therefore, the algorithm must be a fan beam one. Furthermore, a filtered-backprojection algorithm seems highly suitable : it could permit real time acquisition data processing and the reconstruction of a limited image region (the region of interest i.e. the heart in cardiac imaging).

3.3. X-ray source

X-ray emission is achieved by a circular array of 121 flash tubes.

Flash tube principle

In a high vacuum (10^{-6} mm Hg) field effect emitted electrons are extracted from a cathode (K) in a short time and accelerated towards the top of a conic anode (A) to produce X-ray pulse (Fig. 10). The electric arc between the anode and the cathode may be caused by a capacitor discharge or by a high voltage pulse on a trigger electrode. For higher than 200 kV voltage pulses, flash X-ray tubes are connected to a Marx generator (see Fig. 11) : voltage pulses of a large amplitude are generated when capacitors (C) initially charged in parallel are series-connected with the aid of spark gaps (E). If the number of capacitors, or stages, is n, the amplitude of the output pulse of the unloaded Marx's multi-stage circuit is :

$$V_t = n \, |- V|$$

Preliminary results

Some experiments are currently carried out with a flash tube and Marx generator system lent by l'Institut Franco-Allemand of Saint-Louis - France. Some well established characteristics of such X-ray tubes are the following |8|:

- The X-ray pulse duration, measured at full width half maximum is 20 ns.

- The focus diameter is 2-3 mm.

Results have been obtained by using a ten stage Marx generator and scintillator-photodiode detectors. Operating at 280 kV high voltage anode pulse the number of X-ray photons at the mean 140 KeV energy is about 5.10^7 per cm^2 at 1 meter in the axial direction for a corresponding dose of 5 mR per flash. The angular distribution of X-ray intensity was also measured (Fig. 12) the emitted fan beam well covers the 500 mm diameter scan zone.

All these characteristics are appropriate for high speed cardiac imaging.

3.4. Detection

Our laboratories are currently studying and developing wide-spread radioprotection products in particular high efficiency cadmium-telluride polycrystals detectors. These direct charge collecting devices operate at room temperature and their technology is cheap and easy. The main characteristics of such detectors are the following :

- Size	3 x 4 x 15 mm
- Density	5.86 g/cm
- 150 KeV detection efficiency	∿ 60 %
- Expended energy to create an electron-hole pair	4.43 eV
- Collection efficiency (under development)	∿ 50 %

As the current pulse duration is very short it is quite easy to overcome the trail effect of these detectors by doing differential measurements (see Fig. 13).

4 - CONCLUSION -

A new high speed multislice X-ray tomographic system of low cost technology is being studied for cardiac imaging. A circular array of 121 flash X-ray tubes will provide very intense pulsed beams for a total dose of 1,5 R.X-Ray detection will be achieved by a stationnary circular cadmium-telluride multidetector.

This system will allow the production of image of the human heart with qualities that can be compared to the ones produced by existing whole body CT scanners and with a time resolution of 20 ms.

REFERENCES

1 HARELL GS, GUTHANER DF, BREIMAN RS, MOREHOUSE CC, SEPPI EJ, MARSHALL WHJR, WEXLER L. "Stop action cardiac computed tomography" - Radiology 123 : 515-517, May 1977.

2 BERNINGER WH, REDINGTON RW, DOHERTY P., LIPTON MJ, CARLSSON E. - "Gated cardiac scanning : canine studies" - J. Computer-assisted tomography 3(2) : 155-163, April 1979

3 ROBB RA, RITMAN EL, GILBERT BK, KINSEY JH, HARRIS LD, WOOD EH - "The DSR : A high speed three-dimensional X-ray computed tomography system for Dynamic Spatial Reconstruction of the heart and circulation" - IEEE Trans. Nucl. Sci. NS-26 N° 2 : 2713-2717, April 1979.

4 IINUMA TA, TATENO Y, UMEGAKI Y, WATANABE E. - "Proposed system for Ultrafast Computed Tomography" - J. Computer Assisted Tomography 1(4) : 494-499, 1977.

5 BOYD DP, GOULD RG, QUINN JR, SPARKS R, STANLEY JH, HERRMANNSFELDT - "A proposed dynamic cardiac 3-D densitometer for early detection and evaluation of heart disease" - IEEE Trans. Nucl. Sci. NS-26 N°2 : 2724-2727, April 1979.

6 HAIMSON J. - "X-ray source without moving parts for ultra-high speed tomography" IEEE Trans. Nucl. Sci. NS 26 n° 2, 2857-2861, April 1979.

7 ROBB RA, RITMAN EL, HARRIS LD, WOOD EH. - "Dynamic three-dimensional X-ray computed tomography of the heart, lungs and circulation" - IEEE Trans. Nucl. Sci. NS-26 N° 1, Febr. 1979 : 1646-1660.

8 JAMET F, THOMER G. - Flash Radiography -Elsevier Scientific Publishing Company - Amsterdam 1976.

		MAYO CLINIC Rochester USA (3)	National Institute of Radiological Science Chiba JAPAN (4)	University of California San-Francisco USA (5)
Geometry		3-D 180°	2D around 360°	multislice around 180°
X-ray source		28 X-ray tubes	azimuthally swept electron beam	azimuthally swept electron beam
Detectors		fluorescent screen + 28 sets of image intensifiers and video cameras	high speed scintillators	scintillators (BGO) + photomultipliers
	Scan time	10 ms for 28 views	⩽ 10 ms	50 ms
Estimate characteristics	Spatial resolution	~ 1 mm (240 views) ~ 2-3 mm (112 views)	3 - 6 mm	1,6 mm mode C 2,2 mm mode A and B (FWHM)
	Density resolution	~ 1 % (240 views) ~ 2-3 % (112 views)	1 %	7 % - mm mode B 10 % - mm mode A and C contrast detail perceptability)
	Number of slices	240	?	8 (mode A) within 200 ms
	Number of views	28 → 240 (180°) (360°)	?	210 mode A,B, C 420 mode D
	Dose	60 mR (112 views) 2 R (120 volumes)	?	0,26 R mode A,B,C (average skin dose)

TABLE 1 : Main features of under investigation cardiac scanners

X-ray tubes ring diameter	1600 mm
Number of X-ray tubes	121
Mean energy of X-ray photons	120-150 KeV
Electric energy of a single flash	30 J
Axial dose per flash	10 mR
Focus diameter	2-3 mm
Detector ring diameter	1500 mm
Number of detector per ring	1500
Number of rings	2 or 4
Detection efficiency	> 60 %
Rotation speed	~ 50°/sec.
Reconstruction area diameter	500 mm
Section thickness	30 mm
Number of simultaneous slices	2 or 4
Collimator efficiency	50 %
Scan time	30 ms - 60 ms
Limit spatial resolution	3 lines pair/cm
Density resolution (standard deviation for a 200 mm diameter water cylinder and 60 m.sec mode)	0,5 %
Dose (60 ms mode)	~ 1,5 R

TABLE 2 : Characteristics of the proposed multiple flash X-ray tubes high speed scanner.

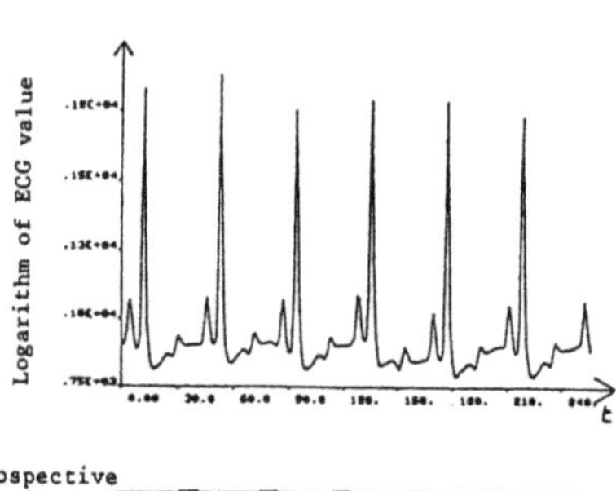

Fig. 1 : Principle of gated CT

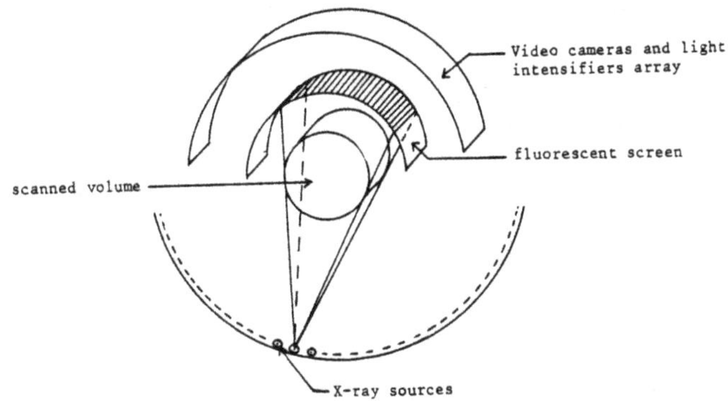

Fig. 2 : schematic drawing of the DSR (from (3))

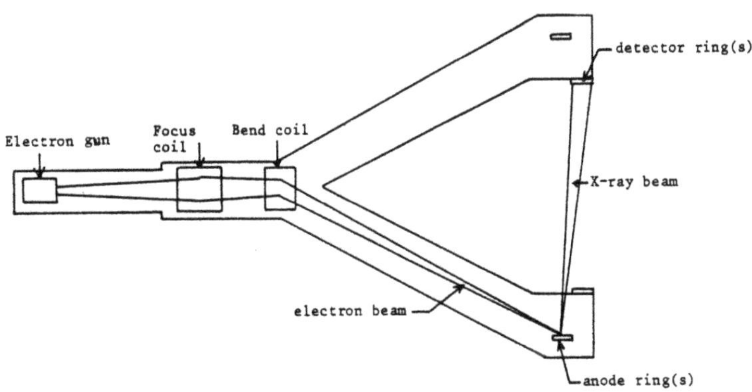

Fig. 3 : Schematic cross-section of a high speed swept electron beam X-ray source scanner (from (5))

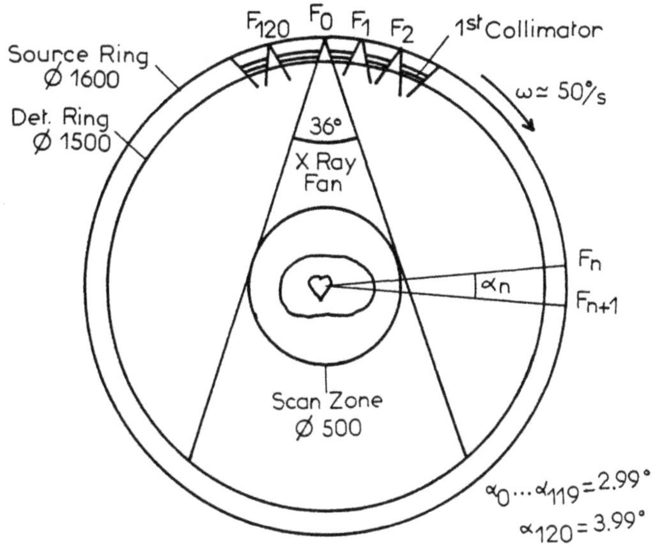

Fig. 4 : Front view of the proposed scanner.

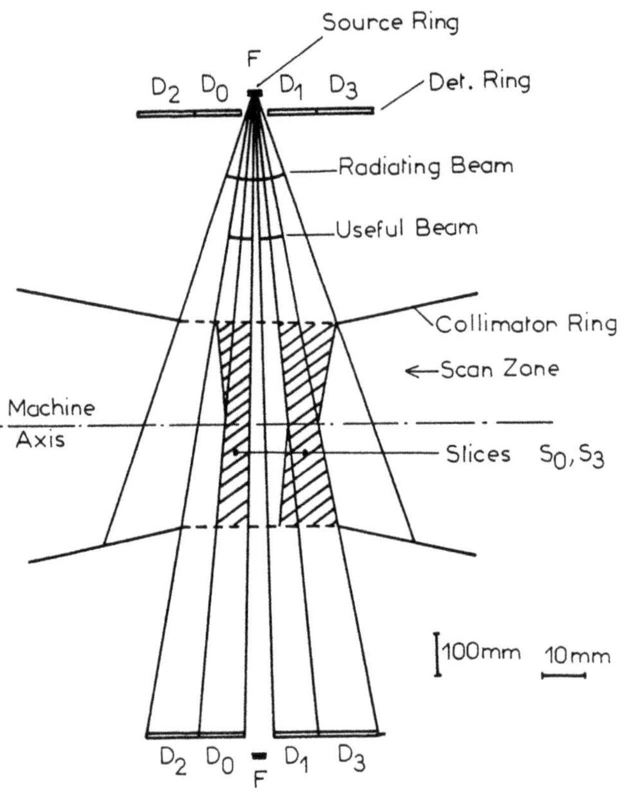

Fig. 5 : Schematic longitudinal cross section showing collimators geometry and the multiple slices.

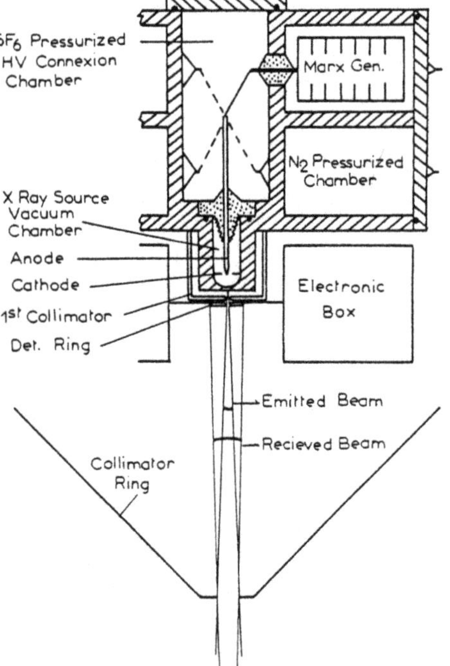

Fig. 6 : Schematic cross section of the whole X-ray emission system.

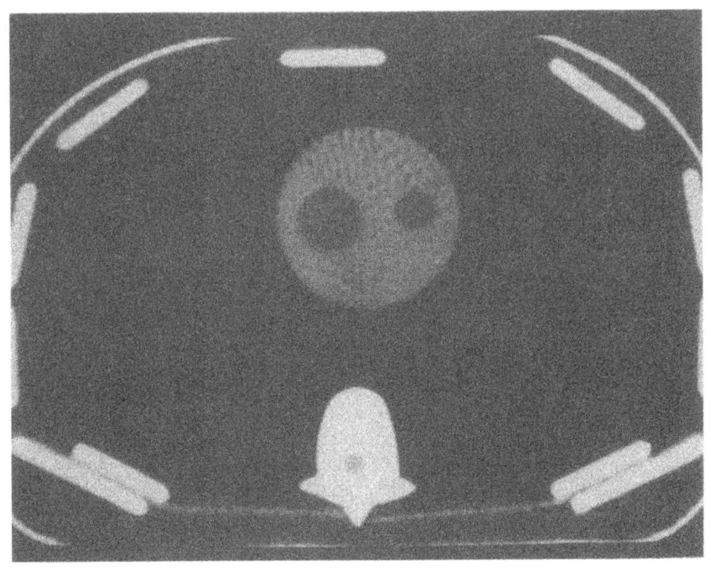

Fig. 7 : Reconstructed image of a thoracic phantom from 192 equispaced views around 360°

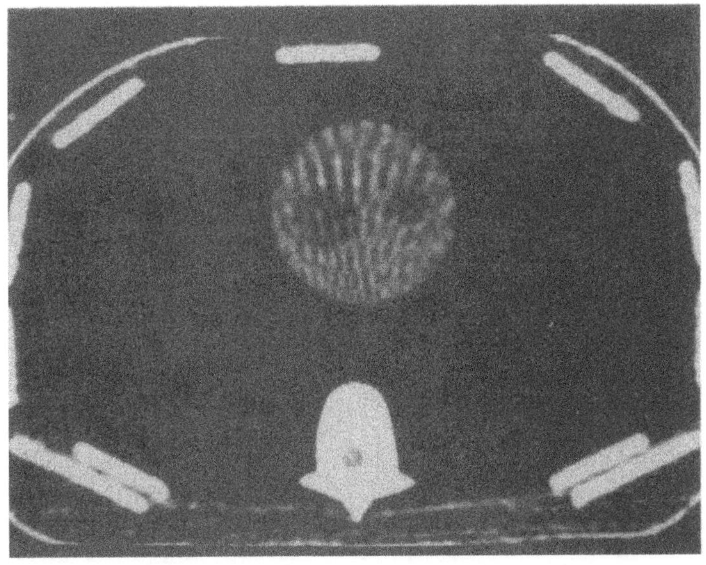

Fig. 8 : Reconstructed image of a thoracic phantom from 96 equispaced views around 360°

Fig. 9 : Relative standard deviation analysis of three zones of the phantom image as a function of the views number.

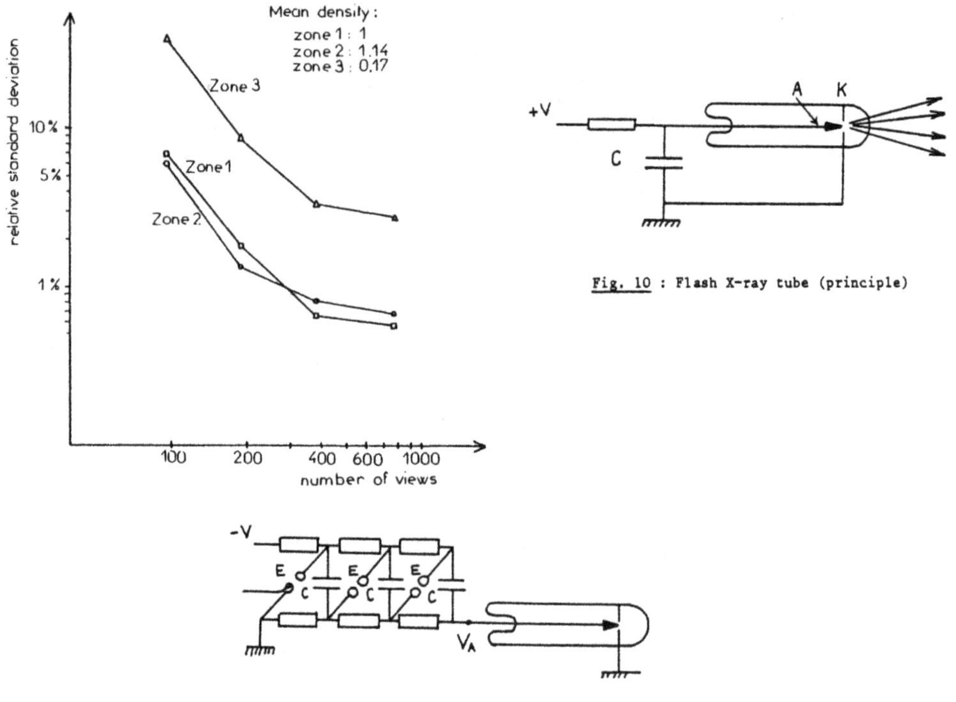

Fig. 10 : Flash X-ray tube (principle)

Fig. 11 : The Marx generator and the flaxh X-ray tube (principle)

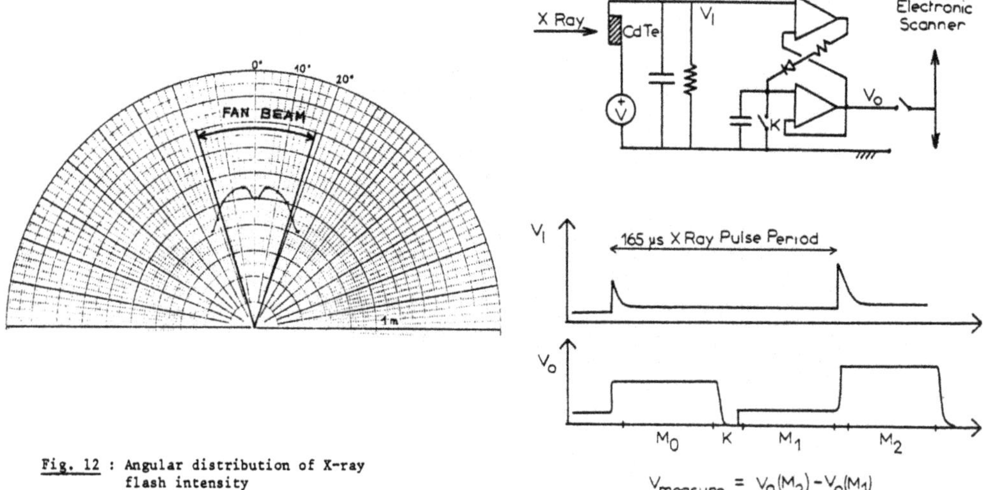

Fig. 12 : Angular distribution of X-ray flash intensity

Fig. 13 : Principle of a detection data acquisition sequence.

APPROACHES TO REGION OF INTEREST TOMOGRAPHY

by

Orhan Nalcioglu
Department of Radiological Sciences
University of California
Irvine, California 92717
U.S.A.

1. INTRODUCTION

The objective of computed tomography is to obtain good quality images while keeping the dose to the patient as low as possible. Unfortunately, the interdependence of patient dose, contrast and spatial resolution puts limitations on the arbitrary variations of these parameters. In other words, one can not change one without affecting the others. In some clinical situations, reconstruction of the whole slice is not needed, especially when a disease is well localized from a previous study and a follow-up scan of the same area is required. If one could scan and reconstruct only the region of interest (ROI) one could increase the spatial resolution within the region of interest and reduce the dose in the outside region. However, it should be remembered that since the same dose-contrast-resolution relation mentioned earlier still applies, in order to improve the resolution within the ROI one would also have to increase the dose in that region. Thus the region of interest tomography techniques could involve a redistribution of the dose within the whole slice if one tries to improve the resolution within the ROI.

The present reconstruction algorithms require the collection of the x-ray projection data of the whole slice even when one is only interested in a small region within the slice. If one does not scan the whole slice, one encounters artifacts of varying magnitude depending on the ratio of the size of the scanned region to that of the whole region. Before we discuss the methods to reduce these artifacts, it would be instructive to see how these artifacts manifest themselves. In Figure 1, we have a mathematical head phantom known as the Shepp phantom. It consists of several ellipses and circles of varying densities. The details of the phantom can be found in reference 1.

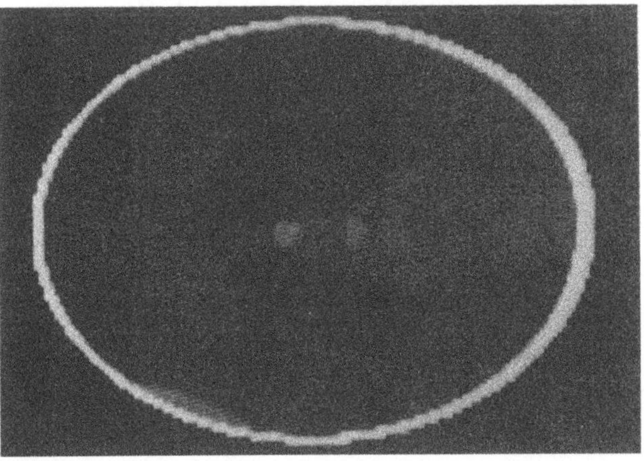

Figure 1. Shepp head phantom

Let us assume that we are interested in a circular region of radius 1.25 cm which is centrally located within the whole slice. A magnified view of the region of interest is shown in Figure 2.

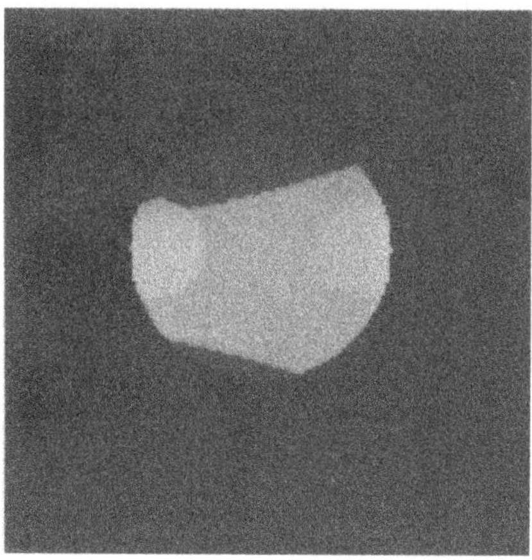

Figure 2. The region of interest (magnified)

If only the ROI is scanned and reconstructed one obtains the image shown in Figure 3. It is seen that the gray levels near the edge of reconstruction region are artificially elevated with respect to the center indicating the severity of the artifacts.

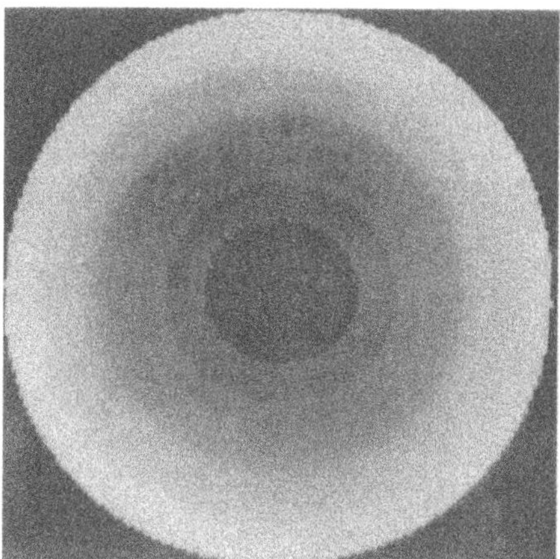

Figure 3. Cupping artifact due to truncation (Reproduced with permission from Proc. SPIE 206: 98, 1979).

The cupping artifact seen in Fig. 3 is similar in appearance to the beam hardening cupping artifact [2] but of different origin. It is due to the fact that the commonly used reconstruction algorithms assume that the whole object is seen from all views whereas in this case one does not cover the whole object but only the region of interest.

Section 2 will be devoted to different methods for the region of interest tomography. A discussion of these methods will be given in Section 3.

2. METHODS

2.1. Spatially Varying Irradiation Scan (SVIS)

This method was proposed by Wagner [3] and makes use of additional data outside the ROI. In the SVIS approach, one irradiates the whole object but with different x-ray intensities. The x-rays which pass through outside the ROI are filtered by means of an absorber before they are incident on the object. The physical implementation of the SVIS is illustrated in Figure 4.

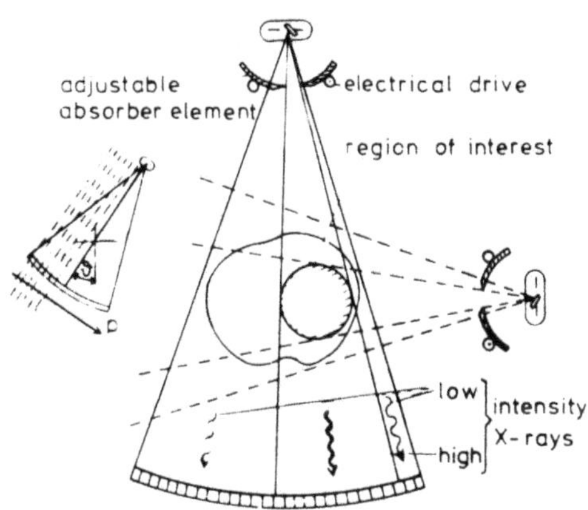

Figure 4. Implementation of SVIS for a rotate-rotate scanner (Reproduced with permission from IEEE Trans. Nuc. Sci. NS-26: 2866, 1979)

Thin filters are placed in front of the x-ray tube so as to reduce the x-ray intensity (or dose to the patient) in the external region. The ROI portion of the x-rays is not subject to this additional filtration and thus get the full exposure. By changing the filter aperture one can vary the size of the region of interest. Before starting the scan, the operator specifies the center and the diameter of the desired region from a priori knowledge. It should be emphasized that if the center of rotation and the center of the ROI do not overlap one would have to move the filters as the x-ray tube rotates. Figure 5 shows two examples of this method.

Since the number of photons which pass through the external region are heavily filtered one gets very noisy images of the external region as shown in Figures 5a and 5b. It is also seen from these figures that the noisy data outside the ROI does not seriously affect the reconstructed image within the ROI. This is due to the fact that the noisy data from the external region enters into the ROI during the convolution process via the tail of the convolution filter. The two images shown in Figs. 5a-5b were obtained with different amounts of filtration and are for different size region-of-interest.

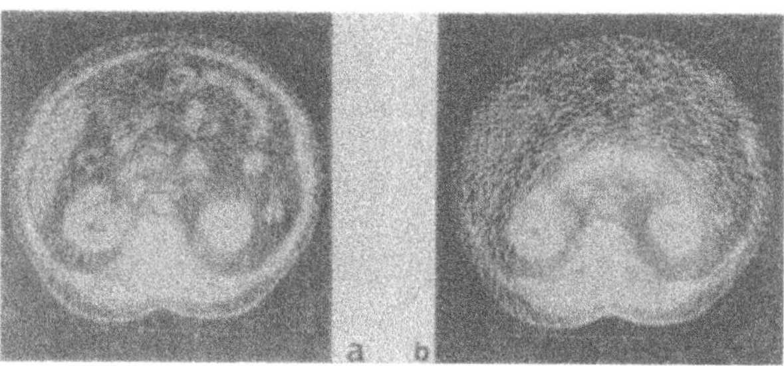

Figure 5. Examples of the SVIS
(Reproduced with permission from IEEE
Trans. Nuc. Sci. NS-26: 2866, 1979)

2.2. Truncation-Extrapolation Technique

In contrast to the previous method, here it is assumed that the data outside the ROI is not available at all. This method was proposed by Wagner [3] and Lewitt [4] independently. A possible implementation scheme proposed by Wagner [3] is shown in Figure 6.

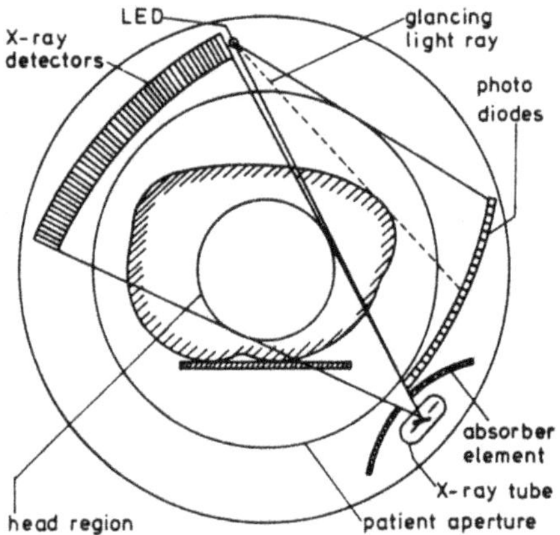

Figure 6. Truncated scanning
(Reproduced with permission from IEEE
Trans. Nuc. Sci. NS-26: 2886, 1979)

The x-rays outside the ROI are completely stopped by means of absorber elements and an optical set up is used to trace the boundaries of the object. The extrapolation is performed as shown in Figure 7.

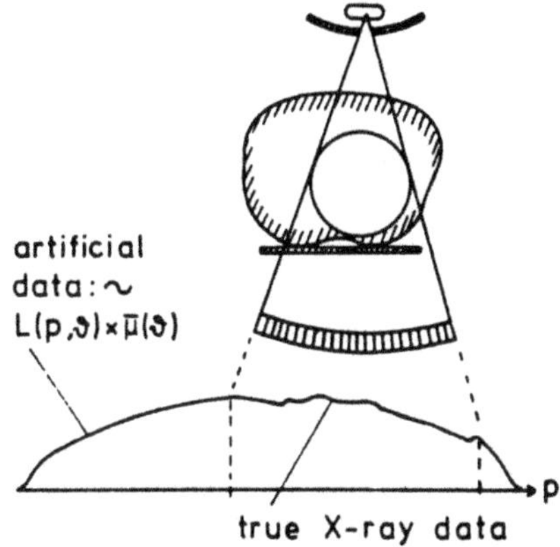

Figure 7. Extrapolation (Reproduced with permission from IEEE Trans. Nuc. Sci. NS-26: 2886, 1979)

The artificial data outside the ROI is obtained by extrapolating the true x-ray projection data to the optically determined object boundary as shown in Figure 7. At certain angles, there are some problems with the optical boundary detection technique due to the nontransparency of the patient couch. In addition, when one has a high density material such as bone outside the region of interest the extrapolation technique would not be able to account for it and this would result in the generation of some artifacts in the ROI.

Figure 8 shows a mathematical thorax phantom. The circular region of interest is also shown in Figure 8.

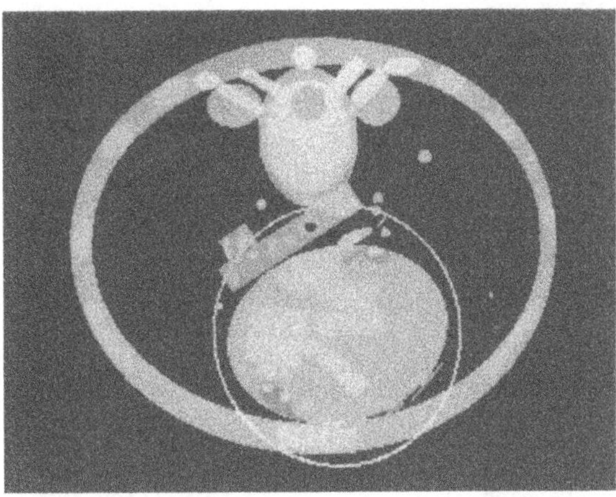

Figure 8. Thorax phantom and the ROI (Reproduced with permission from Med. Phys. 6: 412, 1979).

The next figure shows a density profile through the ROI.

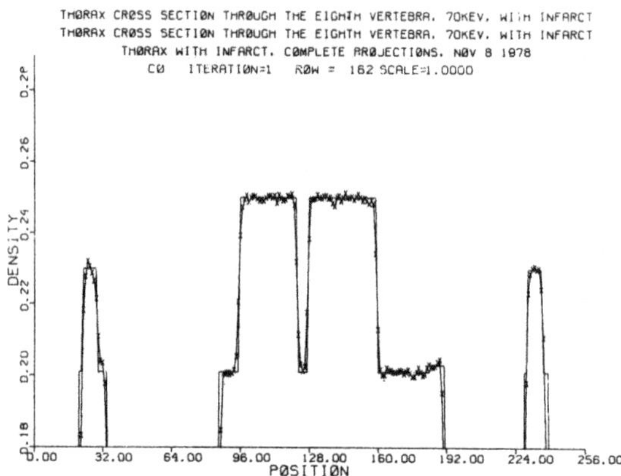

Figure 9. Density profile through the ROI (Reproduced with permission from Med. Phys. 6: 412, 1979).

The flatness of the response in the central region is an indication of constant density of certain areas. If one scans only the region of interest and reconstructs the whole object one obtains the reconstructed image shown in Figure 10.

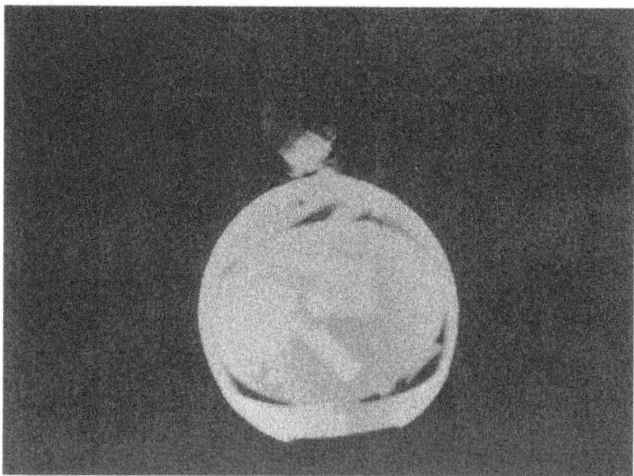

Figure 10. Reconstruction after truncated scanning (Reproduced with permission from Med. Phys. 6: 412, 1979)

This figure shows cupping artifacts similar to the one in Figure 3. A density profile through the same row is shown in Figure 11. The artificial elevation towards the edges is another demonstration of the cupping artifact.

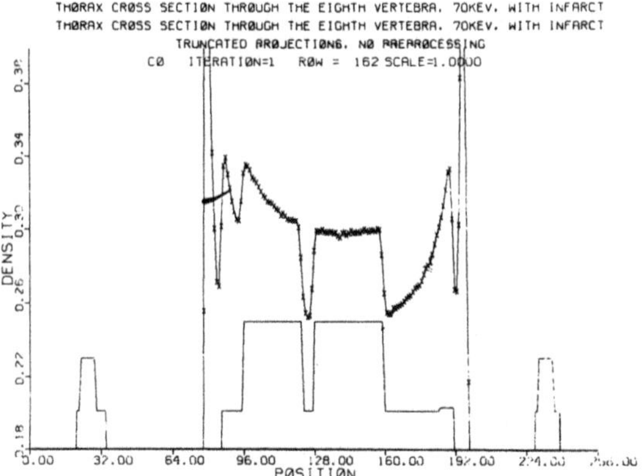

Figure 11. Density profile through the reconstructed image after truncated scanning (Reproduced with permission from Med. Phys. 6: 412, 1979)

The next figure shows the ROI image after the external projection data is artificially extrapolated.

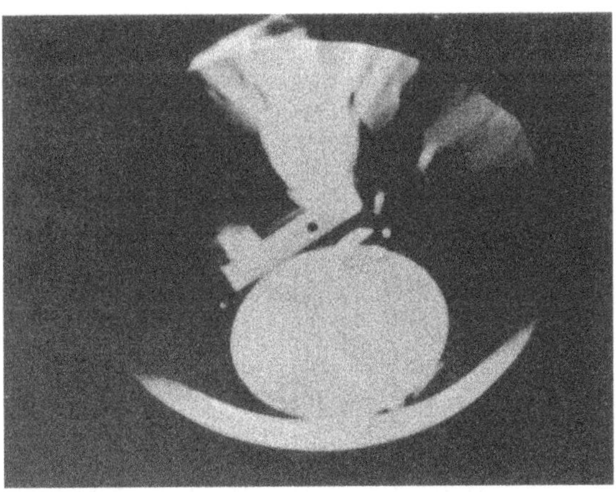

Figure 12. Reconstructed ROI after extrapolation correction (Reproduced with permission from Med. Phys. 6: 412, 1979)

It is seen that most of the cupping artifact has been removed by filling the external projection data artificially. Figure 13 is the density profile through the same row for Figure 12.

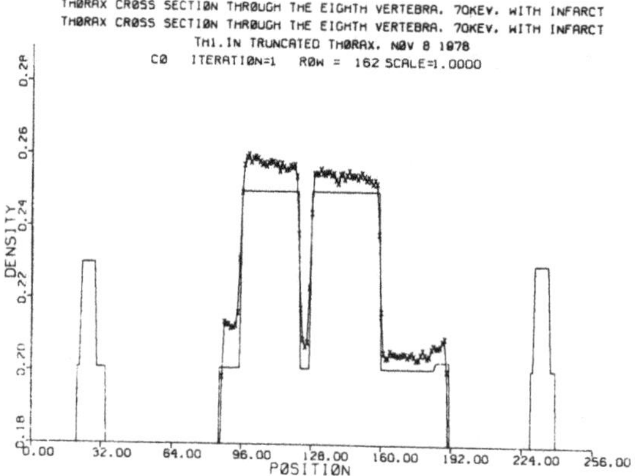

Figure 13. Density profile after correction (Reproduced with permission from Med. Phys. 6: 412, 1979)

The improvement (Figs. 12-13) with a fairly simple extrapolation scheme seems to be quite impressive. The amount of improvement strongly depends on the size of the ROI and the size, position and density of objects outside the ROI. Similar results were also reported by Wagner [3].

2.3. Variable Sampling Technique

In reference [5], Nalcioglu, Sankar and Sklansky have proposed a method which is a combination of the two methods described previously. This method is called the variable sampling and is illustrated in figure 14.

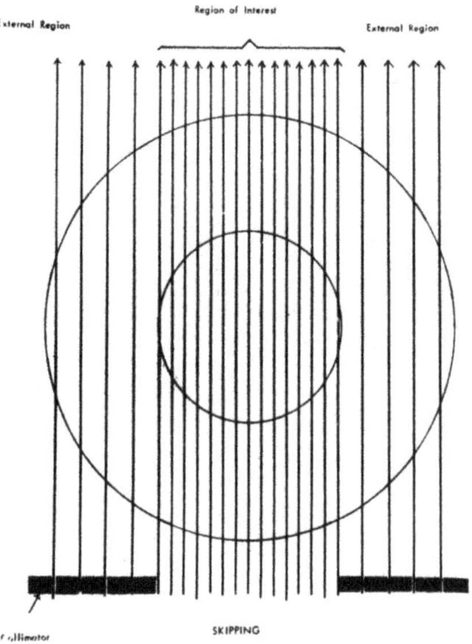

Figure 14. Variable Sampling Scheme (Reproduced with permission from Proc. SPIE 206: 98, 1979)

In this scheme the ROI is spatially sampled using a small sampling interval T_f whereas the external region is sampled coarsely with a sampling interval of T_c. The variably sampled data for a single projection is shown in Figure 15.

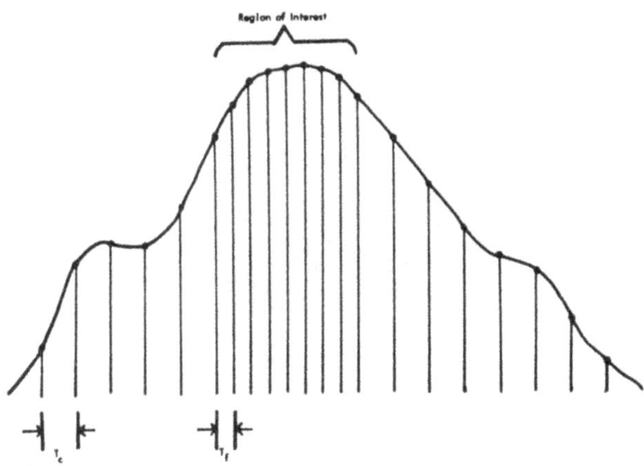

Figure 15. Variably sampled projection (Reproduced with permission from Proc. SPIE 206:98, 1979)

The coarsely sampled external projection data is then linearly interpolated to the same spatial sampling interval as the ROI and this is called the quasi-fine sampling. The projection data shown in Figure 15 looks like Figure 16 after one performs the interpolation.

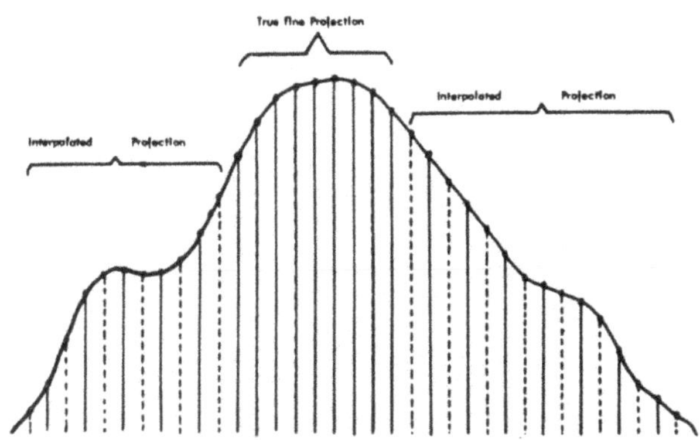

Figure 16. Interpolated projection (Reproduced with permission from Proc. SPIE 206: 98, 1979)

In the next figure, we used the same ROI as shown in Figure 2 and applied the variable sampling technique. The ratio of coarse to fine sampling intervals was 4:1. The image was reconstructed on a 64x64 matrix which translates into a 512x512 matrix for the whole image (the size of the ROI was 1/8th of the whole object).

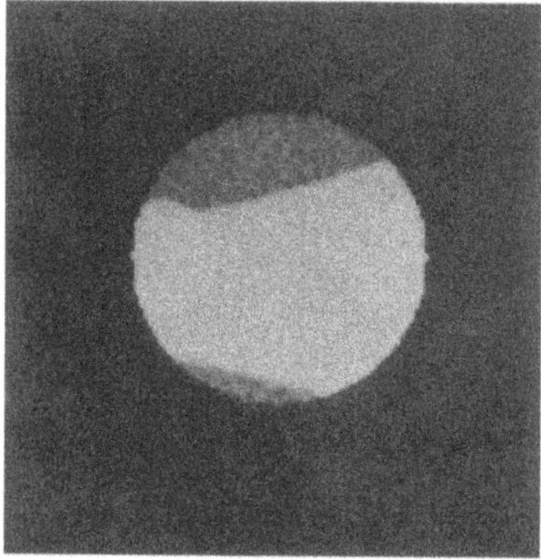

Figure 17. ROI after variable sampling reconstruction
(Reproduced with permission from Proc. SPIE 206:98, 1979)

In addition to the coarse sampling in the external region the number of photons per ray were reduced by a factor of 1000 with respect to the ROI, similar to the SVIS method. A combination of x-ray tube filtration and variable sampling produces region of interest images of high quality. This can be seen by comparing the real ROI (Fig. 2) and the reconstructed one (Fig. 17).

2.4. Differential Reconstruction

A completely different approach to the ROI tomography was proposed by Abele and Erdos [6]. This method, called the differential reconstruction, proves to be quite useful when one is interested in the details within the ROI but not the attenuation coefficients. Even though it is derived differently, the method is very similar to the well known harmonization technique in radiology. In the harmonization technique a blurred (low pass filtered) version of an image is subtracted from itself, thus resulting in the high pass filtration of the original image. These authors derive a convolution filter which is the difference of a standard filter minus a smoothed version of the filter. This process also results in a high pass convolution filter which is later used in the convolution. Figure 18 shows a conventional CT filter (solid line), a smoothed one (dotted one) and the difference of the two.

If one reconstructs a circular disc of unit density using these filters one obtains Figure 19.

It is seen from the density profile in Fig. 19 that the conventional filter reproduces the uniform density distribution adequately. When one uses the differential filter shown in Fig. 18 and reconstructs the same disc one obtains the dashed curve, which happens to be the derivative of the solid curve and hence the name "differential reconstruction".

Abele and Erdos have applied this technique to the ROI reconstruction and have obtained excellent edge images. One can change the behavior of the differential filter by different choices and change the appearance of the reconstructed image. Figure 20 is an example of this method for a real patient. It should be remembered that in this method only the ROI is irradiated.

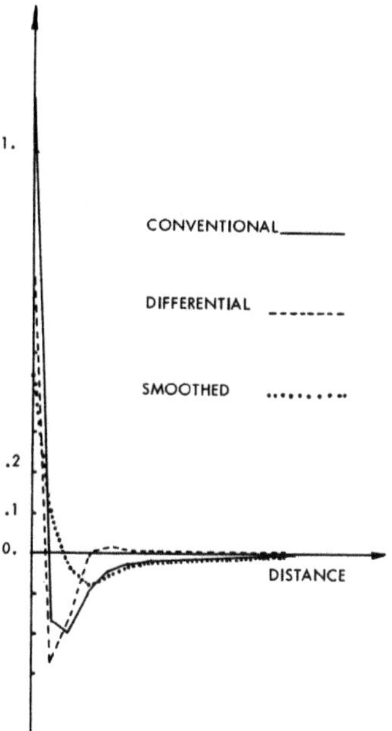

Figure 18. Conventional, smoothed and differential convolution filters (from ref. 6)

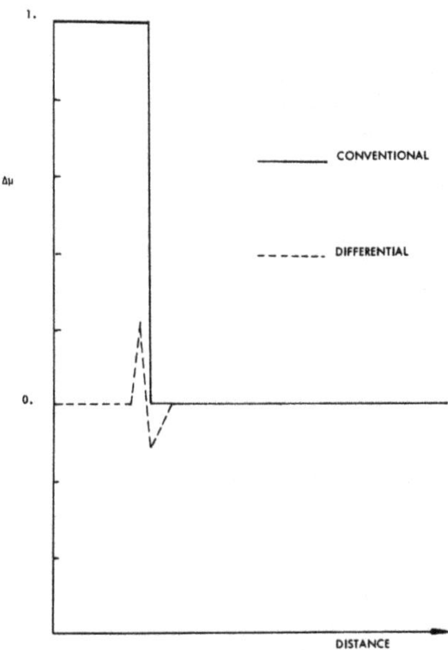

Figure 19. Reconstruction of a disc using conventional and differential filters (courtesy of Dr. Abele).

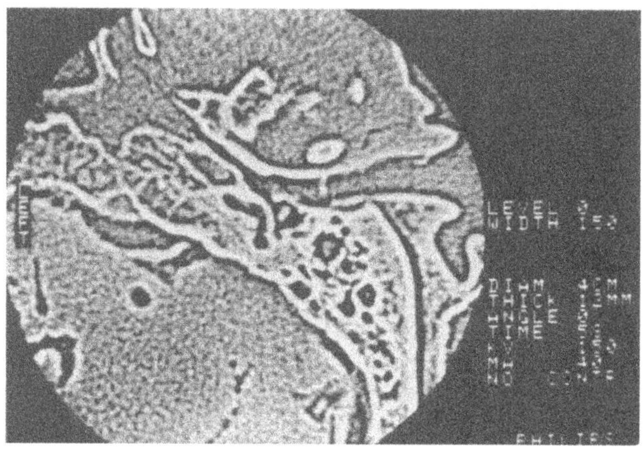

Figure 20. Differential imaging applied to the ROI tomography (courtesy of Dr. Abele)

3. DISCUSSION

In the previous section, we described four different methods for the ROI tomography. The first three are fairly close in spirit in the sense that they try to estimate the external projection data either from noisy or coarsely sampled data. The variable sampling scheme described in Section 2.3 actually approaches the truncation method (Section 2.2) in the limit when the external sampling distance becomes very large. Based on this observation, we have computed point by point error images as a function of coarse to fine sampling ratio. The errorless image was taken to be the image of the ROI obtained by complete fine sampling without any photon noise. The definition of the error image is given by

$$\tilde{\mu}_{ij} = \frac{\mu_{ij} - \mu_{ij}^{(0)}}{\mu_{ij}^{(0)}} \qquad (1)$$

where $\mu_{ij}^{(0)}$ is the reconstructed value of pixel (i,j) for the errorless case and μ_{ij} is the reconstructed value of the ROI image when the external region is sampled coarsely. The error image defined by equation (1) was computed for six different sampling ratios and is shown in Figure 21.

In addition to changing the sampling ratio, the number of photons in the external region were reduced by 1000 in calculating the μ_{ij} (the ROI reconstructed image). From Fig. 21 it is seen that until a ratio of 32:1 (bottom left) is reached the error is quite random in nature. After that point one starts getting elevated densities towards the edges indicating that a certain amount of cupping artifact is starting to build up. This is due to the fact that as one increases the coarse sampling interval one starts missing the skull bone as shown in Figure 1. After missing the high density bone the interpolation of the projection data does not completely recover the projection data in the external region. The nonuniform distribution of the error is due to the nonsymmetric shape of the head phantom (Fig. 1).

Using the data in Fig. 21, we also calculated a mean percentage error per pixel for the whole image by the relation:

$$\%\ \text{error-mean} = \sum_{ij} |\tilde{\mu}_{ij}| \times 100/\#\ \text{pixels} \qquad (2)$$

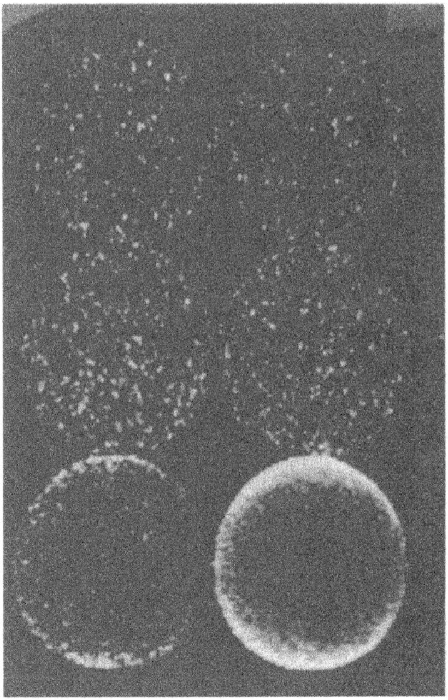

Figure 21. Error images at different sampling rates. Top left 2:1, top right 4:1, middle left 8:1, middle right 16:1, bottom left 32:1 and bottom right 64:1 (T_{coarse}: T_{fine})

The quantity defined in eq. (2) is plotted as a function of T coarse/T fine ratios in Figure 22.

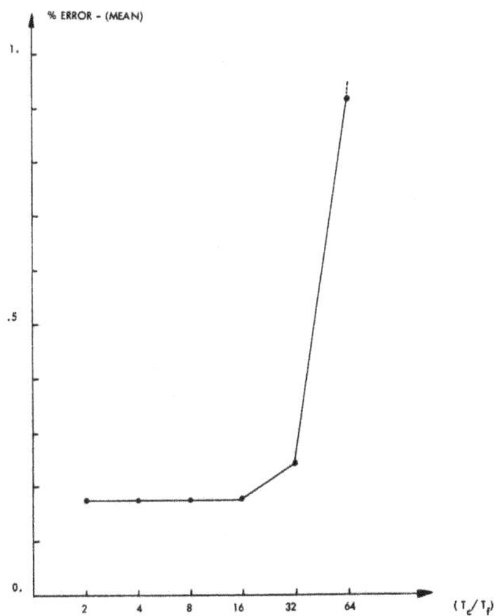

Figure 22. Mean % error per pixel.

It is seen that the % error is fairly constant up to a ratio of 16:1, indicating that the error is mainly due to quantum noise. After that value the error value goes up drastically due to aliasing errors. Depending on the relative density and the size of objects outside and inside the region of interest one could have substantial errors in the reconstructed images if one uses the extrapolation methods, since the error in these images would be given by large T_c/T_f values in Fig. 22. If one has fairly continuous density distribution in the external region the extrapolation technique is expected to work adequately and one does not have to resort to variable sampling. The presence of high density objects outside the ROI is also expected to cause artifacts in the differential reconstruction technique.

ACKNOWLEDGEMENTS

The author acknowledges assistance given by Dr. Sankar in obtaining the variable sampling results presented here. The cooperation given by Drs. Abele and Lewitt are also gratefully acknowledged.

REFERENCES

1. L.A. Shepp and B.F. Logan, "The Fourier reconstruction of a head phantom," IEEE Trans. Nuc. Sci., NS-21:21-43, 1974.

2. O. Nalcioglu and R.Y. Lou, "Post-reconstruction method for beam hardening in computerized tomography," Phys. Med. Biol., 24:330-340, 1979.

3. W. Wagner, "Reconstructions from restricted region scan data - new means to reduce the patient dose," IEEE Trans. Nuc. Sci., NS-26:2866-2869, 1979.

4. R.M. Lewitt, "Processing of incomplete measurement data in computed tomography," Med. Phys., 6:412-417, 1979.

5. O. Nalcioglu, P.V. Sankar and J. Sklansky, "Region-of-interest x-ray tomography (ROIT)," Proc. SPIE, 206:98-102, 1979.

6. M.G. Abele, J.I. Erdos and C.H. Marshall, "High resolution bone structure imaging in CT," NYU Medical Center Report TR-1-1, July 1977 (unpublished).

CODED APERTURE TOMOGRAPHY

by

J. BRUNOL
Institut d'Optique théorique
et Appliquée, Faculté d'Orsay
91406, ORSAY, France.
Hopital Cochin, service des
Radioisotopes.

I. INTRODUCTION

The development of tomographic methods has led to considerable progress in medical diagnosis based on external exploration. Among these examinations, nuclear medicine has a fundamentally functional vocation as opposed to the morphological exploration methods (X-rays, echography). The result is a high diversity in the nature itself of the study (scintigraphy).
An essential distinction can thus be made between static examinations (or quasi-static examinations), dynamic examinations which can be classified in large (lungs, liver) or restricted fields of view (heart, coxofemoral joints ...).
The latter feature directly stems from the specific characteristics of the radiotracers used and of the organs to be examined. Moreover, in the case of low object fields, the resolution must be high to maintain a quality of the image essential for the interpretation. However, the spatial detectors (Anger cameras mainly) covering the 70-600 keV energy range do not achieve very fine resolution. Thus, diversified tomographical methods have been developped in nuclear medecine.
An example is the Emission Computerized Axial Tomography (ECAT) which allows large field static or quasi-static explorations with a resolution of around 1.5 cm, and the tomographic methods in low field allowing 5 mm resolution (either static or dynamic studies). The latter category mainly includes the methods using a multi-pinhole collimator and coded aperture imaging (CAI). The two following results obtained in the cardiac (CAI) and pulmonary (ECAT) fields illustrate the necessity of a diversified combination of tomographic methods.

After attempting to give a brief summary of the reasons why a unique method cannot solve all the problems of nuclear tomography, we shall state the points common to the above techniques before making a more general statement on coding methods.

2. BASIC COMMON PROBLEMS IN NUCLEAR TOMOGRAPHY

One of the characteristic features of these methods (ECAT,CAI, multipinhole) is that they can be broken down (at the level of principles) into two stages :

- The first is a data recording stage (1 or 2-D Poisson Processes). The nature of this recording considerably differs from one method to the other. It should be noted however, that the data can always be read out in terms of non-linear function of 3-D emission data (which are the parameters to be found) and of absorption data which have a part to play here in the generation of undesirable secondary phenomena.

- The second is a reconstruction stage. From the theoretical point of view, the problem raised by the search for a 3-D distribution from the recordings can be outlined as follows

  1. Irrespective of statistical limitations, is there one and only one solution to the problem of mathematical inversion ?

  2. If there is actually a solution, what is the influence of the statistical variability of the recordings on the 3-D emission distribution that is deducted ?

  Practically, the problem must be tackled in different terms. In fact, the existence of a theoretical solution does not guarantee the existence of an algorithm which can be used to find it. The physicist's part is then - and this has been checked for the different methods (including the problem of non-monochromaticity of X-ray in CT scanner) -

1. To find an appropriate mathematical formulation,

2. To find a practical solution to the problem studied,

3. To make an evaluation and to make the best possible correction of the error introduced by approximation (correction of self absorption for instance).

In nuclear or radiologic tomography, these proceedings are justified because the fundamental limitations mainly stem from the statistical problems and from the resolution or from the non-linearity of the detection which introduces larger artifacts than those linked to the residual errors indicated above.

It is the existence of these two stages, which can however be simultaneously achieved due to the introduction of parallel processing units, which has led to the classification of these methods under the heading "Reconstruction methods", as opposed to conventional recordings.

The second characteristic feature which is common to these methods, as far as practical application is concerned, is the existence of considerable statistical fluctuations linked to the low number of available counts. This problem is fundamental in clinical applications because it determines the signal to noise ratio of the reconstructed image and therefore the ability of the method to lead to a significant interpretation to the local emission variations.

Mathematically, the analysis of the statistical fluctuations in the reconstructed image is not an easy problem. Without going into the mathematical details of the analysis, let us nevertheless indicate that :

1. The random character of the image can no longer be considered in terms of Poisson Process as is the case for an ordinary scintigraphical image.

2. Generally speaking, the noise in a point of the reconstructed image depends, in a complex manner, on the set of fluctuations relating to each point of the object. In axial tomography, for a 2-D image and a given total analysis time, the statistical quality of the image obtained will usually be poorer with a recording and an axial reconstruction than for perpendicular conventional imagery. Let us emphasize the fact that the degradation depends on the object studied (or more precisely on the field occupation coefficient) and that, especially as far as the preceeding example is concerned, the statistical quality of the image is the same in both instances for an emissive point and is degraded if emissive objects increasing in size are considered.

These statistical considerations are actually part of the method's multiplex character. It is not without reason that important analogies emerge with Fourier transform spectroscopy, or with similar systems of Girard grating spectometer. We shall now deal with coded aperture imaging.

3. SOME ASPECTS IN CODED APERTURE IMAGING

Coded Aperture Imaging is the direct result of Mertz's and Young's studies in X-ray astronomy. The recording principle consists in placing a code made of transparent and opaque parts, at the selected radiation, between the patient - who has preliminarily been given an injection of a radiopharmaceutical -

and the detector. The code in the first techniques available, and more particularly H.H. Barrett's technique, used a Fresnel zone plate, on or off-axis, resulting in an incoherent hologram-type recording. An analogical optical decoding or reconstruction can be considered, with a certain number of differences as compared to conventional holography. The reconstruction's coherent nature, with the major fluctuations it introduces, the superposition of the different diffracted orders have not made it possible to achieve satisfactory results in practice with these methods.

The second generation methods have eliminated the principle of coherent reconstruction and with it, the quite particular code of the Fresnel zone.

We have, for instance, pointed out that the unique annular aperture linked to a partial deconvolution led to an improved -

1. reconstruction of the combined spatial frequencies selectively reduced by the recording stage,

2. signal to noise ratio in the object space as well as in high frequency spaces which are, it should be noted, the most interesting regions, since they are mainly responsible for the interpretation of the details of the objects under analysis, and therefore for the resolution of the method,

3. tomographical discrimination linked to the external coding or radiations corresponding to the system's broad optical" aperture.

It has consequently become possible to obtain satisfactory results. The field of cardiac-dynamic 3-D imagery has, in particular, shown the real importance of this kind of method.

The information from the different above and underlying planes is not entirely eliminated. Algorithms, similar to those developped by Parker, make it possible, to a certain extent. In any case, in spite of its limitations, the coded aperture imaging justifies dynamic acquisitions and a large magnification makes it possible to achieve the high resolution necessary for cardiac applications, for instance. Moreover, an increased signal to noise ratio is obtained : it is not equal to the square root of the increase in the number of collected photons, but the field occupation coefficient makes it possible nevertheless to reach values between 2 and 3 which correspond to gains in times of analysis of 4 to 9.

It should be pointed out that, if the results obtained for fields low in CAI are very satisfactory as compared with low resolutions and with the poor statistical quality obtained in ECAT, the problem is inverted in the case of larger organs.

Other methods of the CAI type have been developed. In particular Tanaka has proposed a recording method based on the use of a rotating slit aperture : this kind of method makes it possible to more easily obviate a certain tomographical superposition, but it no longer enables rapid dynamic acquisitions. Even though easier to apply, it is of a nature similar to methods using multicoding.

IV. FUTURE DEVELOPMENTS IN NUCLEAR TOMOGRAPHY

The development of nuclear tomography methods is not independent of those of the following three branches

- Study of radiotracers. It is evident that the obtaining of more specific and shorter period tracers should make it possible to improve both the nature of the information extracted from imagery proceedings and to appreciably increase the statistical quality of the results for equivalent examination times.

- Development of acquisition systems (Gamma camera). For a constant signal to noise ratio, an increase in the resolution of the tomographical methods linked to an improved statistical quality of the images is conditioned by more efficient detection systems which are at present in the study phase (intrinsical high resolution, high energy discrimination, large fields ...).

- Development of the power of digital processing systems. The third aspect is probably the most advanced. Extremely rapid parallel processing units are already a reality. Moreover, increased storage and processing capacities should be achieved in the near future (Mostek's 64K x 1 bit Dynamic Memories, end of 1980).

Taking into consideration these probable future developments, the nuclear tomographical methods should undergo a considerable evolution.
As a matter of fact, as previouly indicated, linear-type analyses linked with a-posteriori corrections have often made it possible to push the processing quality over the limits resulting from detection and statistical problems. Thus in the near future, the improvement of the tomographical methods (and their consequences) seem :

- In ECAT to lead to non-linearity corrections of detectors and to the development of a biophysical methodology of the interpretation of the results obtained in slow dynamics

- In longitudinal tomography to lead to reconstructions using methods operating in the Fourier 3-D space (Fourier aperture or high resolution multipinhole collimator),

In the long run, it seems that the problem of linear analysis must be re-examined.

V. CONCLUSION

The current and future problems concerning nuclear tomography methods from the viewpoint of applied physics have mainly been dealt with in the present article. Nevertheless they should not be separated from the aims of improving the understanding of the general and local functioning of the organism. The part played by imagery methods is, in parallel to those of the other technologies implied, to give high performance results. In order to express the nature and the frequencies of the biological interactions, these results must be quantitative. Under these conditions it will become possible to consider much higher performance modelings than those resulting from the actual state of techniques. A development of this kind will undoubtedly be achieved by a thorough reformulation of the notion of compartmented analysis. Such research should from now on be undertaken on the existing premises : failure to do so could lead to disconnecting the physicians preoccupations from the technicians.

REFERENCES

1. L. Mertz and N.O. Young, "Fresnel Transformation of Images", Proc. Internat. Conf. on Opt. Instr., Chapman et Hall, London, 305 (1961)

2. Colloque International sur les Progrès Récents en Spectroscopie Interférentielle, Journal de Physique et Le Radium, 19, (1958).

3. A. Girard, Optica Acta, V.1, 81 (1960).

4. J. Brunol, J. Fonroget, Opt. Commun. V.22, 301 (1977).

5. R.G. Simpson, H.H. Barrett, J.A. Subach et H.D. Fisher, Opt. Eng. V.14, 490 (1975).

6. J. Brunol, J. Fonroget, Opt. Commun. V. 25, 35 (1978).

7. M.Y. Chiu and al., J. Opt. Soc. Am. V. 69, 1323 (1979).

8. R.P. Parker and al., Proc. of The Seventh L.H. Gray Conf., Leeds 13-15 April (1976).

FIGURES

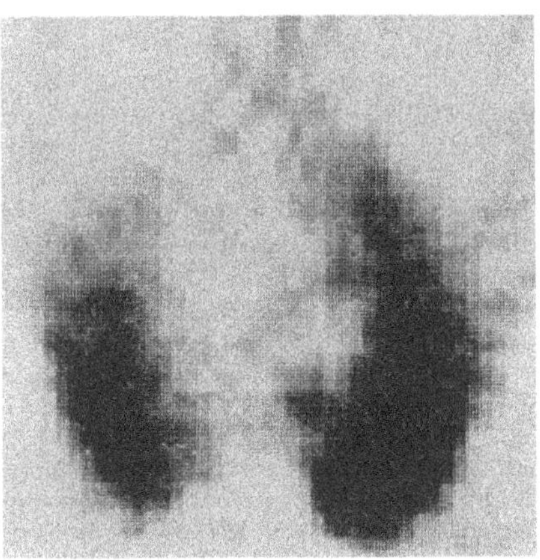

Figure I. Slice of a lung (ECAT) : - Correction of self absorption.
- Noise dependent filtering.

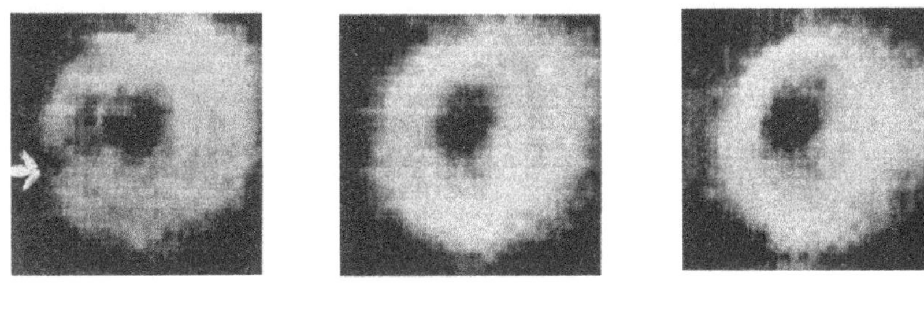

II.1 II.2 II.3

Figure II. (1, 2, 3) Reconstruction of 3 slices of a heart (CAI) :
- Isotope $^{201}T\ell$
- Not gated study
- Defect of fixation (→ II.1)

POSITRON EMISSION TOMOGRAPHY

by
Michel M. Ter-Pogossian, Ph.D.
Mallinckrodt Institute of Radiology
Washington University School of Medicine
St. Louis, Missouri 63110

ABSTRACT

Positron emission tomography (PET), is a tool of major promise in biomedical research and clinical applications, which yields images representing the distribution of a systemically administered positron-emitting radionuclide in transverse tomographic sections of the body of human subjects or experimental animals. The usefulness of PET stems from the fact that some elements of fundamental importance in the investigation biological processes possess radionuclides which decay by the emission of positrons. Most of these radionuclides (^{11}C, ^{13}N, ^{15}O, ^{18}F) decay with half-lives of minutes and must be prepared in the vicinity of the site of utilization. Many molecules of physiological importance have been labeled with these radionuclides. Through the use of these molecules, PET permits the in vivo regional assessment of a number of biochemical processes essential to life. Most PET devices utilize scintillation detectors fitted either with sodium iodide, bismuth germanate or cesium fluoride crystals. A promising improvement in PET consists in the incorporation of photon time-of-flight information in the image reconstruction process. PET images are reconstructed from a large number of measurements and the storage and utilization of this information requires large computer memory capabilities and fast processing systems. State of the art PET devices yield images with the spatial resolution better than 1 cm with a contrast resolution of better than 10% in a period of time of less than 1 minute.

1. INTRODUCTION

Since the middle 70's, positron emission tomography (PET) has emerged as a tool of major promise in the investigation in vivo regionally, and non-invasively, of physiological and pathophysiological processes. Methodologically, PET consists of the systemic administration to the subject under study, of a selected chemical compound labeled with a positron-emitting radionuclide followed by the imaging of the distribution of the radionuclide as a function of time in transverse tomographic sections. From this information, through the application of a suitable model, a number of physiological processes can be studied in vivo. PET draws its usefulness from the synergistic interaction of two components: 1. The imaging process and, 2. the chemical nature of a small number of radionuclides which decay through the emission of positrons.

2. PET IMAGE

The images provided by PET are transverse tomographic sections of the subject's body (human patient or experimental animal) in which the image forming variable is the distribution of a positron-emitting radionuclide. The image reconstruction principle utilized for the formation of the image is identical to that utilized in transmission CT [1]. In PET, the presence of positron-emitting radionuclides is detected through the annihilation radiation generated when electron-positron pairs undergo annihilation in matter with the conversion of their masses into two 511 keV photons emitted nearly co-linearly. By detecting the distribution of the annihilation radiation around the subject, it is possible through the application of algorithms similar to those used in transmission CT to obtain highly quantitative images of the distribution of the radionuclide. The faithful reconstruction of such images imposes suitable angular and linear sampling [2].

The imaging by PET of the distribution of a positron-emitting radionuclide in vivo is considerably helped by some of the physical properties of the annihilation process. The coincidence detection of the annihilation radiation is highly efficient as compared to absorption type collimation utilized conventionally in nuclear medicine, furthermore, it provides a relatively uniform sensitivity between the two detectors operated in coincidence over a large percentage of the distance separating them [3]. The fact that two annihilation photons must be detected to yield a coincidence event permits the easy and accurate correction for the attenuation of this radiation in tissues. Last but not least, the fact that the two coincidence photons are emitted simultaneously permits, through the use of fast detectors, the utilization of time-of-flight in the localization of the event between the detectors. This additional information to the reconstruction process improves its signal to noise ratio [4].

3. "PHYSIOLOGICAL" RADIONUCLIDES AND THEIR USE

Probably the most serendipitous occurrence in the utilization of PET is the fact that four radionuclides which decay through the emission of positrons, namely carbon-11 ($T_{1/2}$=20 min), nitrogen-13 ($T_{1/2}$=10 min), oxygen-15 ($T_{1/2}$=2 min), and fluorine-18 ($T_{1/2}$=110 min), exhibit chemical properties highly useful in biological investigations. The first three radionuclides (^{11}C, ^{13}N, ^{15}O) are major constitutents of living matter and therefore are actively involved in the majority of metabolic processes and the fourth one, ^{18}F, is a particularly useful label for metabolic substrate analogs and of some other molecules useful in biological investiation. For convenience in this text, these isotopes will be called "physiological" radionuclides.

The basic premise in the utilization of PET (at this point, the term is meant to cover the combined use of positron emission tomography and of the "physiological" radionuclides) is the following: Every biological manifestation is preceded and accompanied by regional biochemical activity. Furthermore any form of pathology is either preceded or accompanied by biochemical processes different from the normal. Under the circumstances, the in vivo and regional study of biochemical processes offers a particularly promising tool in the study of normal physiology and disease. The general approach followed in achieving that goal consists in the administration of either a metabolic substrate or of another molecule of fundamental importance in the process to be studied followed by a time course assessment of the distribution of the label as a function of space and time. Through the application of a suitable model most often developed on the basis of in vitro biochemistry, the process under study can, in many instances, be unraveled.

It may appear that the above approach might be compromised or even defeated by the short half-lives of the "physiological" positron-emitting radionuclides. Indeed, their fleeting existence might be too short either for the tracing of the major physiological processes or for the labeling of the needed metabolic substrates and other compounds of interest. Fortunately, it is now well established that the majority of important physiological processes are sufficiently short in their time scale to allow their tracing through the use of the "physiological" radionuclides. Furthermore, in the past two decades, a large number (Table I) of compounds of physiological importance have been labeled with ^{11}C, ^{13}N, ^{15}O, or ^{18}F. This has been often accomplished through the development of ingenious rapid chemical procedures.

TABLE I

SUBSTANCES OF DEMONSTRATED OR POTENTIAL IMPORTANCE IN THE STUDY OF PHYSIOLOGICAL PROCESSES WHICH HAVE BEEN LABELED WITH POSITRON-EMITTING RADIONUCLIDES

Label	$T_{1/2}$(min)	Labeled Substance	
^{11}C	20.3	carbon monoxide	amino acids
		carbon dioxide	amines
		cyanides	nitriles
		alkynes	sugars
		alcohols	sugar analogs
		ethers	hydantoins
		carboxylic acids	nucleotides
		fatty acids	psychoactive drugs
		different macromolecules	butyrophenones
^{13}N	9.96	nitrogen	
		nitrous oxide	
		ammonia	
		amino acids	
		amines	
^{15}O	2.07	oxygen	
		water	
		carbon monoxide	
		carbon dioxide	
^{18}F	110	fluoroethanol	
		spiroperidol	
		fluoroestrogens	
		haloperidol	
		sugar analogs	
		fluorodopa	

The short half-lives of the "physiological" radionuclides impose a number of burdens and limitations upon their use. With the exception of fluorine-18, which, because of its half-life of 110 minutes, can be relatively easily shipped over long distances, the others, carbon-11, nitrogen-13, and oxygen-15 must be prepared in the immediate vicinity of the site of their use, which requires the availability of a cyclotron or of another positive ion accelerator and of chemistry facilities suitable for the handling of large quantities of radioactivity. Furthermore, the labeling of the desired compounds must, in most instances, precede by a short period of time their utilization. In many instances, the fleeting existence of the physiological labels all but rules out their use either because of the impossibility of labeling the desired compound rapidly enough or because of the fact that the physiological phenomenom to be studied is too long with respect to the half-life of the label. In many instances, however, the short half-lives of these labels exhibits distinct advantages. Large doses of activity of these short-lived physiological labels can be administered with concomitant high imaging counting rates with a modest dose of radiation delivered to the patient. Repeated examinations in the subject are practical. From the chemical standpoint, the short half-lives of the labels permits to achieve a higher specific activity of the desired labeled compound than if a longer lived label had been used. This is a precious characteristic in a number of instances particularly in the imaging of saturable receptor sites.

In general, the chemical requirements of PET have stimulated the development of a highly active branch of chemistry with very specific requirements such as rapid labeling procedures, attention given to biological and radiation purity and high specific activity. The vigorous activity of this branch of chemistry has resulted in the labeling of the substances shown in Table I and of their rapid proliferation.

4. PET DEVICES

The imaging instrumentation required for PET consists essentially of a data acquisition gantry and of a computer and peripherals (Figure 1) for data storage, image reconstruction, and display.

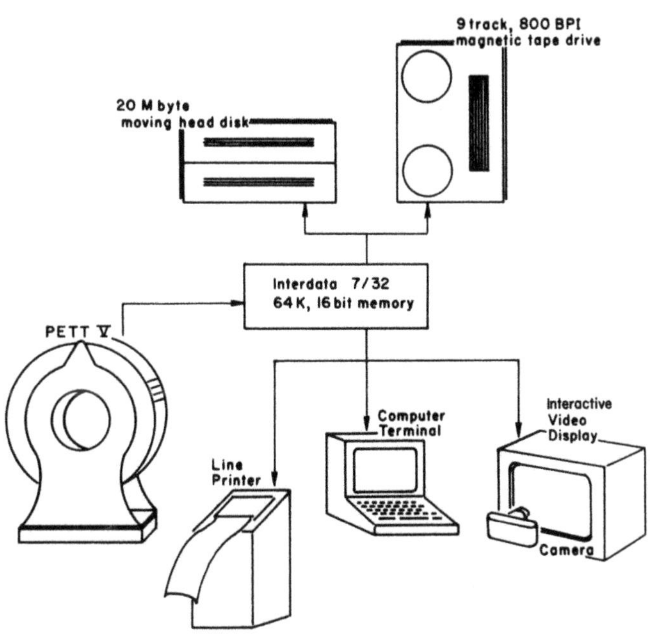

FIGURE 1: Block diagram of a positron emission tomograph (PETT V) [10].

At this time the detectors most often used for PET are scintillation counters because of the requirements of high detection efficiency for the 511 keV annihilation radiation and of fast timing imposed by the need for reduction of random coincidences. The early scintillation detectors used for PET incorporated sodium iodide crystals which later were superceded by bismuth germanate and more recently, some of the desirable characteristics of cesium fluoride were recognized for this purpose [4] (Table II) (Fig 2).

TABLE II

SOME PHYSICAL CHARACTERISTICS OF 3 SCINTILLATION CRYSTALS USED FOR PET

	Cesium Fluoride CsF	Bismuth Germanate $Bi_4Ge_3O_{12}$	Sodium Iodide NaI(Tl)
Density (g/cm^3)	4.64	7.13	3.67
Effective atomic number	52	72	50
Linear attenuation Coefficient at 511 keV (1/cm)	0.44	0.92	0.34
Wavelength of max emission (nm)	390	480	410
Decay constant (nsec)	5	300	230
Gamma scintillation conversion for S-11 photocathode response with respect to NaI(Tl)	0.05	0.08	1
Index of refraction at wavelength of maximum emission	1.48	2.15	1.85

Adapted from:
Harshaw Scintillation Phosphors, 3rd Edition, Copyright 1975 (Courtesy Harshaw Chemical Co.)
H.E. Swanson, M.C. Morris, E.H. Evans, and L. Ulmer: N.B.S. Monograph 25, Sec. 3, 26 (1964)
Author's calculations.

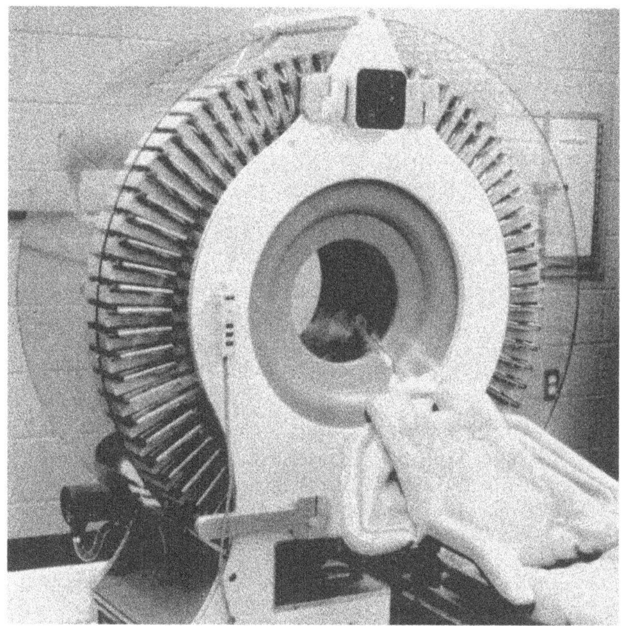

FIGURE 2: Photograph of the data acquisition gantry and patient couch of PETT VI, a positron emission tomograph utilizing cesium fluoride scintillation detectors.

Faithful imaging with PET requires suitable linear and angular sampling of the data and a number of detector configurations (Fig 3) have been tested for this purpose. Early PET systems provided only one slice at a time and utilized either a circular distribution [5] of detectors or a polygonal array incorporating linear and rotational motions of the detectors to increase sampling [3]. Soon multislice capability was incorporated into the latter geometry [6]. The MGH positron camera was adapted [8] for PET through the addition of suitable motions. Most of the more recent devices provide multislice capabilities and utilize a circular distribution of detectors, either stationary [7] or animated by a wobble and rotational motion [9-10].

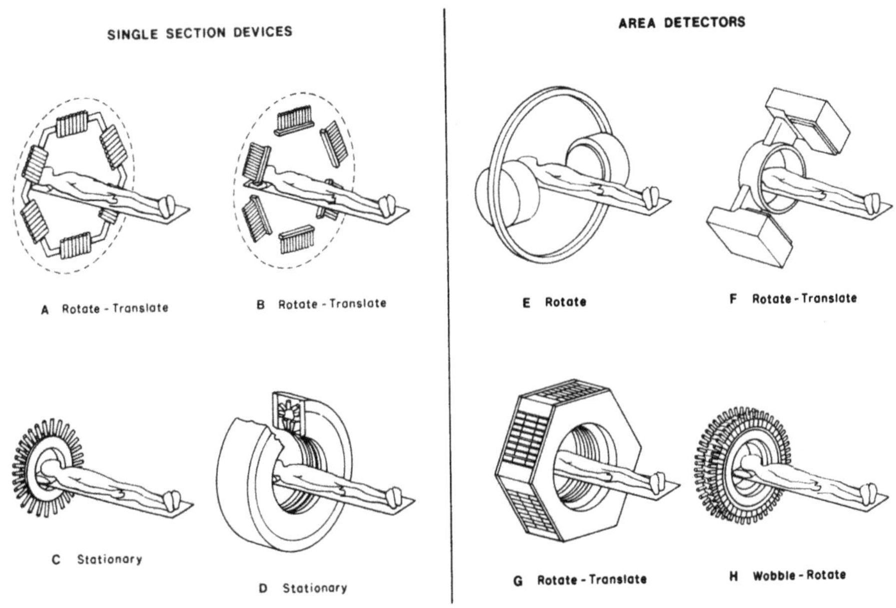

FIGURE 3: Diagrams of configurations utilized for PET data acquisition gantries.

A conservative assessment of the performance characteristics of modern PET devices yields the following figures:

Spatial resolution: about 1 cm in the plane of the section for a section thickness of about 1.5 cm.
Contrast resolution: better than 10%.
Data acquisition temporal resolution: shorter than 1 minute.

It should be noted that in the physiological applications of PET the realistic performance figures may vary considerably according to factors such as physical dimensions of the object imaged, quantity and distribution of the imaging radionuclide, radiation absorption homogeneity of the tissues imaged, etc.

There is little doubt that the above performance figures can be improved within certain limitations, however, through the application of state of the art technology. The spatial resolution of PET devices can probably be improved to a value of about 5 mm, through the utilization of smaller or highly collimated detectors, and with the use of adequate sampling [11]. It seems however difficult to achieve a resolution much superior to 5 mm because of a number of factors which militate against such an improvement. The range of positrons in matter is not negligible and contributes to the unsharpness of the image [12-13]. Another important factor is the divergence of the annihilation photons from colinearity [12-13], which further militates against high resolution. Finally, any increase in resolution must be supported by a rapid increase of counting statistics [12] and the latter requirement is often limited by the patient's permissible dose of radiation.

Improvements in contrast resolution can be achieved by raising the signal to noise ration, either by improving counting statistics or by some other means. A particularly promising approach to achieve the latter is the use of time-of-flight information [4]. Temporal resolution is often limited by the influence of random coincidences and the utilization of faster scintillators such as cesium fluoride relieves considerably this difficulty. It is quite probable that temporal resolution of better than 10 sec can be achieved with doses of radiation to the patient within permissible standards.

The requirements imposed by PET images upon the data display system incorporate the type of interactive capabilities which are generally desirable and available in image display systems designed for other purposes such as transmission CT. These capabilties include region of interest assessment, superimposition of images, zooming, edge detection, image rotation, color capabilities, etc. There is a trend toward firmware implementation of such functions.

5. CONCLUSION

At this time, PET has reached a degree of considerable maturity as a tool. A very large number of labeled chemical compounds of potential usefulness in the application of PET have been synthesized and are available for use. Furthermore, newer compounds with particularly desirable chemical characteristics, such as high specific acitivity are made available at a fast rate. PET instrumentation, quite adequate for a number of physiological studies, is available from several commercial companies. A particularly promising development is the incorporation of time-of-flight information in the reconstruction process.

It appears that one of the major thrusts which will occur within the next few years in PET will be its utilization in physiological investigation and probably also, in clinical practice [14] (Fig 4).

The possible usefulness of PET as an investigative modality has now been widely recognized throughout the world. There are presently over 40 centers with either available PET capabilities or committed to the implementation of this tool.

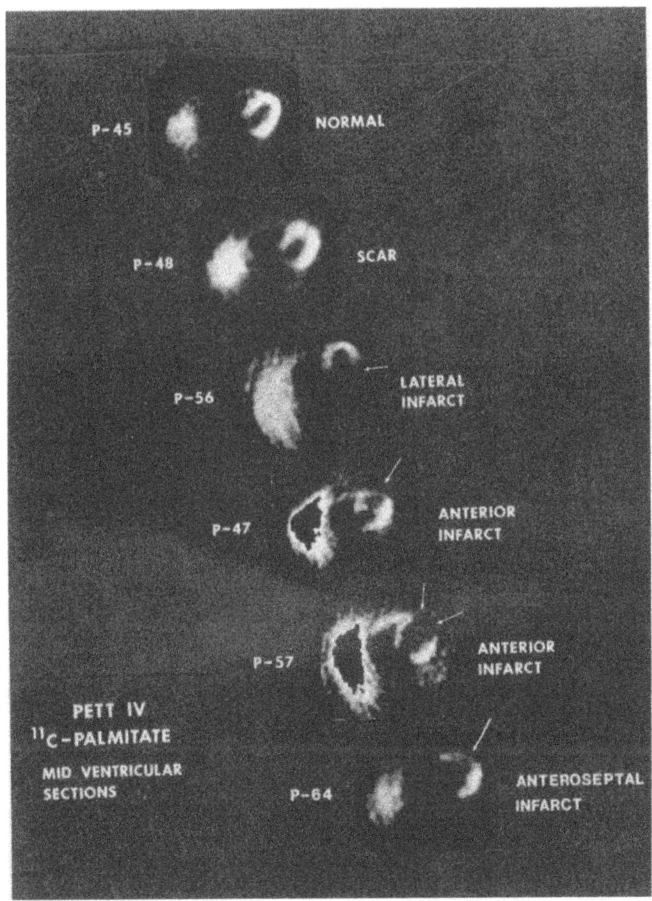

FIGURE 4: PET images of the heart obtained in a series of subjects following the intravenous administration of palmitate labeled with carbon-11. The tomographic sections were obtained by means of PETT IV [6] at approximately the mid-ventricular level in one normal subject and in patients with myocardial infarcts at the loci indicated based on analysis of the images and of the ECG's in each case. The concentration of activity to the left of the heart is that of the liver. (Reproduced by courtesy of CIRCULATION [14].)

REFERENCES

1. M.M. Ter-Pogossian, Basic principles of computed axial tomography, Sem Nucl Med 7:109-127, 1977.

2. R.A. Brooks, G. Di Chiro, Principles of computer assisted tomography (CAT) in radiographic and radioisotopic imaging: Review article, Phys Med Biol 21:689, 732, 1976.

3. M.M. Ter-Pogossian, M.E. Phelps, E.J. Hoffman, et al: A positron emission transaxial tomograph for nuclear imaging (PETT), Radiology 114:89-98, 1975.

4. R. Allemand, C. Gresset, J. Vacher, Potential advantages of a cesium fluoride scintillator for a time-of-flight positron camera, J Nucl Med 21:153-155, 1980.

5. J.S. Robertson, R.B. Marr, M. Rosenblum, U. Radeka, Y.L. Yamamoto, "32 crystal positron transverse section detector," Tomographic Imaging in Nuclear Medicine, edited by G.S. Freedman, Society of Nuclear Medicine, New York, 1973, pp. 142-153.

6. M.M. Ter-Pogossian, N.A. Mullani, J. Hood, C.S. Higgins, C.M. Currie, A multi-slice positron emission computed tomograph (PETT IV) yielding transverse and longitudinal images, Radiology 128:477-484, 1978.

7. C.A. Burnham, G.L. Brownell, A multi-crystal positron camera, IEEE Trans NS-19:201-205, 1972.

8. S.E. Derenzo, T.F. Budinger, J.L. Calhoon, W.L. Greenberg, R.H. Hesman, T. Vuletich, The Donner 280-crystal high resolution positron tomograph, IEEE Trans Nucl Sc NS-26(2):2790-2993, 1979.

9. C. Bohm, L. Eriksson, M. Bergstrom, J. Litton, R. Sundman, M. Singh, A computer assisted ring detector camera system for reconstruction tomography of the brain, IEEE Trans Nucl Sc NS-25:624-637, 1978.

10. M.M. Ter-Pogossian, N.A. Mullani, J. Hood, C.S. Higgins, D.C. Ficke, Design considerations for a positron emission transverse tomograph (PETT V) for imaging of the brain, J Comput Assist Tomogr 2:539, 1978.

11. R.A. Brooks, V.J. Sank, G. Di Chiro, W.S. Friauf, S.B. Leighton, Design of a high resolution positron emission tomograph: The Neuro-PET, J Comput Assist Tomogr 4(1):5-13, 1980.

12. E.J. Hoffman, M.E. Phelps, An analysis of some of the physical aspects of positron transaxial tomography, Comput Biol Med 6:345-360, 1976.

13. S.E. Derenzo, T.F. Budinger, Resolution limit for positron-imaging devices, J Nucl Med 18:491, 1977.

14. M.M. Ter-Pogossian, M.S. Klein, J. Markham, R. Roberts, B.E. Sobel, Regional assessment of myocaridal metabolic integrity in vivo by positron-emission tomography with ^{11}C-labeled palmitate, Circ 61:242-255, 1980.

A NEW TIME-OF-FLIGHT METHOD FOR POSITRON COMPUTED TOMOGRAPHY (P.C.T.)

by

R. ALLEMAND, R. CAMPAGNOLO, P. GARDERET, R. GARIOD, C. GRESSET

C. JANIN, M. LAVAL, R. ODRU, E. TOURNIER, J. VACHER

CENTRE D'ETUDES NUCLEAIRES
Laboratoire d'Electronique et de
Technologie de l'Informatique

85 X - 38041 GRENOBLE Cedex

1. INTRODUCTION

P.C.T. design is complex because many physical, technological or geométrical parameters must be taken into account but it appears that one of the main limitations of the P.C.T. image quality is due to the detection system characteristics.

A time-of-flight technique using a very fast and high stopping power scintillator has been investigated. Cesium-fluoride (CsF) appears to be becoming the detector of choice for this application. The most important aspects of the detection features are discussed and a comparison is made with Bismuth-Germanate (B.G.O.) and sodium-iodide NaI(Tl) scintillators.

The feasibility of a time-of-flight technique combined with a conventional reconstruction method was carried-out with a phantom which was scanned in translation and rotation by a pair of CsF scintillators detectors. Preliminary results are presented and we show the importance of this détection method for the design of high-resolving-time P.C.T.

2. TIME-OF-FLIGHT TECHNIQUE (T.O.F. technique)

In a conventional P.C.T., the time-coïncidence technique consists of détermining the direction of each event by detecting the two 511 Kev annihilation photons emitted 180° apart with two opposing banks of detectors. Thus, the image reconstruction method uses the back-projection of each event over the whole size of the image {1} {2}.

The time-of-flight technique consists of directly determining the localization of each event (Fig. 1). That method supposes that a very fast time-coïncidence technique should be obtained : a time interval of 1 n.sec corresponds to a point source position variation of 15 cm.

G. BROWNELL {3} proposed a time-of-flight system for three-dimensional positron imaging using plastic scintillators. More recently, DUNN {4} used the same technique to directly localize each emitting source without further mathematical processing. A time fluctuation of 180 p.sec (FWHM) was obtained with very fast plastic scintillators and phototubes and by adjustment of the energy threshold to 300 Kev.

3. PRINCIPLE OF THE PROPOSED METHOD

This method consists of combining the advantages of a fast and efficient scintillator with those of the time-of-flight technique. In measuring the time distribution of the events with a far greater accuracy than the transit time of a photon in the object, a gaussian spatial distribution of each event can be determined. The basic difference between the conventional method and the T.O.F. technique is shown in figure 2 {5}. In the first case, the section of the point spread function is of the form $\frac{1}{\rho}$, where ρ is the distance to the point source. In the second case, the point spread function is a Gaussian function with a radial symetry around the oy axis, whose section $G(\rho)$ is given by

$$G(\rho) = \frac{1}{\sqrt{2\pi}\sigma} \frac{e^{-\frac{\rho^2}{2\sigma^2}}}{\rho}$$

where : ρ is the distance to the point source
σ is the standard deviation

Figure 2 shows the information is much more concentrated close to the point source in the T.O.F. technique than in the conventional method, because the information is back-projected on a length only a fraction of the size of the image.

It is important to add that the importance of CsF for P.C.T. design is not limited to the T.O.F. technique. Substantial added advantages relative to the time coïncidence reduction can be expected for high counting rate capability conventional P.C.T. design.

4. COMPARISON BETWEEN DIFFERENT DETECTION METHODS

To make such an evaluation, it is useful to recall some physical aspects of the two 511 Kev photons detection by a time-coïncidence technique.

4.1. Physical limitations of the quality of the P.C.T. image {6}{7}{8}

A scintigraphic image can be characterized by its statistical noise due to the number of detected photons and by its spatial resolution. The optimum perception of the image depends on the size and the contrast of the nodule to be detected. Thus a trade-off must be achieved between the sensitivity and the resolution.

This approach is not sufficient to characterize a P.C.T. image. A large amount of annihilation photons are scattered in tissue. Thus, a scattered coïncidence occurs when an unscattered photon is detected in coïncidence with a scattered photon from the same positron. Random coïncidences are due to the detection of two photons from two independant positrons within the coïncidence time. Typically, true coïncidences represent only a very low fraction of the total counting rate of each detector. Scattered and random coïncidences yield a low spatial frequency background which reduces the contrast of the image and introduces an error for quantitative measurements. The mean value of random coïncidences can be substracted by performing an electronic coïncidence delay, but the associated statistical noise remains.

4.2. Detector characteristics comparison {9}{10}

The main characteristics of the different types of scintillators are summarized in tables 1 and 2. Nuclear characteristics were performed with a Na^{22} source and two opposing XP 2020 phototubes and a 20 mm diameter collimator.

Scattered coïncidences can be reduced by the choice of the geometry of the gantry, the shielding, and by an energy selection. Fig. 3 gives the probability per incident photon (E.= 511 Kev) that the scattered photon ($E'\gamma$) will be directed in a cone whose half-angle is θ. It shows that a good energy resolution detector is needed to eliminate a high amount of scattered events. It is important to add that the energy selection rejects good events corresponding to scattered photons inside the detector itself. Thus, with NaI (Tl) detectors, a low energy threshold (100 to 150 Kev) is usually chosen in order to optimize the efficiency to the detriment of the scattered photons contribution. From this point of view, bismuth-germanate (B.G.O.) is more suitable than NaI (Tl) because the photopeak fraction is higher, but its light yield is only 8 % than that of NaI. It means that the B.G.O. energy resolution is poor (25 % at 511 Kev) and consequently a relatively low fraction of scattered events can be rejected.

Random coïncidences rate is proportional to the time coïncidence. For an ideal system, the time window is determined by the transit time ofa photon in the object. With conventional detectors, the coïncidence resolving time limit is given by the scintillation decay time. This is the major disadvantage of B.G.O. From this point of view, NaI(Tl) is about two times better, but cesium-fluoride (CsF) appears to be the most suitable one.

4.3. Cesium-fluoride characteristics {9}

A 550 p.sec resolving time (FWHM) was obtained with two 1"x1" crystals coupled with two phototubes type XP 2020*, 2 inches in diameter. This means that high counting rate capability can be obtained without pile-up effects and that a time-of-flight technique combined with a reconstruction method can be applied. A detailed nuclear characterization was performed by means of the single photo-electron method {11}. Fig. 4 shows the time distribution spectrum of the light pulse. The decay time is equal to 3.2.n. sec and no long component was found. Fig. 5 gives the time of response for different types of scintillators . The resolving time of CsF is comparable to that of plastic scintillators and the linear attenuation coefficient at 511 Kev is a little better than that of NaI(Tl). Typically, the photoelectron yield was found to be 400 photoelectrons per Mev. More recently, some better results were obtained with doped crystals which were grown by LETI/CRM Laboratory. 15 % more light was obtained with CsI doped sample, but further improvements of CsF properties can be expected with selective doping.

4.4. Associated phototube

A very fast phototube was used for the CsF characterization in order to keep negligeable the timing phototube contribution. Fast commercially available photo-tubes are two inches in diameter and the corresponding spatial resolution for a P.C.T. design would be very poor. A one inch diameter phototube seems to be a good trade-off for a whole body P.C.T. Time measurements were performed with a 1" $\frac{1}{8}$ diameter phototube type P.M. 1982[X] and it was found that its own resolving time was very good on the 15 mm diameter central area. A modification of the electron input optics was carried out and the results obtained with the first prototypes of that new small diameter fast phototube (called PM 1992) are very promising. A 700 p.sec (F.W.H.M.) resolving time was obtained with two prototypes coupled to two encapsulated CsF scintillators among which was a doped CsI. That test was performed with 25 mm diameter and 40 mm long scintillators. The energy threshold was adjusted to 100 Kev.
This size appears to be a good trade off between the detection efficiency and the resolving time for a time-of-flight P.C.T. design, but it is clear that longer scintillators could be chosen for high counting rate capability P.C.T. where time-of-flight information would not be used. The above resolving time figure must be considered as a preliminary result. Some further ameliorations can be expected by using doped crystals with better optic coupling to the phototube and by improving the phototube time response.

5. TIME-OF-FLIGHT TECHNIQUE RESULTS

5.1. Experimentation

Fig. 6 is the schematic draft of the time-of-flight experiment. A cylindrical phantom is moved in translation and rotation between two opposing detectors. The experimental conditions were the following :

- Phantom : 15 cm in diameter with a cold spot 30 mm in diameter and a hot spot 30 mm in diameter (activity ratio = 2)
- Type of radionuclide : ^{68}Ge - activity ratio = 2

- Detectors : . Two phototubes XP 2020 coupled with undoped CsF scintillators($\frac{1}{2}$"x1")
  - . Energy threshold = 100 Kev
  - . Resolving time (F.W.H.M.)= 400 p.sec
  - . Collimator slit : 4 mm
- Sampling : . Linear = 6 mm step to step
  - . Angular : 6° over 360 °
- Number of counts : 7.10^5

5.2. Data handling

Each detected event is stored with an address corresponding to its translation and rotation position and its time-of-flight measurement. Fig. 7 shows a perspective view of a histoprojection with the T.O.F. method. It represents the raw data alond a direction for a uniform phantom 320 mm in diameter. The left part of Fig. 8 shows the same histoprojection after attenuation correction and the right part presents a conventional projection after attenuation correction.
A large memory would be needed for the histogram mode acquisition with T.O.F. technique ; thus the list mode handling is a better approach to optimize the digital hardware.

5.3. Reconstruction method

After attenuation corrections, and possibly measurement corrections, each event of the object O (ρ,θ) is back-projected along its own direction with a Gaussian distribution on the image matrix and the corresponding bidimensional Fourier transform of the back-projected image is $\mathcal{F}_2\left[O(\rho,\theta) * G(\rho)\right] = I(\nu,\varphi)$.

Where ν is the radial frequency and φ the argument.The inverse filter $H(\nu)$ of the point spread function $G(\rho)$ is shown on Figure 9 for different values of the standard deviation σ. $C(\nu)$ is the associated window function which was chosen for the reconstruction.

Thus : $\mathcal{F}_2\left[O(\rho,\theta)\right] = I(\nu,\varphi) \times N(\nu) \times C(\nu) = K(\nu,\varphi)$

and : $O(\rho,\theta) = \mathcal{F}_2^{-1}\left[K(\nu,\varphi)\right]$

5.4. Results

Figure 10 shows the comparison between conventional and T.O.F. methods for a uniform phantom 150 mm in diameter. The dotted curve is the activity density distribution along a diametrical section. Figure 11 establishes the same comparison with a phantom 150 mm in diameter comprising a cold spot 30 mm in diameter and a hot spot 30 mm in diameter (activity ratio = 2).

The statistical noise reduction is clearly illustrated for the activity density distribution along a diametrical section, and, at a lower level, for the noise structure perception of the image and for the outline definition of the spots. Further improvements can be expected in optimizing image reconstruction parameters.

Those results were obtained with a good resolving time and a small diameter object. Comparable improvements can be expected with a lower resolving time and a larger object as would be the case in practice.

6. CONCLUSION

Positron imaging is essentially a method for studying dynamic phenomena (biochemical kinetics and hydrodynamic flow) and positron emitters are characterized by a short life which allows the injection of a high activity. This means that a high counting rate capability is a major feature of the P.C.T.. Furthermore, a high resolving

time reduces the random coïncidence contribution as discussed above. For all these reasons, CsF appears to be the most suitable scintillator.
Its fast decay time permits the generation of time-of-flight information which improves the signal to noise ratio of the image. This advantage is a function of the T.O.F. accuracy. Further developments can be expected along these lines by the use of doped crystals which have better optic coupling and very fast small diameter phototubes. But this technique is strongly dependant on the state of the art in very high speed analog and digital data manipulative methods. As a first step, the importance of CsF is remaining for a P.C.T. design without the use of T.O.F. technique, because the CsF very high counting rate capability is a major advantage for first dynamic studies with short-lived emitters.

Footnote :* Radiotechnique Compelec

REFERENCES

{1} MM. TER POGOSSIAN, M.E. PHELPS, E.J. HOFFMAN and al.
"A positron-emission transaxial tomograph for nuclear medicine imaging (P.E.T.T.) Radiology 114, 1975 : pp. 89-98

{2} M.E. PHELPS, E.J. HOFFMAN, N.A. MULLANI and al.
"Application of annihilation coïncidence detection to transaxial reconstruction tomography"
J. Nucl. Med. 16, 1975 : pp. 210-224

{3} G.L. BROWNELL, C.A. BURNHAM, S. WILENSKY
"New developments in positron scintigraphy and the application of cyclotron produced positron emitters".
Salzburg. August 6-15, 1968, Vienna, I.A.E.A., 1969 : p. 466

{4} W.L. DUNN
"Time-of-flight localization of positron emitting isotopes"
Thesis in Physics, Vanderbilt University, Nashville, TN, 1975

{5} R.E. CAMPAGNOLO, P. GARDERET, J. VACHER
"Tomographie par émetteurs de positrons avec mesure de temps de vol"
Communication au Colloque National sur le traitement du signal, Nice, mai 1979

{6} E.J. HOFFMAN, M.E. PHELPS
"An analysis of some of the physical aspects of positron transaxial tomography" Comput. Biol. Med. 6, 1976 : pp 345-370

{7} T.F. BUDINGER, S.E. DERENZO, G.T. GULLBERG, R.H. HUESMAN
"Trends and prospects for circular ring positron cameras"
I.E.E.E. Trans. Nucl. Sci. N.S. 26 n° 2, 1979 : pp 2742-2745

{8} M.E. PHELPS, E.F. HOFFMAN, SUNG-CHENG HUANG, D.E. KUHL
"Design considerations in positron computed tomography"
I.E.E.E. Trans. Nucl. Sci. N.S.26 n° 2, 1979 : pp 2746-2751

{9} R. ALLEMAND, C. GRESSET, J. VACHER
"Potential advantages of a cesium-fluoride scintillator for a time-of-flight positron camera"
J. Nucl. Med. 21, n° 2, 1980 : pp. 153-155

{10} R. ALLEMAND, R. GARIOD, M. LAVAL, E. TOURNIER
"Etat actuel et évolution des tomographes à positrons"
20ème Colloque de médecine nucléaire de langue française, BORDEAUX, Sept.1979

{11} M. MOSZYNSKI, C. GRESSET, J. VACHER, R. ODRU
"Properties of CsF, fast inorganic scintillator in energy and time spectroscopy". To be published in the Journal of nuclear instruments and methods

FIGURE CAPTIONS

Fig. 1 Principle of the time-of-flight method

Fig. 2 Basic difference between the conventional method and the T.O.F. technique

Fig. 3 The probability per incident photon ($E\gamma$ = 511 Kev) that the scattered photon ($E'\gamma$) will be directed in a cone whose the half angle is θ.

Fig. 4 Time distribution of the light pulse of a 5 mm thick CsF sample

Fig. 5 Time of response for different types of scintillators

Fig. 6 Schematic draft of the time-of-flight experience

Fig. 7 Perspective view of an histoprojection with the T.O.F. method. It represents the raw data along a direction for a uniform phantom 320 mm in diameter

Fig. 8 Comparison between the data acquisition obtained with the T.O.F. technique and those of conventional method

Fig. 9 Variation of the theoretical inverse $H(\nu)$ as a function of the spatial frequency ν, for different values of the standard deviation σ and variation of the window function $C(\nu)$.

Fig. 10 Comparison between conventional and T.O.F. methods for a uniform phantom 150 mm in diameter. F.W.H.M. resolution = 400 p.sec . The dotted curve is the activity density distribution along a diametrical section

Fig. 11 Comparison between conventional and T.O.F. methods for a phantom 150 mm in diameter with a cold spot (Ø 30 mm) and a hot spot (Ø 30 mm) (activity ratio = 2).
The dotted curve is the activity density distribution along a diametrical section

Table 1 and Table 2

Physical and nuclear characteristics of different types of scintillators NaI(Tl), B.G.O., CsF and plastic scintillators NE 104.

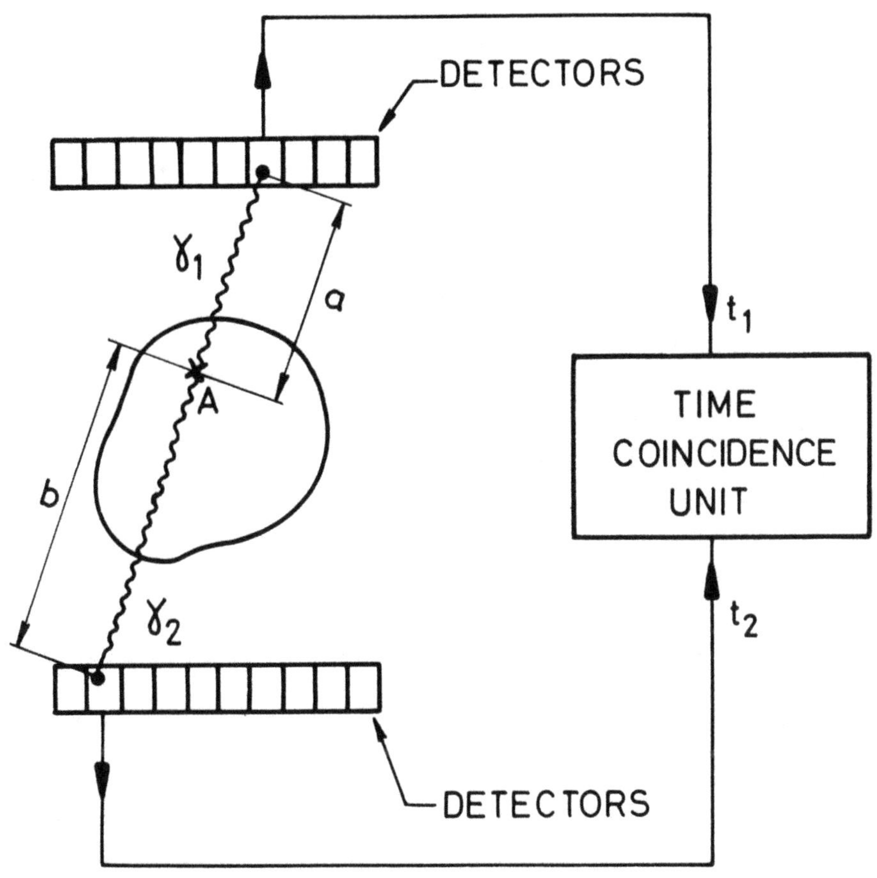

$$b - a = c\ (t_1 - t_2)$$

PRINCIPLE OF TIME-OF-FLIGHT METHOD

Fig. 1 : Principle of time-of-flight method

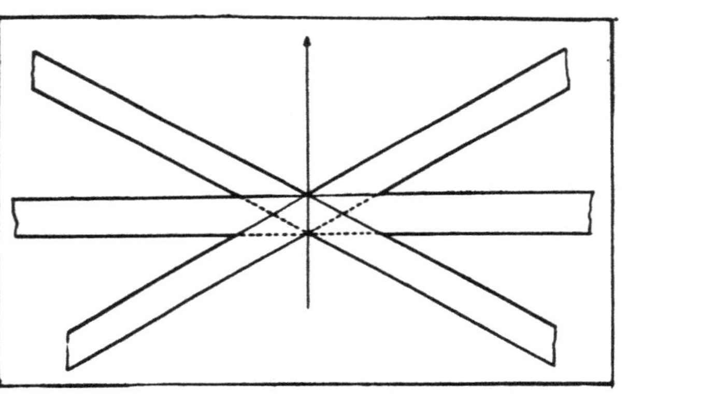

CONVENTIONAL
BACK-PROJECTION

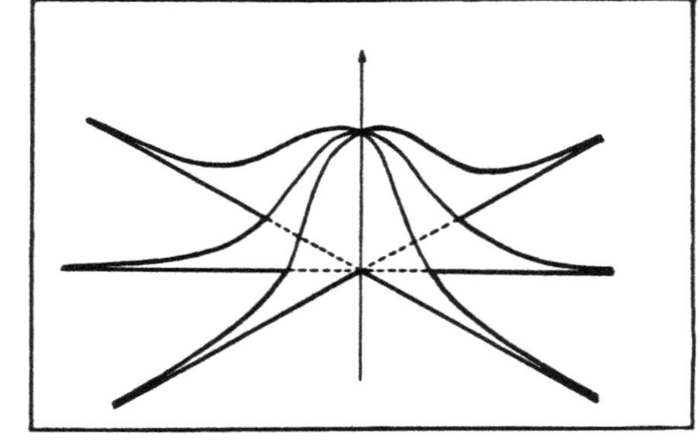

BACK-PROJECTION
WITH TIME-OF-FLIGHT (TOF) METHOD

$G(\rho) = \frac{1}{\rho}$

POINT SPREAD FONCTION

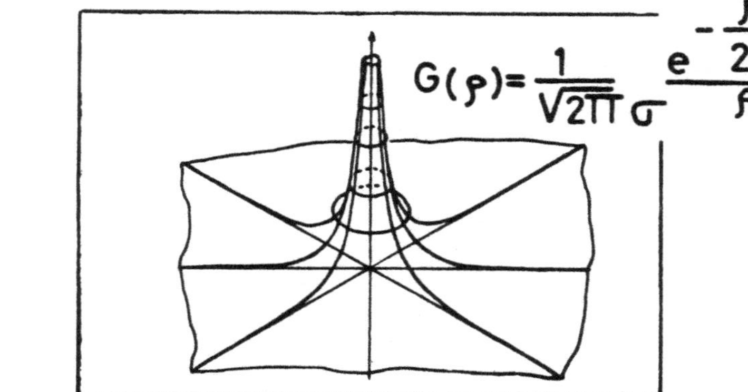

$G(\rho) = \frac{1}{\sqrt{2\pi}\,\sigma} \frac{e^{-\frac{\rho^2}{2\sigma^2}}}{\rho}$

POINT SPREAD FONCTION
WITH "TOF" METHOD

Fig. 2 : Basic difference between the conventional method and the T.O.F. technique

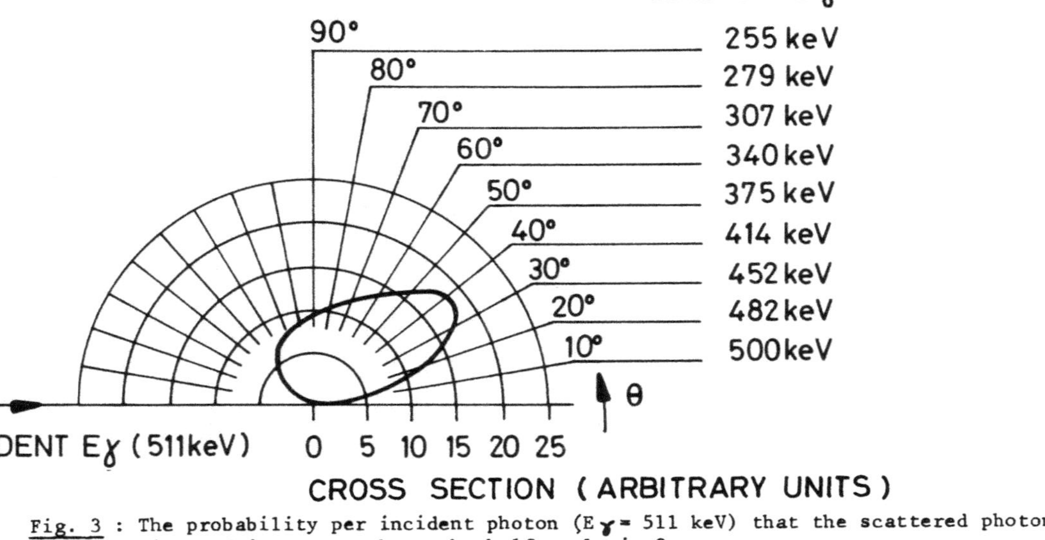

Fig. 3 : The probability per incident photon (E_γ = 511 keV) that the scattered photon (E'_γ) will be directed in a cone whose the half angle is θ.

THE PROBABILITY PER INCIDENT PHOTON (E_γ = 511 keV) THAT THE SCATTERED PHOTON (E'_γ) WILL BE DIRECTED IN A CONE WHOSE THE HALF ANGLE IS θ.

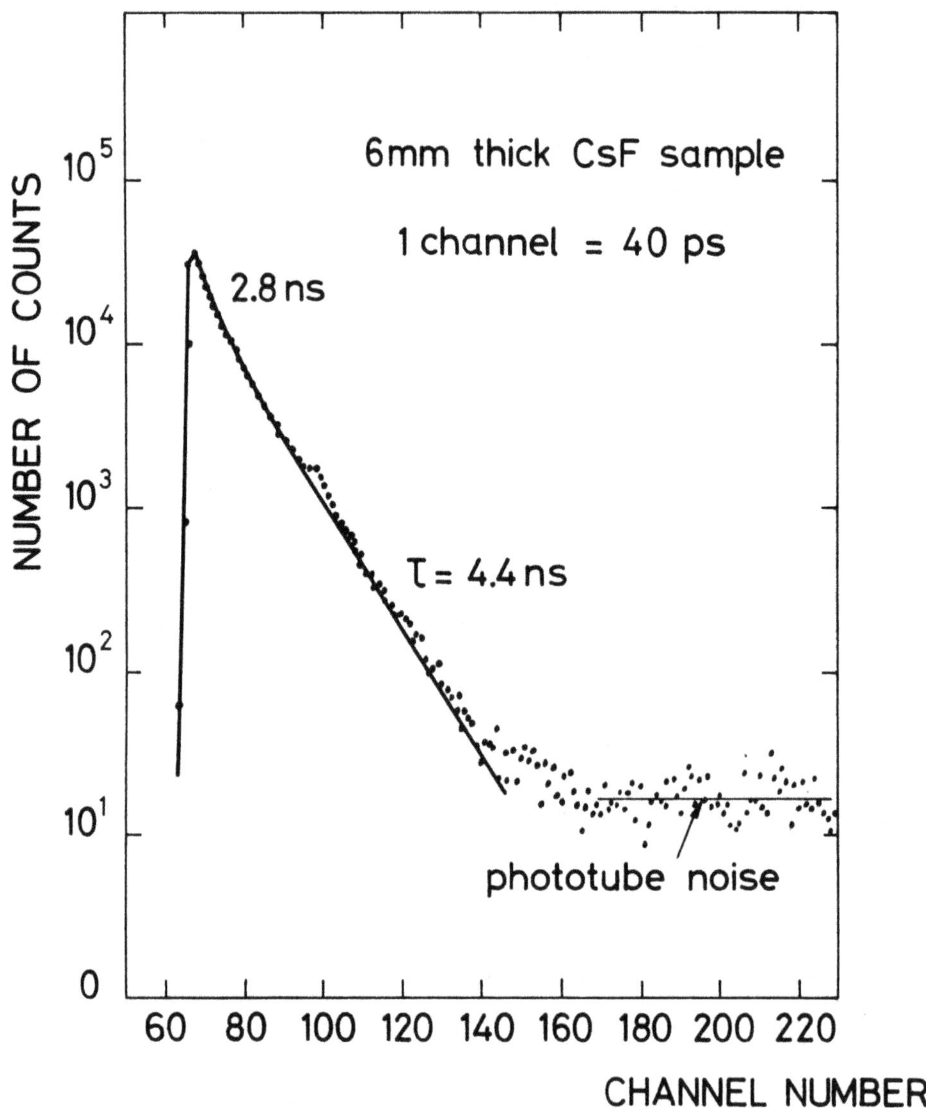

Fig. 4 : Time distribution of the light pulse of a CsF sample

TIME DISTRIBUTION OF THE LIGHT PULSE OF A CsF SAMPLE

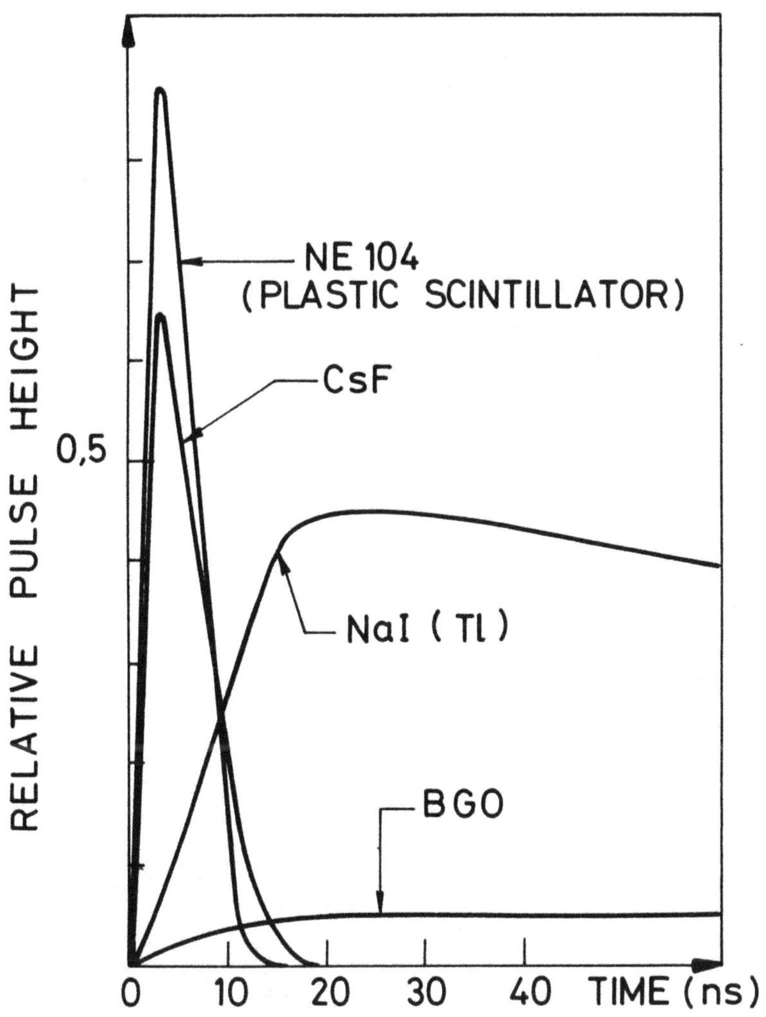

Fig. 5 : Time of response of different scintillators

TIME OF RESPONSE OF DIFFERENT SCINTILLATORS

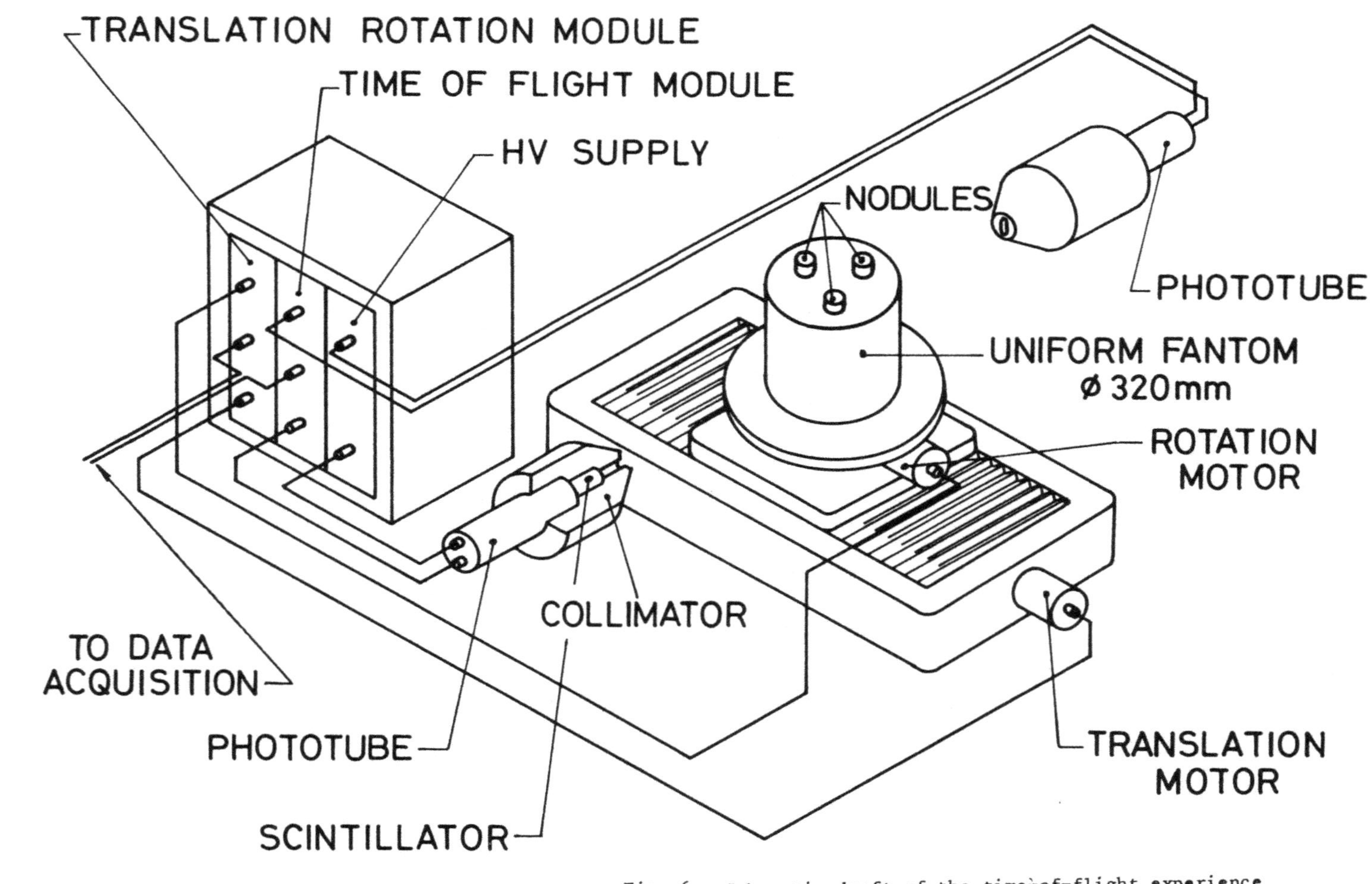

Fig. 6 : Schematic draft of the time-of-flight experience

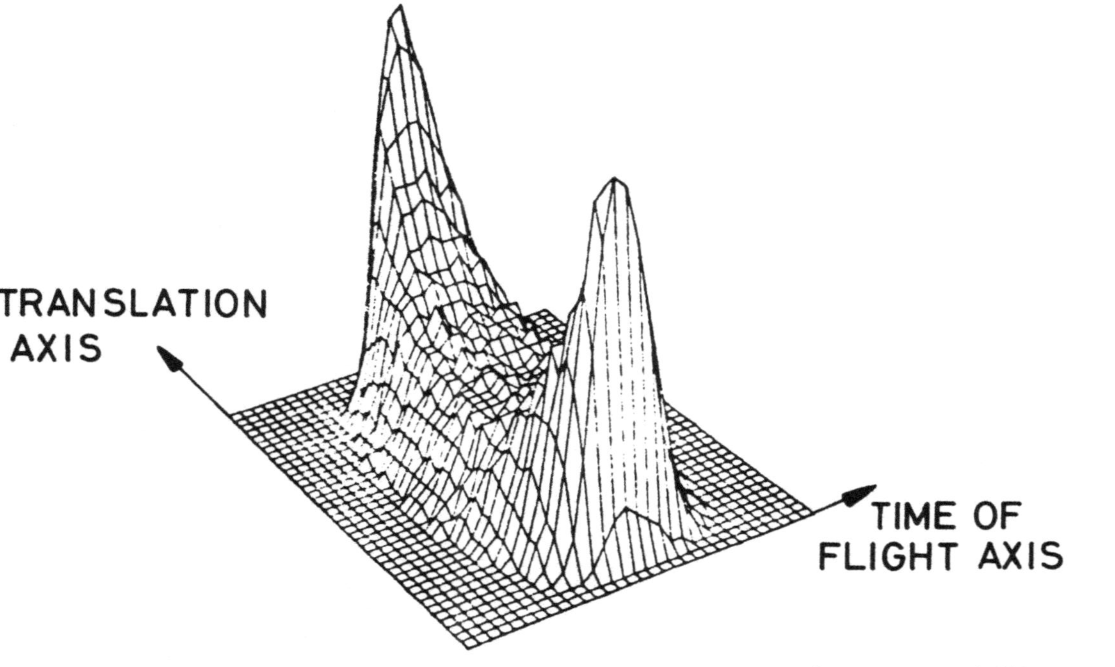

Fig. 7 : Time of flight method = raw data along a direction for a uniform fantom Ø 320 mm

TIME OF FLIGHT METHOD = RAW DATA ALONG A DIRECTION
FOR A UNIFORM FANTOM Ø 320 mm

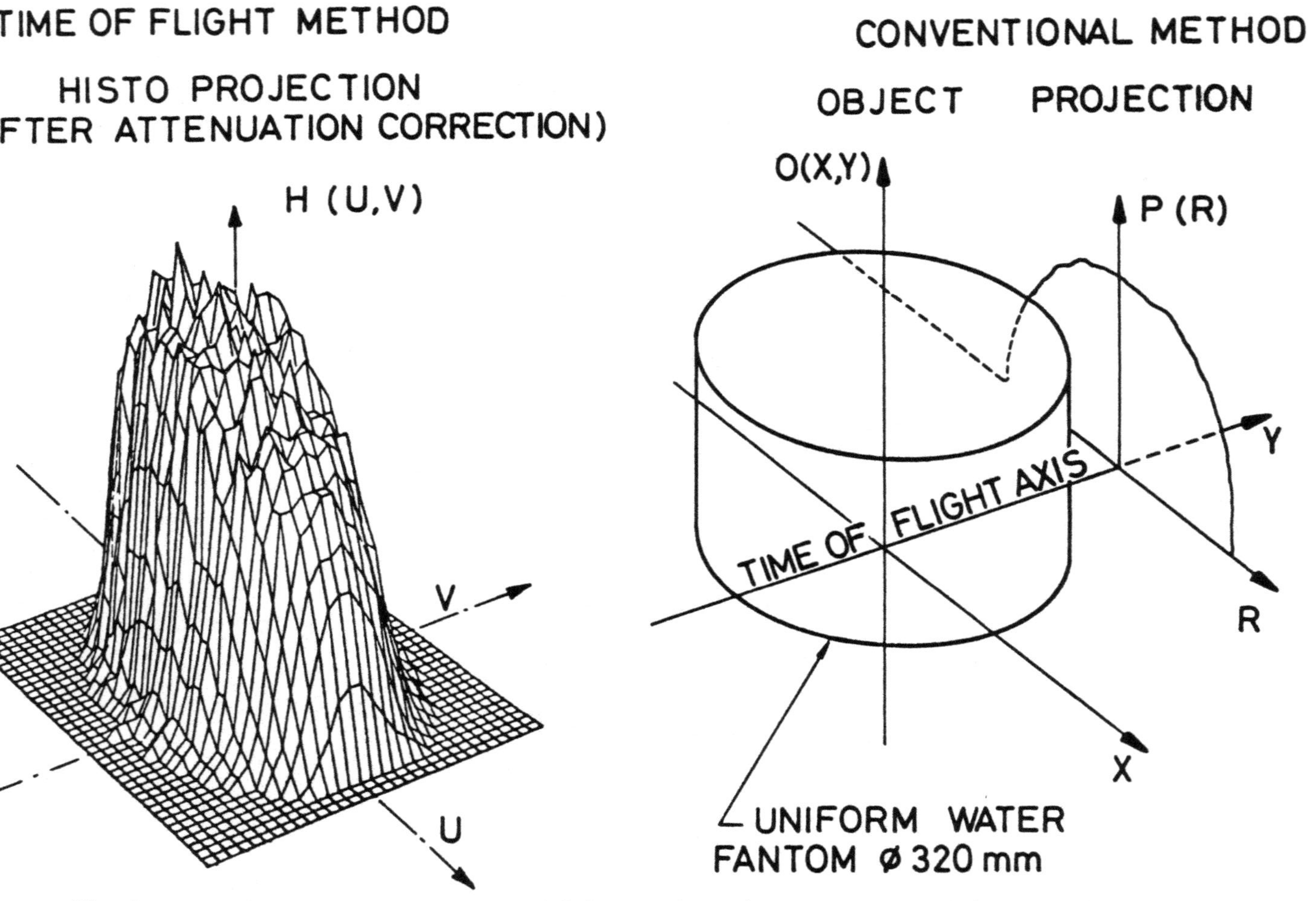

Fig. 8 : Comparison between the data acquisition obtained with the T.O.F. technique and those of

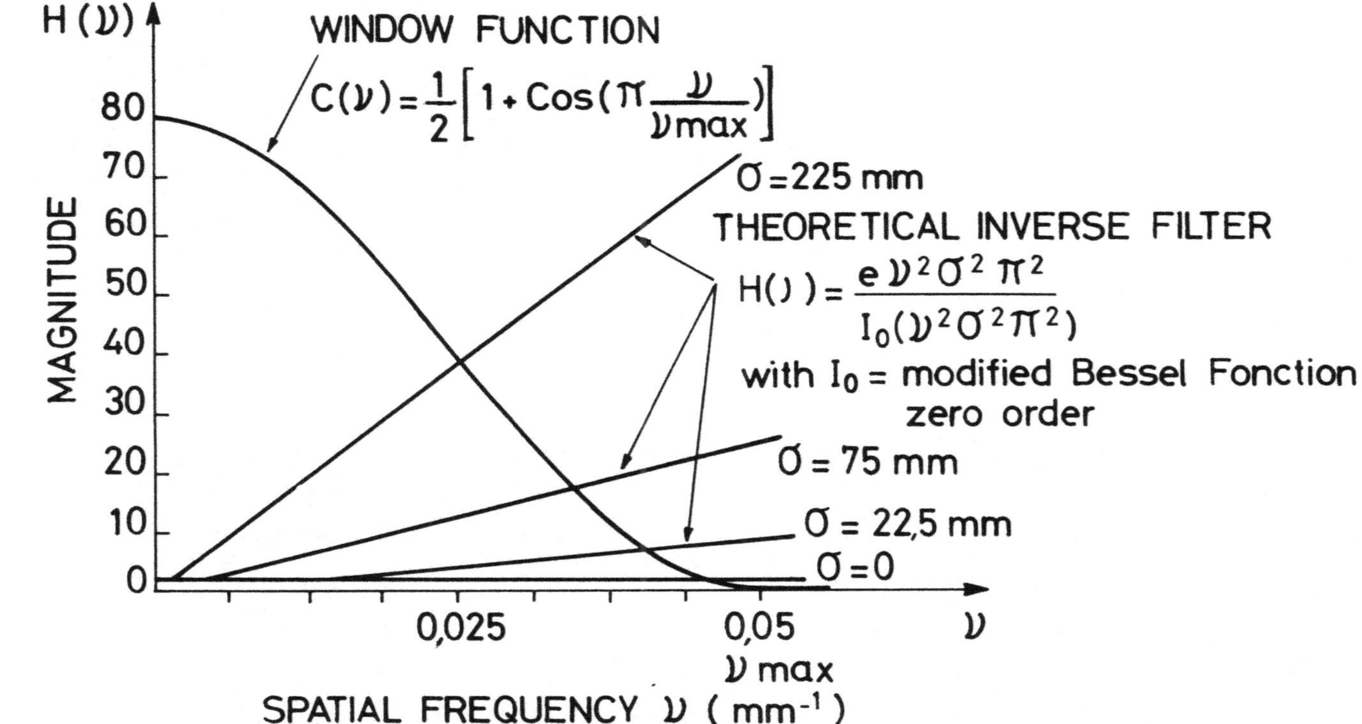

Fig. 9 : Variation of the theoretical inverse $H(\nu)$ as a function of the spatial frequency ν, for different values of the standard deviation σ and variation of the window function $C(\nu)$.

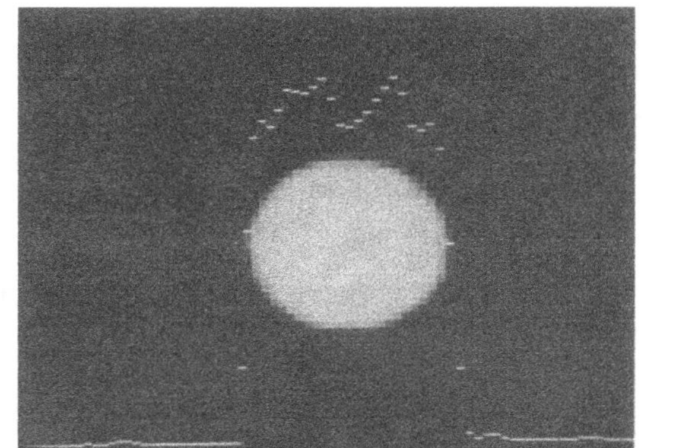

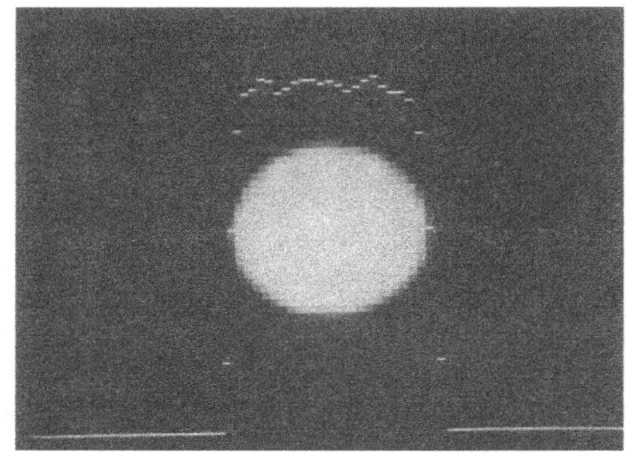

Fig. 10 : Comparison between conventional and T.O.F. methods for a uniform phantom 150 mm in diameter

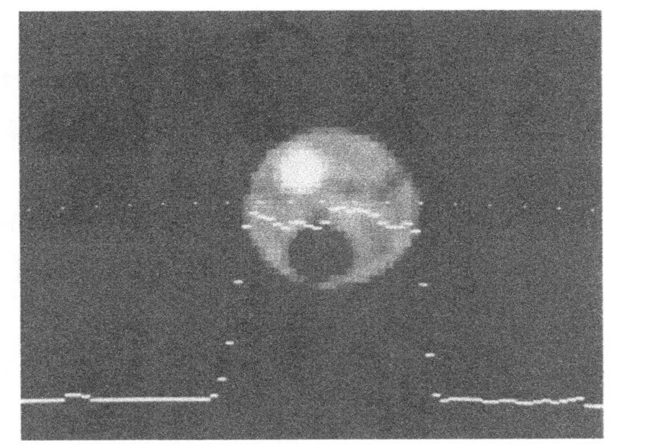

CONVENTIONAL METHOD

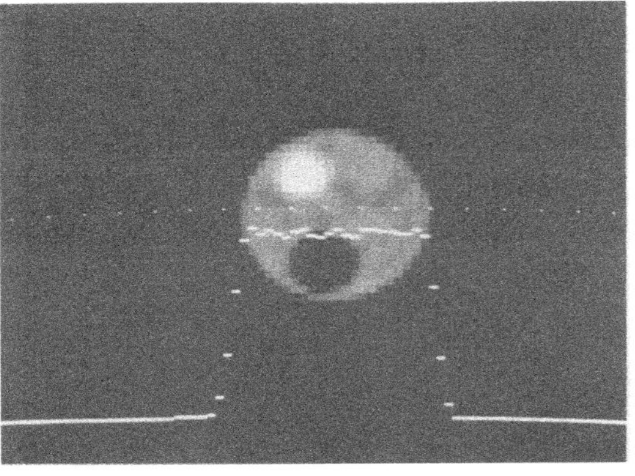

TIME OF FLIGHT METHOD
FWHM TIME RESOLUTION : 400 ps

Fig. 11 : Comparison between conventional and T.O.F. methods for a phantom 150 mm in diameter with a cold spot (Ø 30 mm) and a hot spot (Ø 30 mm)

COMPARISON BETWEEN
TIME OF FLIGHT METHODS

FANTOM Ø 150mm WITH COLD SPOT Ø 30 mm
AND HOT SPOT Ø 30mm (ACTIVITY RATIO = 2)

COMPARISON BETWEEN NaI (Tl), $Bi_4Ge_3O_{12}$, CsF, AND Ne-104				
	NaI (Tl)	$Bi_4Ge_3O_{12}$	CsF	Ne - 104
DENSITY	3.67	7.13	4.61	1.03
ATOMIC NUMBERS	11, 53	83, 32, 8	55, 9	1, 6
LINEAR ATTENUATION COEFFICIENT AT 511 keV (cm^{-1})	0.34	0.92	0.39	
SCINTILLATION PEAK WAVELENGTH nm	413	480	390	406
INDEX OF REFRACTION AT PEAK WAVELENGTH	1.78	2.15	1.48	1.58
DIMENSIONS OF THE CRYSTALS: DIAMETER AND HEIGHT	1 1/4" x 1"	4/5" x 1 1/4"	1" x 1"	1 1/4" x 1"

Table 1

COMPARISON BETWEEN NaI (Tl), $Bi_4Ge_3O_{12}$, CsF, AND Ne-104				
	NaI (Tl)	$Bi_4Ge_3O_{12}$	CsF	Ne - 104
RELATIVE SCINTILLATION OUTPUT (%)	100	8	3.7	29
ENERGY RESOLUTION AT 511 keV (%)	10	25	35	No Photoelectric Effect
SCINTILLATION DECAY TIME (nsec)	230	300	5	2,0
COINCIDENCE RESOLVING TIME (FWHM) FOR A 100-keV THRESHOLD (nsec)	2.0	3.4	0.55	0.52
RELATIVE SINGLE COUNTING RATE (%) FOR THE SAME VOLUME OF SCINTILLATOR	100	178	118	13
PHOTOPEAK FRACTION	0.3	0.8	0.3	

Table II

SAMPLED APERTURE TECHNIQUES FOR HIGH RESOLUTION ULTRASOUND TOMOGRAPHY

Steven A. Johnson
Department of Bioengineering
University of Utah
Salt Lake City, Utah 84112

ABSTRACT

This paper reviews two new imaging techniques which depend upon sampling the ultrasound pressure signal at many places on an aperture. The predicted performance of these new methods is compared with well known and standard ultrasound techniques such as those found in focused piston transducer B-scan systems and phased array imaging systems. These new methods show promise for improved resolution and qualitative tissue characterization. The first of these techniques, synthetic focusing, is analogous to the seismic imaging methods known as seismic migration used in geophysical exploration for petroleum. The relationship of this method to acoustical holography will be discussed. The second sampled aperture technique, diffraction tomography, is a first-order perturbation method for finding inverse solutions of the wave equation in the interior of a region from measurements on its boundary. The method holds promise for reconstructing ultrasonic refractive index, attenuation, and specific impedance. Both new methods are capable of producing images with resolution of about one wavelength.

1. INTRODUCTION

Medical ultrasonic imaging has shown steady growth and has become a reliable clinical tool. Nevertheless, the present clinical ultrasound scanners do not provide quantitative images of tissue parameters. Furthermore, the resolution of many clinical scanners is below the theoretical limit. The advent of computers with high computation speeds at reasonable costs and the success of X-ray computed tomography have prompted the search for corresponding qualitative ultrasound reconstruction techniques. In this paper we explore two methods which hold promise for providing improved resolution and qualitative measurement.

2. DESCRIPTION OF TRADITIONAL SYSTEMS

Some of the earliest ultrasonic imaging methods made use of a fixed focused piston transducer with or without an attached lens or curved reflecting surface to provide a fixed focal length. These transducers are mounted on angle sensing arms to provide information on beam direction. Some skill and artistry is required by the operator in using this method, since the transducer is scanned by hand. The beam direction and pulse arrival times are combined by a controller to provide a registered image on a cathode ray tube for viewing and photographing. Many of today's ultrasound B-scanners are based on these techniques.

Recently, the use of annular arrays (i.e., so-called bull's eye transducers) have been proposed and tested to overcome the fixed focus limitations of earlier schemes (D. Dietz, et al.). Although, in general, annular arrays only focus along a line perpendicular to their face, a two-dimensional image may be produced by mechanical translation or rotation of an annular array. Some of these systems operate at, so-called, "real-time" rates of 15 or more scans per second. When used with solid-state scan converters, these images provide sufficient time resolution for circulatory system imaging and can show pulsating changes in vessel diameter. The requirement for uniform received echo waveform for point target at all distances may not be met with a fixed focus transducer for two reasons: First, lateral resolution is optimum only in a certain depth of field zone containing the focal point, and second, the series of nulls and 180° phase reversals which occur along the axis of symmetry of the beam path for each component frequency may (especially for narrow band signals) produce echo distortion except in the focal depth-of-field zone.

Pulse shape (i.e., waveform) uniformity and focal depth of field can be improved sufficiently by use of annular arrays to warrant their use in many applications. Nevertheless, in their customary mode of operation, annular arrays, with time variable delay line focusing, do not provide the optimum solution to pulse shape uniformity, depth of field, and maximum lateral and depth resolution requirements. The reason for this shortcoming is found in the mathematical impossibility of focusing the transmitted waves at more than one point on the symmetry axis. That the scattered waves may be dynamically focused for a single transmitted signal for all points along the symmetry axis by time variable delay lines on the receiver channels is true enough, but the transmitted waveform may not be dynamically focused. Thus, the scattered waves from each point along the symmetry axis do not have a uniform pulse shape. Even an attempt to transmit a plane wave is not a perfect solution because of the periodic phase reversals associated with a piston transducer [P. R. Stephanishen, 1971]. One method of preserving scattered pulse shape for all ranges would be to transmit a wave which is focused for a particular range and simultaneously focus the receiver delay lines on this point and repeat these two steps for every range increment. However, this method is time-consuming. A more elegant and time-efficient method is synthetic focusing, which we will describe in more detail later. We note also that synthetic focusing may be used with annular arrays to improve their performance.

Linear phased arrays or so-called beam steering arrays have demonstrated improved depth of focus and time resolution [N. Bom, *et al.*, 1973]. Scan times of 30 fields per second are possible with linear phased arrays by the use of electronic beam forming and beam scanning (i.e., beam steering) techniques. The small size and flexibility of linear arrays simplify their application to many areas of the body in comparison to mechanical scanners and is one reason for their increased popularity. Although a linear array is capable of transmitting and receiving a beam within a wide scan range (typically 60° to 90°), the same limitations on focusing apply along each individual beam direction as applies in the case of annular arrays. In other words, receiving dynamic focusing is possible, but the transmitted beam is fixed by laws of physics to focus only one point per transmission. Some workers have simply ignored this problem in the design of their scanners, and yet images produced by their equipment are quite good in comparison with earlir methods and represent a big improvement over some mechanical scanners. Equipment built by other workers tries to overcome this problem by use of interlaced transmitter focal ranges [F. L. Thurstone, *et al.*, 1974]. Improved lateral and especially depth resolution could probably be attained with this equipment if synthetic focusing techniques were used.

3. SYNTHETIC FOCUSING METHOD

During the time of development of X-ray CT acoustic imaging, workers sought to develop ultrasound imaging techniques which would provide improved resolution over conventional B-scan techniques. The Mayo group very early advocated and demonstrated a technique which combined sampled operations, analog waveform digitizing, and digital image computation techniques, which they termed synthetic focus imaging [S. A. Johnson, *et al.*, 1975]. The method was later extended to arbitrary aperatures [S. A. Johnson, *et al.*, 1978]. Resolution was improved by incorporating convolution kernels and apodizing techniques [S. A. Johnson, *et al.*, 1978, 1979] and by direct inversion [S. J. Norton, *et al*, 1978]. It was soon demonstrated that this technique is related to seismic imaging technique [S. A. Johnson, 1978, 1979]. A close mathematical relationship to X-ray CT has been demonstrated by use of the principle of back projection along equal propagation time surfaces [S. A. Johnson, *et al.*, 1979; S. A. Johnson, *et al.*, 1978]. The latter observation has been noted by others and is responsible for an alternate name, "reflection tomography", for synthetic focusing [S. J. Norton, June 1978; G. Wade, *et al.*, 1978]. It is significant that "real time" synthetic focus imaging has been demonstrated [P. D. Corl, *et al.*, 1978].

The mathematics for synthetic aperture imaging may be derived by reference to equation 1. Let P_k define a measure of the probability for acoustic amplitude scattering or reflection toward the detector aperture from picture element k when illumination from each transmitter element in the array aperture, measured at picture element k, is normalized. The probability for energy scattering is the square of P_k. For the case of a very narrow pulse of ultrasonic energy, P_k is given by

$$P_k = \left| \sum_{m=1}^{N} \sum_{j=1}^{N} \sum_{i=t-w}^{t+w} \sum_{z} V_{z,j,m} R_{j,k} T_{k,m} K_{i-z} \right| \quad (1)$$

where $V_{i,j,m}$ is the ith voltage sample from the jth array element when the mth array element was used as the transmitter. $R_{j,k}$ is the receiver-range azimuth illumination normalization factor between the kth picture element and the jth array element. Thus, $R_{j,k}$ is independent of time, but is an approximate function of some power of the magnitude of $\vec{r}_{j,k}$ (where $\vec{r}_{j,k}$ is the vector from array element j to picture element k), and of the cosine of the angle between $\vec{r}_{j,k}$ and $\vec{n}_j$ (the unit vector normal to array element j). Thus, $R_{j,k}$ may be written

$$R_{j,k} = \left[\exp\left(\int_k^j \alpha(s)ds\right)\right]\left[\int_k^j ds\right]^q\left[\vec{n}_j \cdot \vec{S}_{k,j}\right]^{-1} \quad (2)$$

where α is the attenuation coefficient along the ray path connecting k and j, q is a rational number from 0.5 for cylindical waves to 1.0 for spherical waves, and $\vec{S}_{k,j}$ is the unit tanget vector at j of the ray which passes from k to j. $T_{k,m}$ is the corresponding transmitter function between the kth and m^{th} array (transmitter) element. Thus, $R_{j,k}$ and $T_{k,m}$ affect the energy normalizations referred to in the definition of P_k. N is the number of array elements. The factor K_{t-i} is a kernel function for performing convolution or cross correlation operations on the raw data $V_{i,j,m}$. If $V_{i,j,m}$ is of the appropriate pre-transmitted form or post-received processed form, then K_{t-i} may be of the form of a delta function $\delta_{o,t-i} = \delta_{t,i}$. The limits $t \pm w$ are related to the transmitter pulsewidth t_w, which is less than some arbitrary bracketing interval t_B which contains the transmitted pulse of width t_w.

Then,

$$t = \left(\int_m^k \frac{ds}{U(s)} + \int_k^j \frac{ds}{U(s)}\right)\frac{1}{\Delta t}, \quad (3)$$

and,

$$w = t_w/2\Delta t \quad (4)$$

where Δt is the sampling interval time between successive samples in the digitized signal, and U is the effective velocity of sound in the insonified medium. The two line integrals are taken along the rays connecting transmitter m to k and k to receiver j, respectively.

An example of the benefit of using proper transmitted CT kernel-like waveforms and apodization for data derived from linear arrays has been shown [S. A. Johnson, _et al._, 1978, 1979]. It is seen that the wings of the point response function (image of single scattering point) are of a much lower value with the use of apodization. It is also obvious that the Tanaka-Iinuma kernel produces the best suppression of wing artifacts (looks like a bow tie) and concentric ring segment artifacts. Since most array imaging schemes produce damped sine wave signals, the implications for possible improved resolution may be significant.

Synthetic focusing has been extended to allow for arbitrary source and detector geometries, arbitrary waveforms, and arbitrary a priori distributions of attenuation and refractive index [S. A. Johnson, et al., 1978]. One formulation of this extension is based upon the inversion of a matrix which described the data collection process in terms of the incident acoustic field, the object, and the detectors [S. A. Johnson, et al., 1978]. Such an imaging matrix may often be inverted by iterative techniques such as the well known ART method [J. F. Greenleaf, et al., 1975]. A comparison of the convolution-back projection formulation of synthetic focusing as given by equations 1 through 4 above and the matrix inversion formulation has been made [S. A. Johnson, et al., 1979]. In this study, images produced by the matrix inversion method (which uses an ART type algorithm) appear slightly better than images fom the convolution-back projection method. Images of wire targets have been obtained experimentally with resolution near one wavelength using the synthetic focus algorithm of equation 1 [S. A. Johnson, et al., 1978].

The relationship between the synthetic focus technique and acoustical holography can be seen by examination of equation 1. If a single frequency is transmitted, then equation 3 for the round trip time selects the appropriate phase shift as would be calculated by single frequency holography theory.

4. DEVELOPMENT OF DIFFRACTION TOMOGRAPHY

The mathematical elegance of X-ray CT and the corresponding clinical usefulness of cross-sectional images of quantitative tissue X-ray attenuation prompted the Mayo Group [J. F. Greenleaf, et al., 1974; J. F. Greenleaf, et al., 1975] and other researchers [P. L. Carson, et al., 1977; G. H. Glover, 1977] to explore the feasibility of ultrasound transmission computed tomography. The initial effort produced images of ultrasound attenuation from amplitude data [J. F. Greenleaf, et al., 1974] and were followed later with refractive index images from propagation time data [J. F. Greenleaf, et al., 1975]. These techniques made the assumption that the ultrasound beams traveled in straight lines and is a fair assumption in the breast where variations of acoustic speed are usually less than 5 percent. An effort was made to improve image resolution by the use of ray tracing and use of curve path algebraic reconstruction techniques. It was found that use of curved ray algorithms produced improved reconstruction of gross-shape and dimension, but resolution was only slightly improved (resolution remained near about 10 wavelengths of the central spectral peak of the transducer combination) [R. K. Mueller, et al., 1979].

The lack of greatly improved resolution using curved ray algorithms is due to the comparable wavelength of acoustic energy with respect to the details to be resolved. Thus, resolution in ultrasound tomography is diffraction limited, unlike X-ray CT where resolution is governed by the detector resolution and number and completeness of projections. Similar resolution problems were known in the field of optics, and solutions had been suggested by Wolf [E. Wolf, 1969] and others [K. Itawa, et al., 1975]. These techniques make use of approximate solutions to the Helmholtz wave equation by use of perturbation theory. The first-order perturbation solution to the pressure field variable in the wave equation is similar to the well known Born approximation [E. Wolf, 1969]. The Rytov approximation is the first order perturbation solution to a new wave equation obtained by a complex logarithmic transformation of the pressure field and often provides a superior solution for objects with both small scattering centers and varying refractive index [K. Itawa, et al., 1975]. The Mayo group explored the possibility of applying these techniques to their breast cancer detection and imaging program; a portion of their investigation has been published [S. A. Johnson, et al., 1978]. Independently, workers at the University of Minnesota also explored and proposed similar perturbation techniques [R. K. Mueller, 1978] The original opical techniues [E. Wolf, 1969; K. Iwata, 1975] required the use of plane wave illumination. The use of circular or spherical wave fronts would be of great value for medical applications to allow use of multiple sources for higher speed data collections. First-order perturbation solutions to the wave equation for spherical wave illumination have been derived for circular detection data collection geometry by University of Utah workers [J. Ball, et al., 1979] and for linear detector data collection geometry by University of Minnesota workers [R. K. Mueller, 1978]. Experimental images of test objects using plane wave diffraction tomography has been reported by Kaveh [M. Kaveh, et al., 1979]. This field seems likely to remain fertile for years to come as practical diffraction limited solutions and inverse solutions to problems of multiple acoustic parameter (e.g., refractive index, absorption, acoustic impedance, nonlinear properties, etc.) imaging are sought.

The plane wave methods described above have theoretical significance, nevertheless, they have the following practical difficulties:

1. Plane wave transmitting transducers do not produce plane waves unless they are infinite in extent. Thus, finite extent "plane wave transducers" introduce artifacts in received signals.

2. Building an ultrasound scanner based on plane wave algorithms requires large bulky quasi plane wave transducers and slow mechanical rotation. Steering of plane waves for rapid scanning by electronic multiplexing is difficult.

Diffraction tomography based on plane waves does have the advantage of a relatively simple and fast algorithm based on the fast Fourier transform.

The difficulties of constructing a scanner based on plane waves may be overcome by use of spherical waves:

1. Any finite spherical transducer can produce spherical waves. Increasing the size of the transducer increases the strength of the waves.

2. A scanner based on spherical waves can be compact and fast because of the larger number of compact transmitting transducers which may be employed. Electronic switching of transmitters for rapid scanning is easily accomplished.

Until recently, no algorithms existed (that we know of) for inverting the diffraction tomography problem for spherical wave insonification. This condition has been rectified by the algorithms developed at Utah in the past year [J. Ball, et al., 1979; F. Stenger, et al., 1979]. We present here only an outline of the more extensive derivation given in the preceding references.

Sound excitation in a stationary medium with spacial variation of local density P and compressibility κ is described by

$$\left(\nabla^2 - c^{-2}(\vec{r})\,\frac{\partial^2}{\partial t^2}\right)P(\vec{r},\ t) = 0 \tag{5}$$

Here $P(\vec{r},\ t)$ is the sound pressure, and $c(r) = \left(\kappa(\vec{r})\rho(\vec{r})\right)^{-1/2}$ denotes the local sound velocity in the medium.

Assuming $P(\vec{r},\ t) = u(\vec{r})\ e^{j\omega t}$, we obtain the Helmholtz equation for u,

$$\left(\nabla^2 + c^{-2}\omega^2\right)u = 0 \tag{6}$$

We define the useful function for variation in speed of sound from a constant value.

$$f(\vec{r}) = \omega^2\left(c^{-2}(\vec{r}) - c_o^{-2}\right) \tag{7}$$

where c_o is the speed of sound of the medium surrounding the body (so that $f(\vec{r}) = 0$ on exterior of body. Combining the above equations, we obtain for $k = 2\pi/\lambda$.

$$\nabla^2 u + k^2 u = fu \tag{8}$$

Let

$$w \simeq \log \left(u/u_o\right) \tag{9}$$

be the Rytov approximation. Then for the case of a spherical wave source, the amplitude at $\vec{r}$ for source at $\vec{r}_s$ is given by the Green's function,

$$G_1\left(\vec{r}, \vec{r}_s\right) = \frac{e^{ik|\vec{r} - \vec{r}_s|}}{|\vec{r} - \vec{r}_s|} \tag{10}$$

where $\vec{r}_s$ is the source position and $\vec{r}$ is the measurement position. Then the above equations yield a solution for $w\left(\vec{r}_s, \vec{r}\right)$.

$$\begin{aligned} w\left(\vec{r}_s, \vec{r}\right) &= G_1 \, \ell n\left(u/G_1\right) \\ &= \iiint_{\vec{R}<\vec{a}} f(R) \frac{e^{ik\{ |\vec{r}_s - \vec{R}| + |\vec{r} - \vec{R}|}}{4\pi |\vec{r}_s - \vec{R}| \, |\vec{r} - \vec{R}|} d\vec{R} \end{aligned} \tag{11}$$

where $\vec{R}$ is dummy integration variable and $\vec{a}$ is radius of sphere which contains the body.

The expression for $w\left(\vec{r}_s, \vec{r}\right)$ involves a triple integral. This is reduced to a double integral over the tomographic plane by the method of stationary phase. The new double integral equation is then transformed to a matrix equation by orthogonal function expansions.

$$w_i = H_{ij} f_j \tag{12}$$

The resulting matrix equation is solved by multiplying the "data vector" w_i by an inverse matrix H_{ij}^{-1} to obtain the image vector" f_j.

In the method above which we propose (see [Stenger and Johnson, 1979] for details), the matrix to be inverted is sparce and of block diagonal form and, therefore, once the sparce inverse is computed, the coefficients may be stored for computing new images from new data.

As described above, there is no focusing of energy normal to the tomographic plane, i.e., the images are somewhat blurred in the vertical direction. In order to make the tomographic plane narrow (i.e., to make a compact 3-D image point response function), we propose two alternate solutions:

1. Use a synthetic focusing algorithm with a two-dimensional array to focus the phase of all transducer elements in a column normal to the tomographic plane. Sum all these elements to provide a composite phase and amplitude

for the column of elements. Apply the two-dimensional diffraction tomography algorithm to the new synthetically focused composite data.

2. Using a one-dimensional array, obtain a set of two-dimensional images at multiple parallel closely spaced vertical intervals. Transform this set of images into a set of vertically focused images (an algorithm to accomplish this transformation has been developed at the University of Utah).

5. CONCLUSION

The theoretical basis of synthetic focusing and diffraction tomography as high resolution ultrasound imaging techniques has been presented. Some experimental work has been performed with simple test objects which indicate that these techniques will provide improved resolution when applied to imaging in vitro and in vivo objects. Further experimental work remains to test these techniques with tissues and to improve the data collection speed through the use of electronic multiplexing and parallel data pathways. The quantitative accuracy of the images should be improved by solving wave equations which contain terms which more accurately model acoustic processes. Such research hold promise of producing significant improvement in diagnostic value of ultrasonic imaging.

ACKNOWLEDGMENTS

We acknowledge the support and collaboration of Dr. James F. Greenleaf, Mayo Clinic, in the evaluation of the synthetic focus technique while Dr. S. A. Johnson was at Mayo Clinic. The experimental data described in the text was obtained at Mayo. The support of Earl H. Wood and Erik Ritman, consecutive directors of the research unit at Mayo, where the synthetic focus work was performed, is appreciated. Professors Frank Stenger and James Ball played a vital role in developing the spherical wave ultrasound insonification, diffraction tomographic theory described in the text. Discussions with Dr. Michael J. Berggren and Professor Douglas A. Christensen is also appreciated. The secretarial help of Mrs. M. Swenson and Mrs. R. Eichers of the Electrical Engineering Department at the University of Utah is appreciated. Work at Mayo Clinic was supported by National Institute of Health grants RR-00007, HL-04664, and HL-5K04-10070. Continuing support at the University of Utah is provided by American Cancer Society grant PD7-110 and by NIH grants 5R01 CA 23430 and K04 HL 00687. The author expresses appreciation to the National Science Foundation and to Dr. Jack Sklansky, the U.S. cochairman of the National Science Foundation sponsored "U.S.-France Seminar on Biomedical Image Processing", for the invitation to present this seminar paper in Grenoble, France, May 26-31, 1980.

REFERENCES

Ball, J., Johnson, S. A., and Stenger, F., "Explicit inversion of the Helmholtz equation for ultrasound insonification and spherical detection", Acoustical Imaging, Vol. 9, Plenum Press, New York, from the Ninth International Symposium on Acoustical Imaging, Houston, Texas, December 3-6, 1979.

Bom, N., Lancee, C. T., van Swieten, G., et al., "Multiscan echocardiography part I: technical description", Circulation, Vol. XLVIII, pp. 1066-1074, November 1973.

Carson, P. L., Shabason, L., Dick, D. E., et al., "Tissue equivalent tissue objects for comparison of ultrasound transmission tomography by reconstruction and pulse echo imaging", National Bureau of Standards Second International Symposium on Ultrasonic Tissue Characterization, Gaithersburg, Maryland, June 13-15, 1977.

Corl, P. D., Kino, G. S., DeSilets, C. S., et al., "A digital synthetic focus acoustic imaging system", in: Metherell, Alex: Acoustical Holography, Plenum Press, New York, Vol. 8, 1978.

Dietz, D., Parks, S. J., and Linzer, M., "Expanding-aperture annular array", National Bureau of Standards Third International Symposium on Ultrasonic Imaging and Tissue Characterization, Gaithersburg, Maryland, June 1978.

Glover, G. H., "In-vivo measurement of ultrasonic refractive index distibutions in human breasts with time-of-flight tomography", National Bureau of Standards Second International Symposium on Ultrasonic Tissue Characterization, Gaithersburg, Maryland, June 13-15, 1977.

Greenleaf, J. F., Johnson, S. A., Lee, S. L., et al., "Algebraic reconstruction of spatial distributions of acoustic absorption with tissues from their two-dimensional acoustic projections",. Acoustical Holograpy., Vol. 5, Philip S. Green, Editor, Plenum Press, New York, pp. 591-603, 1974.

Greenleaf, J. F., Johnson, S. A., Samayoa, W. F., et al., "Algebraic reconstruction of spatial distributions of acoustic velocities in tissue from their time-of-flight profiles", Acoustical Holography, Vol. 6, Newell Booth, Editor, Plenum Press, New York, pp. 71-90, 1975.

Iwata, K., and Nagata, R., "Calculation of refractive index distribution from interferograms using the Born and Rytov's approximations", Japanese Journal of Applied Physics, Vol. 14, Supplement 14-1, 1975.

Johnson, S. A., Greenleaf, J. F., Duck, F. A., et al., "Digital computer simulation study of a real-time collection, postprocessing synthetic focusing ultrasound cardiac camera", Acoustical Holography, Vol. 6, Newell Booth, Editor, Plenum Press, New York, pp. 193-211, 1975.

Johnson, S. A., Greenleaf, J. F., Rajagopalan, B., et al., "High spatial resolution ultrasonic measurement techniques for characterization of static and moving tissues", National Bureau of Standards Second International Symposium on Ultrasonic Tissue Characterization, 1979.

Johnson, S. A., Greenleaf, J. F., Rajagopalan, B., et al, "Algebraic and analytic inversion of acoustic data from partially or fully enclosing apertures", in: Metherell, Alex: Acoustical Holography, Plenum Press, New York, Vol. 8, 1978.

Johnson, S. A., Greenleaf, J. F., Tanaka, M., et al., "Quantitative synthetic aperture reflection imaging with correction for refraction and attenuation: application of seismic techniques in medicine", Proceedings of the 1978 San Diego Biomedical Symposium.

Kaveh, M., Mueller, R., Rylander, R., Coulder, T. R., and Soumekh, M., "Experimental results in ultrasonic diffraction tomography", Acoustical Imaging, Vol. 9, Plenum Press, New York (in press).

Mueller, R. K., "A new approach to acoustic tomography using diffraction techniques", in: Metherell, Alex: Acoustical Imaging, Plenum Press, New York, p. Vol. 8, 1978 (in press).

Mueller, R. K., Kaveh, M., and Wade G., "Reconstruction tomography and applications to ultrasonics", Proceedings of the IEEE, Vol. 67, No. 4, April 1979.

Norton, S. J., and Linzer, M., "Tomographic reconstruction of reflecting images", National Bureau of Standard Third International Symposium on Ultrasonic Imaging and Tissue Characterization (presented June 1978).

Stenger, F., and Johnson, S. A., "Ultrasonic transmission tomography based on the inversion of the Helmholtz wave equation for plane and spherical wave insonification", Applied Math Notes, Vol. 4, No. 3-4, December 1979.

Stephanishen, P. R., "Transient radiation from pistons in an infinite planar baffle", Journal of the Acoustical Society of America, Vol. 49, No. 5, pp. 1629-1638, 1971.

Thurstone, F. L., and Von Ramm, O. T., "A new ultrasound imaging technique employing two-dimensional electronic beam steering", in Green, P. S.: Acoustical Holography, Plenum Press, New York, Vol. 5, pp. 249-259, 1974.

Wade, G., private communication in 1978. A preliminary experiment using plane waves was performed as early as mid-1976 by G. Wade, S. Elliott, J. Khogeer, G. Flesher, J. Eisler, and D. Mensa, at the University of California at Santa Barbara.

Wolf, E., "Three-dimensional structure determination of semitransparent objects from holographic data", Optic Communication, Vol. 1, No. 4, pp. 153-156, September-October 1969.

"Development of high resolution ultrasound imaging techniques for detection and clinical assessment of cardiovascular disease", National Institutes of Health, Public Health Service, Deparment of Health, Education, and Welfare, Report No. NIH-NHLBI-NO1-HV-7-2928, May 1978.

SEGMENTATION OF TOMOGRAPHIC IMAGES

by
Ruzena Bajcsy

Computer and Information Science Department
The Moore School of Electrical Engineering
University of Pennsylvania
Philadelphia, PA 19104
U.S.A.

ABSTRACT

The objective of this paper is to show what the current techniques in image processing, artificial intelligence, and computer graphics can do in computed tomography. More concretely, we wish to show that given the tomographic data what can be done in order to:

a) improve the spatial resolution
b) improve the visualisation of the data
c) improve the identification of anatomic structures

Thus, we shall not deal with different hardware, nor with various reconstruction algorithms. We shall assume that the data is given and ask what can be done from there on. Examples, documenting each of the above points, will be presented.

1. Introduction

In the past five years a rapid spread of CT Scanners through the medical establishment has also generated a large amount of pictorial data which in turn is begging for intelligent processing. Today we are witnessing the 3-D generation of X-ray CT Scans with improved spatial resolution, speed of scanning, flexibility of taking slices in different orientations, etc. Various head holders have been developed for a better registration of the physical image and its object [29, 6]. In addition to the X-ray CT Scans, we see more and more emission tomographic machines available [27], thus generating complementary data to the X-ray CT Scans.

In view of this overwhelming reality of the quantity and quality of image data, we in the image processing, computer graphics and artificial intelligence community are asking how our technique can be used for some improvements. In this paper we shall present some approaches that have been taken by ours and other laboratories in the effort of improving:

a) the spatial resolution, in particular in the Z coordinate
b) the visualisation of the data
c) the identification of anatomic structures.

The relevant literature is vast and in spite of honest effort to cover all the grounds we may have missed some.

What follows will be a presentation of the points a). through c)., in that order. At the end we shall venture some future efforts in these areas.

2. The Spatial Resolution

The fundamental limitation on spatial resolution stems from the trade-off between the dose of radiation (safety) and the sensitivity of detectors. The standard detectors currently are scintilation counters and as Hounsfield [14] points out, the current resolution is close to theoretical limits.

Other detectors have been considered such as Xenon [9], which do allow thinner sections, 3 mm. as opposed to the standard 12 mm. [21, 22, 31], however these detectors are not as sturdy as the scintilation counters. Chu and his colleagues have experimented with Cadmium Telluride (Cd Te) as an X-ray detector. These detectors are stable and easy to handle and have high detection efficiency. Their efficient conversion of energy to charge permits high spatial resolution. Unfortunately, due to polarization, the tailing of noise is high. There are also variable leakage currents and long 'memory'. In view of all these disadvantages, it is improbable that these detectors will be practical for CAT Scanners.

So far we have considered only collinated beams. Another way to improve the spatial resolution is to have fan-beam geometry[31], and finally cone-beam geometry. In comparison to collinated beams, the cone-beam allows a more compact experimental lay-out; in comparison to a fan-beam, requires fewer exposures and hence a lower radiation dose.[24] However, the reconstruction algorithm for a cone-beam is a challenging problem computationally. For review see [8].

A different approach to improving the spatial resolution in between the slices was taken by Glenn and his colleagues.[10] They have taken multiple, overlapped 8 mm. sections. This data was then deconvoluted and displayed 1 mm. thin sections. Of course this implies increased data collection and thereby increased dose.

We have considered this problem in our laboratory as well. There are two basic solutions for increasing the spatial resolution in between slices:

a) using interpolation in between slices
b) taking some additional measurements.

The interpolation technique is based on the assumption that geometric structure between two consecutive slices is continuous. This approach has been used by us,[4], (see Figure 1) as well as by Herman [12], and Brooks at al. [5], for reconstructing the three-dimensional anatomic structure.

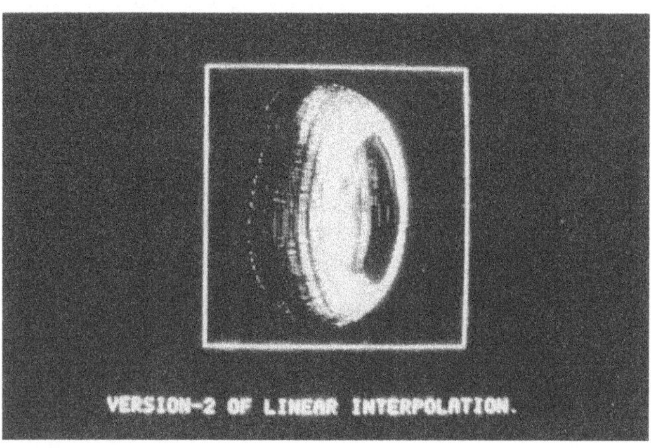

FIGURE 1

The interpolation technique could be aided by the anatomy atlas, so that certain obvious discontinuities in the structure are recorded. The disadvantage of this method is, however, that in general it is an approximation only to the reality.

The second method requires taking more measurements (X-rays) but has the advantage that the reconstruction process is more data driven than knowledge driven.

Consider the following case:

Assume that in addition to the tomographic slices we take two orthogonal X-rays (see Figure 2 a,b). Assume also that for now we are interested only in reconstructing the bone structure. Then the X-ray has (due to the film) the high spatial resolution, while the tomographic slice represents the estimate (the average) of the geometry in the volume as shown in Figure 2c.

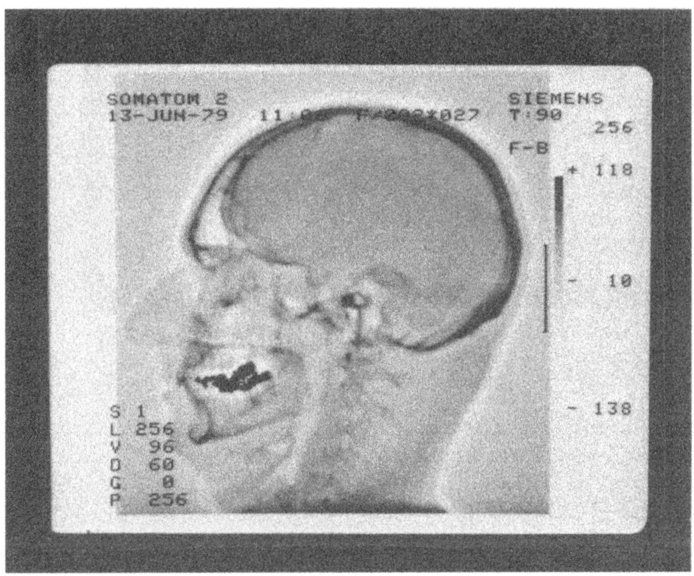

FIGURE 2a

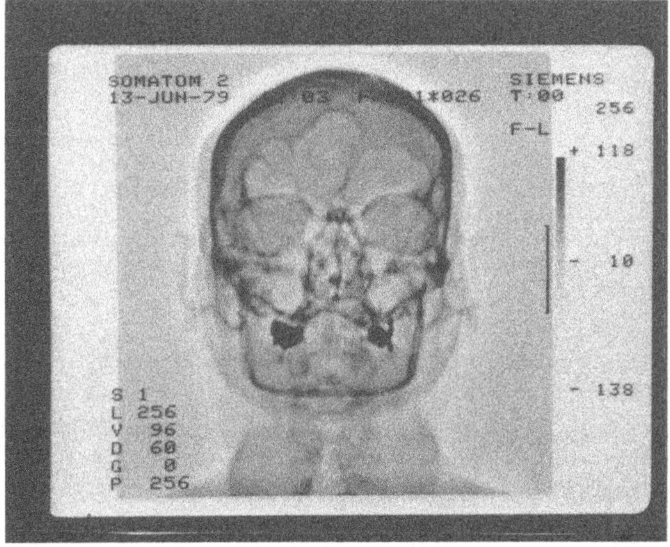

FIGURE 2b

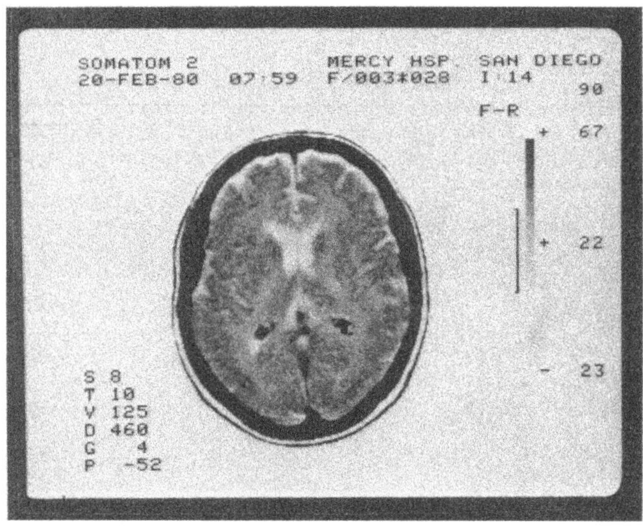

FIGURE 2c

The process of reconstructing goes as follows:

1) find the continuous structures in both X-rays

2) project them onto the tomographic volume, thereby creating boxes of continuous structures

3) within each box we can proceed two ways:

   3a) interpolate using the tomographic slice and checking for each row or column with the two X-rays

   3b) apply the reconstruction algorithm [23] on the two X-rays and if ambiguity occurs check for continuity principle with the tomographic slice.

Bourne [4] has shown that if the difference between two slices is unambiguous, than one can reconstruct the slice from the two projections. Basically, his algorithm employs the assumption about coherency of objects under reconstruction, which measured from slice to slice. Currently we are investigating [28] what the constraints are which can be detected from the individual X-rays, (continuous structures), which in turn will reduce the ambiguity. Examples of some reconstructed slices based on the above idea are presented in Figure 3.

The advantage of this method is that from an additional two X-rays one can improve the spatial resolution in between slices at best with the resolution of the X-ray, at worst with the resolution of detectable discontinuities on the X-rays.

This technique is very attractive in view of the Siemens machine which will provide automatically the topographic maps, which are nothing more than just two orthogonal X-ray projections, as shown in Figures 2 a,b.

3. Visualisation of the Data

The essence of computerized tomography is non-invasive visualisation of the internal

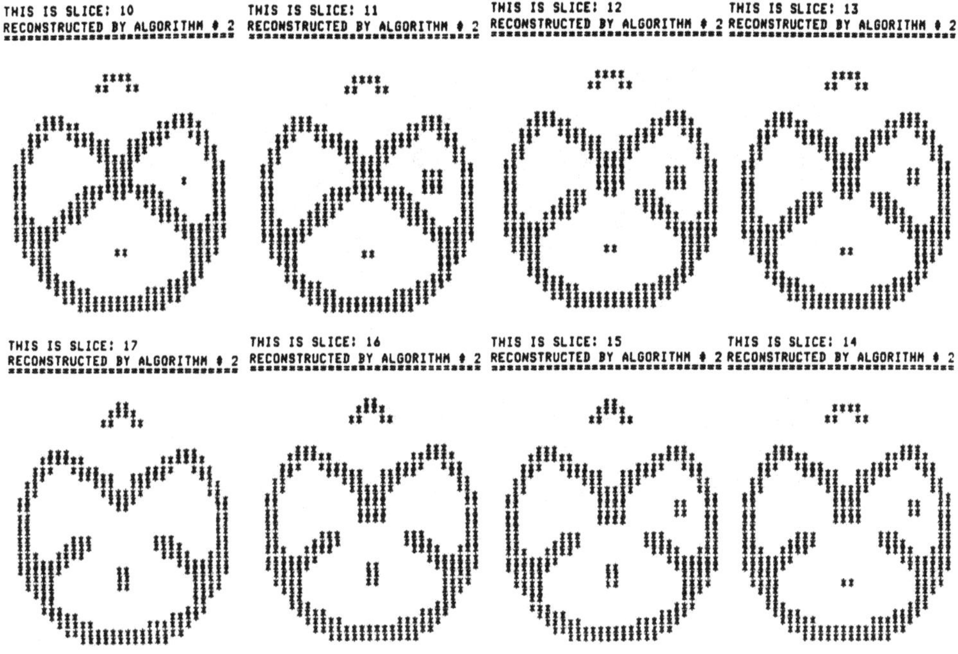

FIGURE 3

structures of the human body. Thus the application of the computer graphics technique is just a natural thing to do with this data. Hounsfield already in 1976 was concerned with the picture quality of the CT Scans. The first thing that comes to mind is an interactive graphics-image processing system which enables the user to selectively enhance various structures using different gray values or focussing on spatially distant structures, and to perform various computation on them such as area average and standard deviation, and perhaps others. Such systems have been developed in various tomographic centers. Just to mention a few: Glenn et al. [11], Philipson [25], Anderson et al. [1], etc. As a sample of what these standard graphic image processing systems provide we cite Huang et al. [15], the system called CTIP - an on-line image-processing software package.

The system:

a) eliminates the head holder or scanning bed from the scan image

b) evaluates CT member distribution in a scan image

c) separates the region of interest in a scan picture

d) extracts the boundary of a cross section

e) computes the mass, center gravity, inertia tensor for anatomical components

f) analyses a density histogram of the region of interest in a CT Scan

So far this is processing of the 2-D data. Since the usual scans provide a series of transaxial slices through the body, it is only natural to consider all the slices in their 3-D form. The first thing that researchers attempted to do was perform orthogonal cut views, [10, 19, 22, 17, 3]. See Figure 4.

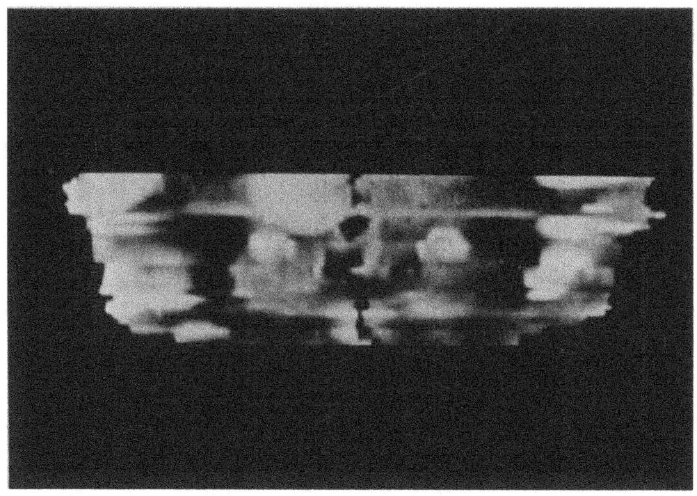

FIGURE 4

Having the 3-D data available, we can visualise it with proper shading, perspective, and hidden line elimination. There are few laboratories which have done this,[see for example, 13 and 4]. In addition to just simple display, one can manipulate the data, for example rotate, extract different anatomic structures, cut in half, etc. [see 12, 4, 18], as it is shown in Figures 5, 6, and 7.

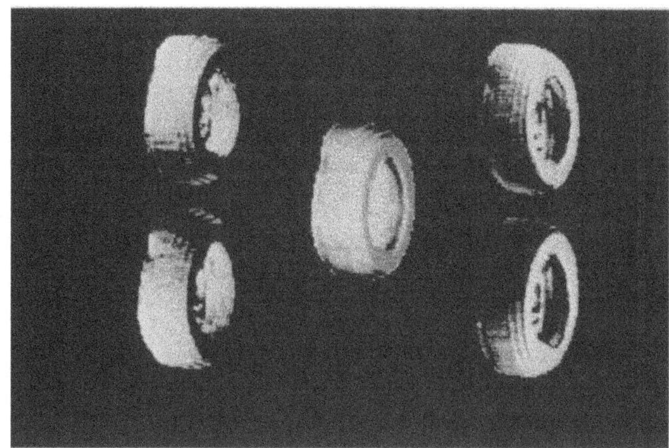

FIGURE 5

The big question remains how useful the 3-D object visualization will be for clinical usage since the current clinicians are not trained and used to viewing 3-D objects as opposed to the cross sections. Herman, [13], reports that in some special cases for surgery of a deformed spine the 3-D visualization turned out to be essential.

4. The Identification of Anatomic Structures

The tomographic images would be useless if we could not identify what we see in those

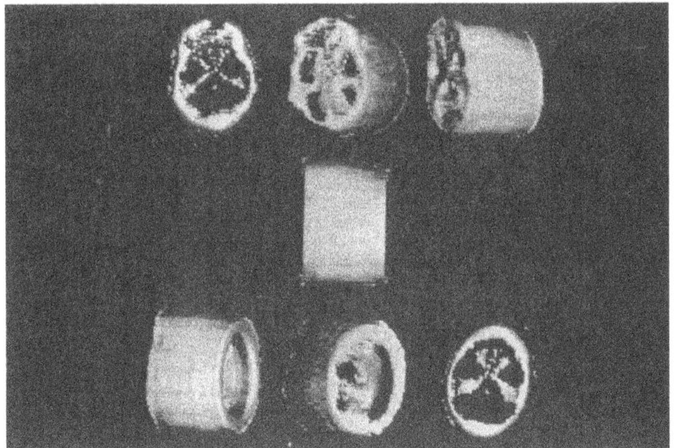

FIGURE 6

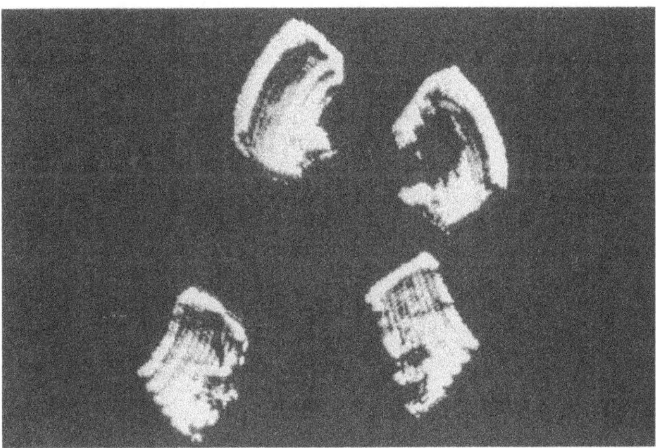

FIGURE 7

images and their meaning. Every radiologist who looks at the CT Scans identifies some anatomic structures. We observe that the radiologist doing so is using his/her knowledge of the anatomy which helps him/her to delineate the boundaries (even if they are noisy) of anatomic structures. In order to partially or fully mimic this behavior by computer one has to give the computer similar knowledge about the anatomy as the radiologist has. This fact led us to implement a computerized anatomy atlas of the brain. [16]

The atlas is a data base of digitized serial sections of the human brain, where every structure is labeled by its corresponding anatomic label, as it is shown in Figure 8. In addition, every structure is associated with a vector of typical values and deviations for the X-ray absorption, and the values of glucose consumption for eventual application on scans obtained from the machine PETT 5. A software package has been developed using Vector general, graphics display, and the computer PDP 11/60 for manipulating individual slices as well as the whole 3-D brain. Examples of the 3-D structures are shown in Figure 9.

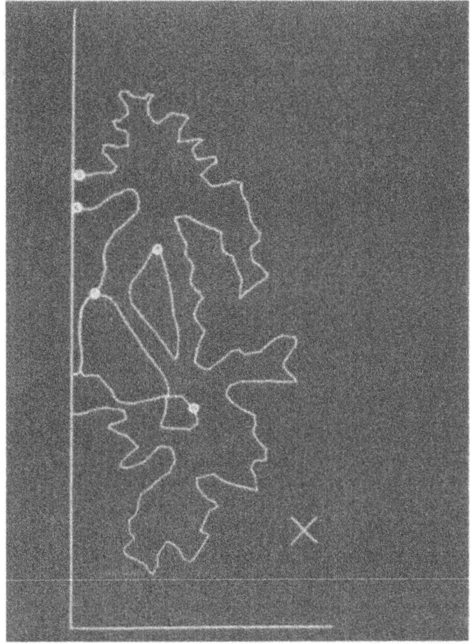

FIGURE 8

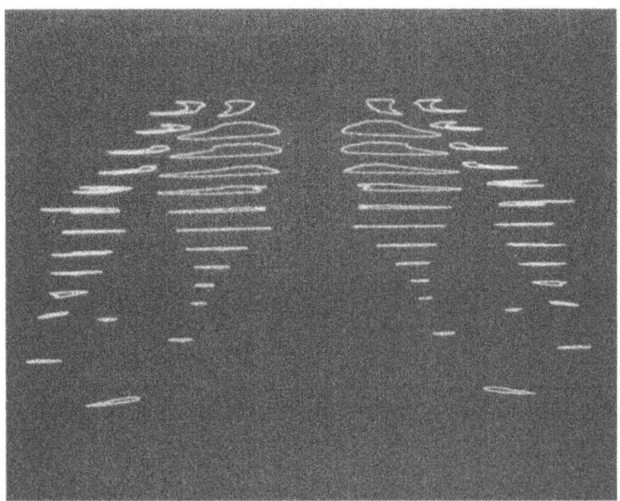

FIGURE 9

Although the computerized atlas may be justified in its own right, for example, for educational purposes,[20], our goal is to use it for guidance in the recognition of anatomic structures. Similar approaches have been taken by Ballard et al.,[2], for identification of ribcage, heart and abdominal organs. Also Selfridge et al., [26], have used a priori anatomic knowledge for boundary detection of various organs.

Our method is automation of what Gado et al.[32], has presented, that is, automatic recognition of anatomic structures found in CT Scans and overlay of them on CT Scans. What follows will be the description of our method:

Consider the input data, for example from the PETT machine as it is shown in Figure 10. The first task is segmentation. This process is composed of the following steps:

1) measurement of the histogram

2) dividing the histogram into n number of buckets, where n is an input parameter. These buckets are chosen on the basis of the largest differences between the local minimum and maximum in the histogram

3) using these buckets, threshold the picture

4) apply region growing and generate description of the region; such as:

   -center of gravity
   -the enclosing rectangle
   -gray value and its statistics

Then the next task is to generate a similar description of the appropriate slice for the anatomy atlas, such as is shown in Figure 11.

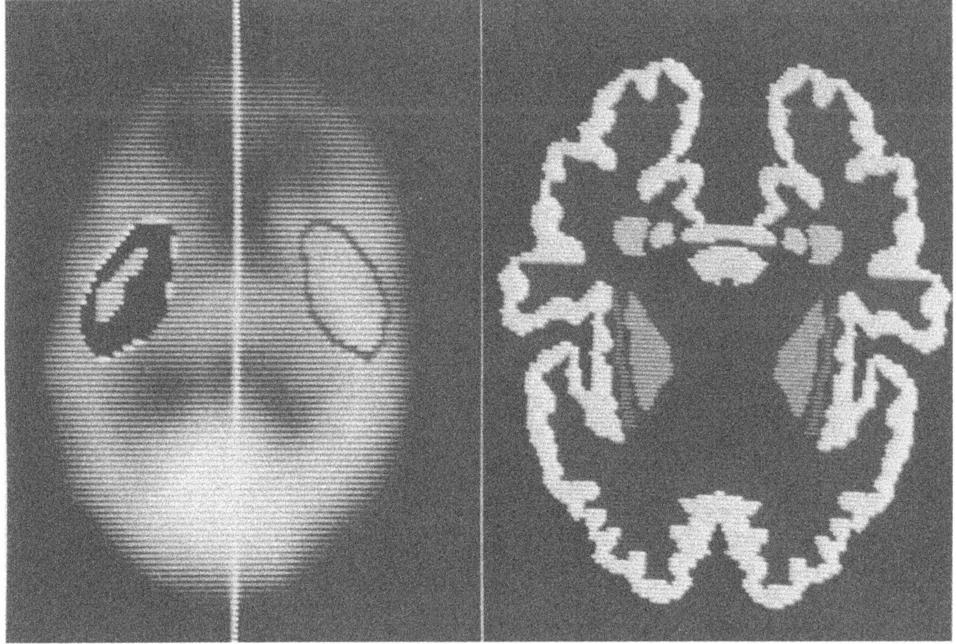

FIGURE 10 FIGURE 11

Once we have the two descriptions, we perform the matching. The matching process is currently under development.

5. Conclusion

As we have outlined in the introduction, the proposal of this paper was to analyse the quality of the data generated by the CT Scanners and see how we can improve it by the state of the art techniques from image processing, computer graphics, and the artificial intelligence resources.

We have concentrated on three issues: how to improve spatial resolution in between two consecutive slices of X-ray CT Scans, what can be done for better visualization of the 3-D data of the CT Scans, and finally how we can aid the radiologist in the recognition process of anatomic structures from the CT Scans.

We have reported some of the most exciting results in these areas in our laboratory as well as in other centers. While there is going to be continuous effort on improving the resolution of the data in the displays, we feel that the future research contribution from the computer vision community will come in finding various representational schemes of 3-D objects (parametricisation) which will enable us to compare the morphology obtained from the CT Scans in more quantitative fashion than it is so far.

ACKNOWLEDGEMENTS

This work was supported partially by:

NIH Grant NS 10939-07 and

NSF Grant MCS-7807466

REFERENCES

1. Anderson, W.H., Chang, C.H.J., Tarlton, M.A., Fritz, S.L., Dwyer, S.J.III, "An Interactive Computer Graphics System for the Computed Tomographic Breast Cancer" (CT/M), Proceeding of COMPSAC 79, Chicago, November 1979, pp. 350-354.

2. Ballard, D.H., Shain, U., Schudy, R.B., "Anatomical Models for Medical Images", Proceedings of COMPSAC 79, Chicago, November 1979, pp.565-570.

3. Bajcsy, R., Winston, I., "A Computer System for Reconstruction and Display of the Macrostructure of the Brain from Radiographs of Serial Sections", BIOSYGMA 1978, April 1978, Paris, France.

4. Bourne, D.A., "Three Dimensional Picture Processing Using Partial Information", Master Thesis, University of Pennsylvania, Philadelphia, December 1978.

5. Brooks, R.A., Weiss, G.H., Talbert, A.J., "A New Approach to Interpolation in Computed Tomography", Journal of Computed Tomography, 2(5), 1978, pp. 577-585.

6. Brown, R.A.,"A Stereotactic Head Frame for Use with CT Body Scanners",Investigative Radiology, Vol. 14, July-August 1979, pp. 300-304.

7. Chu, D., Kaufman, L., Hosier, K., Hoenninger,"An Evaluation of Cadmium Telluride Detectors for Computer-Assisted Tomography", Journal of Computed Tomography, 2(5), 1978, pp. 586-593.

8. Colsher, J.G., "Iterative Three-Dimensional Reconstruction from Tomographic Projection", Computer Graphics Image Processing 6, 1977, pp. 513-537.

9. Fenster, A., "Split Xenon Detector for Tomochemistry in Computed Tomography", Journal of Computed Tomography, 2(3), 1978, pp. 243-252.

10. Glenn, W.V. Jr., Johnson, R.J., Morton, P.E., Dwyer, S.J., "Image Generation and Display Technique for CT Scan Data, Thin Transverse and Reconstructed Coronal and Sagittal Planes", Investigative Radiology,Vol. 10, Sept.-October, 1975, pp. 403-416.

11. Glenn, W.V. Jr., Johnston, R.J., Morton, P.E., Dwyer, S.J., "Further Investigation and Initial Clinical Use of Advanced CT Display Capability", Investigative Radiology, Vol. 10, September-October, 1975, pp. 479-489.

12. Herman, G.T., Lier, H.K.,"Three-Dimensional Display of Human Organs for Computed Tomograms", Computer Graphics and Image Processing, Vol. 9, 1979, pp. 1-21.

13. Herman, G.T., Lecture at Drexel University, Philadelphia, May 1980.

14. Hounsfield, G.N., "Picture Quality of Computed Tomography", American Journal of Roentgenology, 127 : 3-9, 1976.

15. Huang, H.K., Weiss, P., Kraft, H.H., Heidtman, B., "CTIP- An On-Line CT Image Processing Software Package", Proceedings of COMPSAC 79, Chicago, November 1979, pp. 355-361.

16. Karp, P., Bajcsy, R., Stein, A., "Computerized Anatomy Atlas", Workshop on Data Structure and Picture Processing, California, August 1980.

17. Lee, C., "Orthogonal Cut View Generation for CT Scanned Data", Proceedings of COMPSAC 79, Chicago, November 1979, pp. 362-365.

18. Lemke, H., Stiehl, H.S., Scharnweber, H., Jackel, D., "Applications of Picture Processing, Image Analysis and Computer Graphics Techniques to Cranial CT Scans" Proceedings of Conference on Computer-Aided Analysis of Radiological Images,

20-21 June 1979, Newport Beach, California.

19. Leonardi, M., Barbian, V., Fahis, G., Penco, T., "Sagittal CT of the Orbit", Journal of Computed Tomography, 1(4), 1977, pp. 511-512.

20. Livingston, R.B., Wilson, K., The Human Brain: Structures and Organization, University of California, La Jolla, 1976.

21. Maravilla, K.R., Pastel, M.S., Kirkpatrick, J.B., "White Matter of the Cerebellum Demonstrated by Computed Tomography: Normal Anatomy and Physical Principles" Journal of Computed Tomography, 2(2), 1978, pp. 156-161.

22. Maravilla, K.R., "Computer Reconstructed Sagittal and Coronal Computed Tomography Head Scans: Clinical Applications", Journal of Computed Tomography, 2(2), 1978, pp. 189-198.

23. Minerbo, G., Sanderson, J., "Reconstruction of a Source from a Few Projections: Two or Three", Los Alamos Scientific Laboratory, University of California, March 1977.

24. Minerbo, G., "Maximum Entropy Reconstruction from Cone-Beam Projection Data", BioMedicine, Vol. 9, 1979, pp. 29-37.

25. Philipson, L., "Software Development on the EMI Head Scanner Computer Programs", BioMedicine 10, 1979, pp. 162-171.

26. Selfridge, P.G., Prewitt, J.M.S., Dyer, C.H.R., Ranade, S., "Segmentation Algorithms for Abdominal Computerized Tomography Scans", Proceedings of COMPSAC 79, Chicago, 1979, pp. 571-577.

27. Ter-Pogossian, M.M., Mullam, N.A., Hood, J.T., Higgins, C.S., Ficke, D.C., "Design Considerations for a Positron Emission Transverse Tomograph (PETT V) for Imaging of the Brain", Journal of Computed Tomography, 2(5), 1978, pp. 539-544.

28. Villafana, T., Lee, H.S., Lapayowker, M.S., "A Device to Indicate Anatomical Level In CT", Journal of Computed Tomography, 2(3), 1978, pp. 368-371.

29. Williams, D., Forthcoming Master Thesis, University of Pennsylvania, Philadelphia, September 1980.

30. Yaffe, M., Fenster, A., Johns, H.E., "Xenon Ionization Detectors for Fan-Beam Computed Tomography Scanners", Journal of Computed Tomography, 1(4), 1977, pp. 419-428.

31. Gado, M., Hanaway, J., Frank, R., "Functional Anatomy of the Cerebral Cortex by Computed Tomography",Journal of Computer Assisted Tomography, 3(1), 1979, pp. 1-20.

TECHNOLOGY AND BIOMEDICAL APPLICATIONS OF AUTOMATED LIGHT MICROSCOPY

By

Kenneth R. Castleman, Ph.D.
Jet Propulsion Laboratory
California Institute of Technology

Pasadena, California 91103
U.S.A.

ABSTRACT

Digital processing of light microscope images has proved to be a powerful tool for several medical research and diagnostic applications. The acquisition of high quality digital images of microscope specimens requires a carefully designed and implemented mixture of optical, electronic and computer technologies. Image noise level, resolution, magnification and photometric and geometric linearity must all be considered together in the system design. During the processing one should pay careful attention to specimen preparation, spatial and optical density calibration and to the illumination spectrum. This produces digital images of high quality and greatly improves the performance of the processing algorithms.

The technology of automated light microscopy is beginning to move into the practice of clinical medicine. White blood cell differential counters are commercially available, and several hundred units are in use. Clinical prototypes exist for automated chromosome analysis (karyotyping), automated muscle biopsy analysis and automated cervical cancer (Pap smear) screening. Several applications in tissue section analysis are under study. With the continued rapid development of image sensing and integrated circuit technology one can expect continued infusion of automated light microscope technology into clinical medicine and medical research.

1. INTRODUCTION

The light microscope has been a popular source of images for digital processing for over 20 years. The medical applications include the analysis of blood cells, chromosomes, cervical (Pap smear) cells and muscle and nerve fibers. One of these applications, the white blood cell differential counter, has reached the point that commercially produced machines are in routine clinical use. Automated chromosome, Pap smear and muscle biopsy analysis have progressed to the point of prototype clinical systems currently under test. Other applications have clinical systems under development or are being used in medical research applications (Figure 1).

Many of the microscope image analysis applications involve classic optical pattern recognition, that is, finding, measuring and classifying the objects (cells, fibers, etc.) on the slide. Along with optical character recognition these development efforts have produced many contributions to the discipline of pattern recognition. Many now standard techniques were first applied to microscope images and then integrated into the theory and practice of the field of pattern recognition.

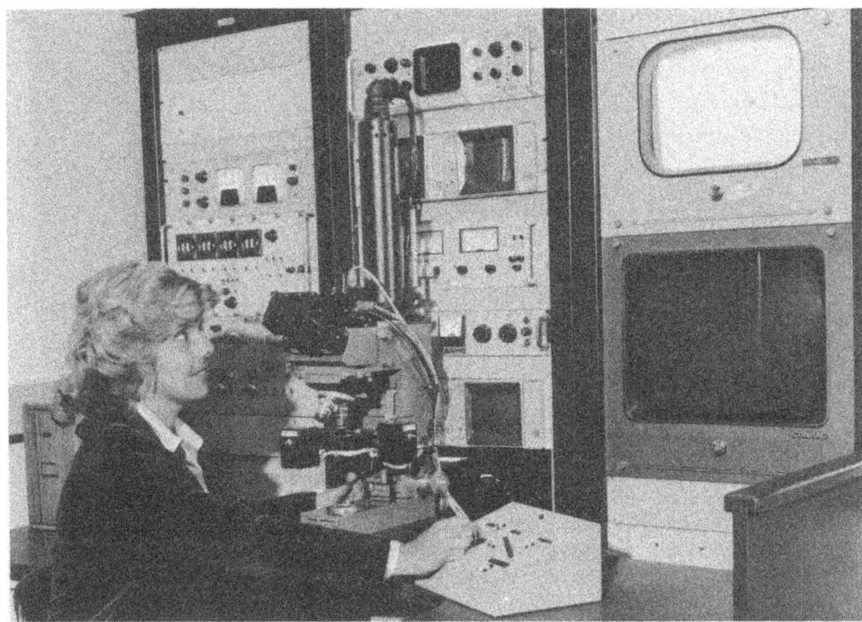

Figure 1. This automated light microscope system, developed at the Jet Propulsion Laboratory, has been used for research and algorithm development for chromosome, muscle biopsy, and Pap smear analysis and for lung microstructure studies.

2. THE APPLICATIONS

The light microscope image analysis problems that have reached successful solutions seem to have three things in common. First, they grow out of a real medical need. This is often a need for a faster, less expensive, more accurate or more quantitative diagnostic test. Second, the solution must be theoretically possible. Often an analysis can be done to show whether or not the intrinsic statistical parameters and the existing resolution, speed and cost limitations will permit a successful solution. Third, the solution must be technologically achievable in light of available hardware and algorithm performance. Only in recent years have the capabilities of commercially available automated microscopes begun to approach the performance required by some of these applications. Stepping stages, for example, are only now achieving the combination of small step size, high stepping speed and mechanical rigidity required for automated chromosome analysis and other applications.

3. THE SOLUTIONS

The final system that results from a successful application of microscope image analysis is usually a compromise developed among three different viewpoints, those of the physician, the mathematician and the engineer. Medical people initially define the problem. In many cases the problem is basically the automation of a diagnostic test currently performed manually. Such tests have developed, over time, to make the best use of the human technician's eye and brain. This naturally involves subjective judgements at a very fundamental level.

The mathematician must abstract from this a problem, posed in objective analytical terms, which is soluble with available analytical techniques. This redefinition of the problem must be compatible with the underlying medical need and minimize the required departure from current laboratory practice. More radical solutions will not meet with medical acceptance.

Finally, the engineer must implement an acceptable solution to the problem within the limitations of available hardware and algorithms. The implementation must not only perform well at reasonable cost, but it must be embraced and accepted by the medical personnel that operate it and use its output.

Rather than a three stage process as outlined above, the development of a successful system involves compromise in a continuing interaction between the three points of view. Overemphasis on any one viewpoint will result in a medically irrelevant or inadequate system.

4. THE TECHNOLOGY

Obtaining high quality digital images of microscopic specimens is not as simple as it might appear. When a human peers through the eyepieces he not only can focus up and down through the specimen with the fine focus knob, but he can also accommodate focus with the lens of the eye. A planar image sensor, however, can do neither, and the resulting images often appear less sharp. Mechanical vibration during the digitizing process can degrade the image. Shading caused by nonuniform illumination, unless severe, goes unnoticed by the human eye but can have disastrous effects on image segmentation algorithms.

Internal reflections in the optical path can cause glare and hot spots in the image. Glare undermines the system's ability to quantify optical density. High resolution, proper pixel spacing and parfocality of the various images can only be maintained simultaneously if the optical interface between microscope and digitizing camera is carefully designed. Geometric linearity requires careful optical and camera design. Both geometric and photometric accuracy can only be maintained with careful and frequent calibration.

5. THE FUTURE

Significant technological advances are affecting the field of microscopic image analysis. New computer architectures specifically designed for digital image processing are being developed. These include parallel image processing systems (PIPS) with multiple processors to handle many pixels at once, and real time image processing systems (RTIPS) that process pixels sequentially at video rates. Several PIPS architectures have been developed. As with any new computer technology the theory and techniques used to design algorithms are lagging behind the hardware development. Thus, it may be some time before the true potential of these machines is demonstrated.

The RTIPS suffer to a lesser degree from a lack of theoretical background since they implement more traditional algorithms, such as convolution for example. Their performance varies, however, depending on the task they are asked to perform. Tasks that lend themselves to line-by-line pixel access can be accomplished at remarkable speed. Tasks inherently requiring random access to pixels, however, can run very slowly. Thus RTIPS will probably be limited to those applications where the algorithms are, or can be made to be, line-by-line in nature.

6. CONCLUSION

With the rapid advances in image processing hardware technology and the ever-growing need for quantitative medical testing, we can expect more microscope image processing technology in clinical laboratories and medical research. It will be particularly interesting to watch as the body of background knowledge grows up around PIPS and RTIPS technologies. Some truly remarkable performance can be expected from these advanced machines. The conventional image processing system, with its single computer and inherent flexibility, will probably remain valuable for feasibility studies and algorithm development for a long time. We will probably see new computer architectures developed specifically for particular problems. Thus hardware and algorithm design will then be integrated into a single effort.

7. ACKNOWLEDGEMENT

This paper presents research conducted, in part, at the Jet Propulsion Laboratory, California Institute of Technology, and supported, in part, by Contract NAS7-100 from the National Aeronautics and Space Administration.

ADVANCES IN THE PROCESSING OF LARGE BIOMEDICAL DATA BASES USING SPECIALIZED COMPUTERS, IMPROVED DEVICE TECHNOLOGY, AND COMPUTER-AIDED DESIGN

B. K. Gilbert, L. M. Krueger, and T. M. Kinter

Biodynamics Research Unit, Department of Physiology and Biophysics, Mayo Foundation, Rochester, MN 55901

ABSTRACT

Many new requirements for the computer processing of large biomedical data bases have arisen during the past decade which exploit the creation of images via computed tomography, the processing of images generated by conventional radiographic techniques, the simulation of large biological systems, and the processing of x-ray crystallographic measurements of biological macromolecular structures. These requirements for ever increasing computational power are motivating advances in the computers which carry out the processing. Several important trends in the technology and design of processors relevant to the biomedical environment will be described, including the newest approaches to computational tasks at various complexity levels, the use of advanced device technology to improve performance, and the growing reliance upon computer-aided design methods to lower development costs for new processor designs.

1. INTRODUCTION

The past decade has witnessed a rapid growth in the use of computer techniques for the processing of large data bases arising from biomedical applications. These tasks include the modelling of molecular structures from x-ray crystallographic data, the simulation of biochemical processes, and the creation of images by means of x-ray, ultrasound, and emission computer-assisted tomography (CT). Simultaneously with the advent of CT techniques, a variety of image processing applications have also arisen, either in support of CT imaging or as independent techniques for the enhancement of projection radiographic images and ultrasound images generated by, e.g., ultrasound sector scanners [1-3]. These new approaches to biomedical research and clinical diagnosis are becoming increasingly reliant on the availability of powerful computational resources which, however, are frequently too costly for routine usage, as when a large scientific computer must be employed at a cost of several thousand dollars per hour to process x-ray crystallographic data. In some cases, the computational resources required to attack certain types of research problems are larger than presently available, and must therefore be developed de novo. For each type of problem, the range of options for achieving the requisite cost-effective computation is evolving rapidly with advancing computer technology.

Initial feasibility studies in the development of a new method for computerized processing of large biomedical data bases are usually performed with the aid of general-purpose mainframe computers or minicomputers using higher level language computer programs (e.g., FORTRAN or PASCAL), a technique which may be suitable indefinitely if the data processing is in a research environment and if the amount of data to be processed is small. However, when the processing task is eventually refined to the level of an independent tool or a portion of a larger technique, operational considerations frequently preclude the execution of these algorithms on all but the most cost-effective hardware configurations dedicated to a narrow range of functions. Three fundamentally different and continually evolving approaches to the development of special-purpose computers for a wide range of data processing tasks will be described, categorized according to the number of computational and bookkeeping operations which must be executed per second to assure an acceptable turnaround time with respect to the human observer: 1) computational tasks requiring up to 10^7 operations per second (assigned at present to mainframe computers and minicomputers); 2) tasks requiring 10^7 and 10^8 operations per second (such tasks presently can be executed only on large mainframe computers); and 3) tasks requiring computational rates greater than 10^8 operations per second (these tasks are not presently executable on any available general-purpose or special-purpose computers). Following a discussion of possible processor implementations in each of these speed regimes, recent and near-future advances in integrated circuit technology will be discussed, as will the use of special software packages, called computer-aided design systems, to speed the engineering development of new machine architectures.

1.1. Low Computational Demand Tasks

During the past few years, tasks requiring from 3×10^5 to 10^7 logical and arithmetic operations/second have been assigned either to mainframe computers, or where possible, to the largest minicomputers, frequently augmented by commercially available "programmable array processors". Available in a variety of designs, these special-purpose devices are capable of executing up to 10^7 arithmetic and bookkeeping operations per second under the supervision of a general-purpose host minicomputer. Although most current array processors execute all primitive arithmetic and numerical functions except division, they are generally optimized for a small subclass of special operations, e.g., the FFT "butterfly" used to compute the Fast Fourier Transform. Costs of these special-purpose array processors in 1980 vary from $10-$150,000, depending upon their level of sophistication and throughput capabilities; in addition, the more expensive units employ floating point arithmetic, while the less costly designs employ fixed precision arithmetic. A combined minicomputer array processor combination is capable of executing from five to ten million operations/second, with primary emphasis on arithmetic functions.

Driven by the advancing digital device technology, the use of large mainframe computers and/or minicomputers augmented with array processors to achieve computation rates up to 10^7 operations/second will be replaced by so-called "microprocessors" possessing considerable computational capability [4-7]. The "single component" microprocessor, which has been described extensively [4-5], will play an increasing role for computation of fixed precision operands and eventually floating point operands [7] up to rates of approximately 2×10^6 operations per second. The most recent generations of single-component microprocessors operate directly on 16-bit or even 32-bit operands, contain on-board read only memory (ROM) and random access memory (RAM), and can directly access the address space of large blocks of solid-state digital memory. These devices execute a large, sophisticated set of assembly language instructions predetermined by the component vendor, including single-instruction arithmetic and inter-register operations on full width operands. Each succeeding generation of these devices has exhibited increasingly more powerful logical and arithmetic capability; the very newest employs 32-bit operands in its internal structure, though the input/output pathways retain a sixteen bit width as a result of pin count limitations on the integrated circuit packages [5]. Using advanced integrated circuit packages with at least 80 input/output pins, one vendor is expected to produce sample quantities of a truly 32-bit processor by early 1981. At present, the slow internal logic gate propagation delays of these devices limit their minor cycle clock rates to 4-8 MHz (every major instruction is executed in several consecutive small segments, each denoted as a minor cycle), enabling them to execute instructions at the rate of $2.5\text{-}3.0 \times 10^5$ major instructions per second. These devices are made possible by advances in the art of integrated circuit fabrication which allows placement of 50,000 to 100,000 logic gates on a single 3 x 3 mm silicon "chip"; this high device density is referred to as very large scale integration (VLSI). The low per-unit costs and the availability of support aids for the development of hardware systems and computer programs based around these single component VLSI microprocessors allows them to execute rather complex arithmetic and logic functions in a cost-effective and straightforward manner. These features, combined with a rapidly increasing availability of microprocessor-oriented high level compilers for the PASCAL and FORTRAN languages, will permit VLSI microprocessors to supplant the use of minicomputers for a wide variety of biomedical data processing algorithms [7].

1.2. Medium Computational Demand Tasks

A new generation of programmable array processors is currently evolving which will fulfill requirements for computation in the range of 10^8 to 10^9 operations/ second. Exploiting architectures understood conceptually for some time but not physically realizable in 1970s array processors, these devices will either be user-programmable, or will be supplied with a vast armamentarium of vendor-prepared subroutines which can be employed as desired by the user. The pressures for development of such devices are arising principally from the earth resources management programs for the processing of high resolution multispectral imaging satellite data; from oil and minerals exploration groups for the processing of seismic data; and from the military for the real-time analysis of moderate bandwidth microwave and radar signals and the rapid solution of large systems of algebraic or differential equations. Unlike present array processors which are optimized for a specific computation such as the FFT "butterfly" operation, the next generation of array processors will possess completely general architectures. With the availability of appropriate software design support aids, and when operated in conjunction with general-purpose host computers, these devices will be capable of executing a wide variety of image and array processing tasks, and will be capable of solving large systems of algebraic equations by inversion or iteration. These same processors will be programmed to solve systems of differential equations using a variety of well-known closed form and iterative methods, and will be capable of simulation and modelling tasks as well. The biomedical community will recognize the benefits of such technological advances without the provision of support for their development costs.

The architectures of the new array processors are fundamental to their computational and programming flexibility. An example of one promising design [8] is depicted in Figure 1. Sixteen distinct arithmetic, control, external communications, and memory modules are connected in parallel to one another through a large digital crossbar network. The crossbar simultaneously allows the outputs of any one or more of the modules to be connected under stored program control to the inputs of any one or more of the other modules for a duration as short as a single cycle of the system clock, or for as long as desired. The inputs and outputs of every module are equipped with data holding registers, creating in effect a parallel multiprocessor which is completely reconfigurable under software control during every clock cycle. It is of interest that the input and output data registers contribute a so-called "pipeline" capability to the design; a complicated numerical operation is said to be "pipelined" when it is subdivided into a number of sequential hardware subunits, with each executing only a portion of the total computation and separated from the others by intermediate data registers. The effective throughput of a process divided into "n" pipelined stages is generally n times greater than if pipelining is not employed. In addition, each of the arithmetic subunits depicted in Figure 1 executes a number of related instruction types; for example, the multiplier unit can perform 8, 16, or 32-bit integer multiply or multiply-accumulate operations, bit reversals, magnitude comparisons, and so on.

Although the computational strengths of the parallel pipelined multiprocessor architecture of Figure 1 have been understood for many years, a substantial obstacle to its physical realization has been the device complexity of the switch shown schematically in the lower portion of the diagram. Efficient crossbar interconnection networks, i.e., those providing data pathways of multi-bit width through the network, are only now becoming cost-effective for small array processors by implementing the elements of the crossbar with custom designed high performance large scale integrated circuits (LSI). If implemented in the appropriate high-speed logic (see below), overall machine clock frequencies of 50 MHz are feasible, with each processor subunit executing an entire operation in one to three clock cycles; in addition, individual processor subunits are themselves amenable to pipeline design, allowing a completed result to emerge from each subunit during every machine cycle. The processor of Figure 1 will execute operations on 8, 16, or 32-bit integer operands, or, with some degradation in throughput, on 64-bit floating point operands.

In the theoretical limit, which is never achieved in practice, the processor should support a maximum of 3.5×10^7 64-bit floating point arithmetic operations per second, a maximum of 1.1×10^8 32-bit fixed precision arithmetic operations per second, or a maximum of 5×10^8 8-bit fixed precision arithmetic operations per second.

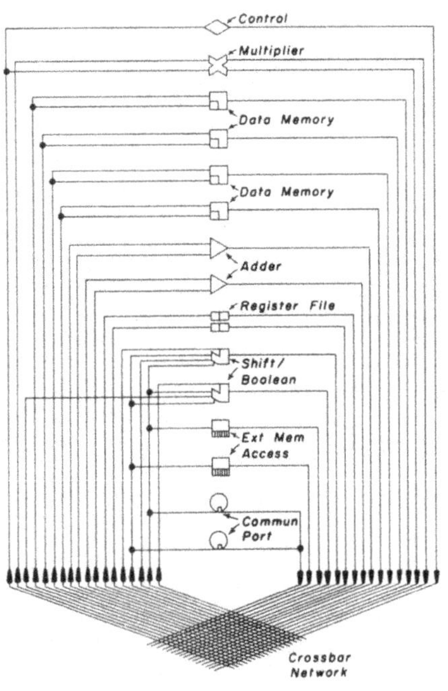

Figure 1 An advanced design for a programmable array processor. Sixteen computational and communications subprocessors are connected in a parallel structure through a large crossbar switch network. A single microcoded control unit provides operating instructions during each clock cycle for all computational, communications, and crossbar substructures. (Reproduced with permission from [8])

The designs of present and future generation array processors emphasize arithmetic operations and input/output functions rather than data dependent branch operations. Limited capability for branch execution is not critical for a processor intended to execute array-oriented arithmetic manipulations on large blocks of data, since with the exception of a few algorithms developed by artificial intelligence specialists, image and signal processing algorithms are heavily computation dependent, are easily pipelined, and rarely deviate from a predetermined set of numerical substeps. It is frequently the case that the larger the image data base to be processed, the lower is the percentage of data dependent branch operations. Nonetheless, a minimal provision for data dependent decisions can be incorporated into the control unit of the array processor, which will in most cases be sufficient for execution of the types of computational algorithms for which such a processing architecture is intended.

During the 1970s many attempts were made to develop computationally powerful processors by interconnecting large numbers of inexpensive single component microprocessors into a network which could partition a large computational task into sections, and then execute each section on one or more of the microprocessors. Several examples [9-11] have demonstrated that the synchronization and communication requirements of a large number of semi-independent but low performance processors frequently increase rapidly with the number of processors in the network. As a result, the individual processors consume much of their capability satisfying the network communications protocol. It is increasingly apparent that an alternative approach will be easier to implement and will demonstrate extremely high throughput and improved cost/performance ratios in comparison to those of the microprocessor network. In the alternate method, a moderate number of extremely high-speed arithmetic, memory, and input/output processor modules possessing no autonomous operational capability whatsoever are operated under the lockstep control of a few system control units, which orchestrate both the step-by-step operations of each processing unit and the interactions of all processor subsections operating conjointly [8]. While this approach may appear to be an architectural "step backward" to designs proposed in the 1960s, it represents instead a return to a potentially powerful technique which was fundamentally sound but for which neither the hardware technology nor the software support aids were then available for its total exploitation. The array processor design of Figure 1 exploits such a control structure, which will also be employed in the highly parallel special-purpose processors described in the next section. Undeniably, a few instances have been identified in which a network of independent, self-controlling subprocessors is absolutely mandatory, generally when "fail-soft" or "fail-safe" system operation is an overriding concern. Even in such specialized cases, the most recent designs represent strenuous efforts to minimize the total number of subprocessors, with a maximum comfortable number of such subunits of approximately sixteen. Computing power is maintained at high levels by making each subprocessor as powerful as possible [12,13], either by an augmentation of its parts count or by the use of a faster digital technology; problems of interprocessor communications are thereby circumvented to the maximum possible degree [12].

The control units of processors such as those depicted in Figure 1 operate by prestoring the control signals for every step of a process, and for each element of hardware in an arithmetic unit, in a large control memory composed of very wide words containing many bit positions. Each control signal for every cycle of the system clock is stored as a "one" or "zero" bit in this memory. Frequently the "grain size" of these instructions is so fine that even a single integrated circuit in the arithmetic unit may have one or several columns of bit positions in the control memory dedicated exclusively to its operational management. The preparation of these microcode control programs is very tedious, since for each cycle of the system clock the designer must encode a wide row of "ones" and "zeros" corresponding to all required control signals for the entire processor. Fortunately, during the past few years special computer programs called meta-assemblers have been developed which, via a computer terminal, permit the designer to define with great rapidity an entire assembly language for his processor, to prespecify default conditions for each bit in the microprocessor control word (often several hundred bits in width), and then to prepare functional programs using the newly defined assembly language; all default conditions, special formats, subroutine call statements, and so on, are automatically handled by the meta-assembler. Figure 2 depicts the output from one such software package. Note the rows of multi-character alphabetic letter groups, representing the assembly language instructions, interspersed with rows of ones, zeros and X's (the X's represent "don't care" conditions which are defined during the final stages of the assembly procedure). With the support of such software aids, the generation of microcontrol code is considerably simplified.

Although the meta-assemblers described in the prior paragraph are of considerable assistance to the machine designer, they do assume a knowledge of the processor architecture more detailed than that possessed by most potential users. The ability to communicate with special-purpose parallel processors of the type depicted in Figure 1 in a higher level language such as FORTRAN is nearly mandatory. However, FORTRAN was developed for sequential computers which execute one arithmetic operation at a time, and hence is not able to control many processing steps simultaneously. Fortunately, higher level languages are now becoming available which 1) employ a highly structured syntax, thereby compelling the programmer to prepare his program in a block-by-block, top-down form; and 2) contain special syntactic structures which facilitate the definition and subsequent execution of several simultaneous subtasks. Concurrent PASCAL is such a language; however, PASCAL is recently developed and not yet completely stabilized. It is thus of considerable interest that the U. S. Department of Defense is presently developing a standard high level structured concurrent computer language, called ADA, which is similar to concurrent PASCAL and which will be very rigorously defined. A special-purpose parallel processor of the type depicted in Figure 1 will become considerably more valuable to its ultimate users if an appropriate compiler is available which can convert program statements written in a structured, parallel processing language such as concurrent PASCAL or ADA into microcode optimized for that processor.

```
MPC-1 CONTROL ROM

0090 ALIGN 16
     ;**  CONVOL1 CONVOLVES PROFILE DATA AND WRITE INTO PM1  **
0090 CONVOL1:        NUM CON1L1 & IF INV,PDR,CJP & PRSHF      ;TEST PDR
0090 0000100101101010 00011XXXXXXXXXXX XXXXXXXXXXXXX1XX XXXXXXXXXXXX
0091                NUM & IF & ACK & LOADREG
0091 0000000000000000 01110XXXXXXXXXXX XXXXXXXXXXXXXXX1 011111X1XXXX
0092                NUM & IF & IORLD & M1PM1BS & PMCTRINC
0092 0000000000000000 01110XXX1XXXXXXX XXXX1XXXXXXXXXXX XXXX1XXXXXXX
0093                NUM & IF & IORLD & M1PM1BS & PMCTRINC
0093 0000000000000000 01110XXX1XXXXXXX XXXX1XXXXXXXXXXX XXXX1XXXXXXX
0094                NUM & IF & IORLD & M1PM1BS & PMCTRINC
0094 0000000000000000 01110XXX1XXXXXXX XXXX1XXXXXXXXXXX XXXX1XXXXXXX
0095                JUMP CONVOL1 & IORLD & M1PM1BS & PMCTRINC
0095 0000100100000000 00011XXX1XXXXXXX XXXX1XXXXXXXXXXX XXXX1XXXXXXX
0096 CON1L1:         NUM CONVOL1 & IF INV,PMF,CJP         ;TEST PMF
0096 0000100100001001 10011XXXXXXXXXXX XXXXXXXXXXXXXXXX XXXXXXXXXXXX
0097                NUM D#28 & IF ,,LDCT & ACK & PRSHF & OKSHF
0097 0000000111000000 01100XXXXXXXXXXX XXXXXXXXXXXXX1XX XXXXXX11XXXX
0098                NUM & IF & PROCLR & LOADREG
0098 0000000000000000 01110XXXXXXXXXXX XXXXXXXXXXXX1XX1 011111XXXXXX
0099 CON1L2:         NUM & IF & PROCLR & IORLD & M1PM1BS & PMCTRINC
0099 0000000000000000 01110XXX1XXXXXXX XXXX1XXXXXXX1XXX XXXX1XXXXXXX
009A                NUM & IF & PROCLR & IORLD & M1PM1BS & PMCTRINC
009A 0000000000000000 01110XXX1XXXXXXX XXXX1XXXXXXX1XXX XXXX1XXXXXXX
009B                NUM & IF & PROCLR & IORLD & M1PM1BS & PMCTRINC
009B 0000000000000000 01110XXX1XXXXXXX XXXX1XXXXXXX1XXX XXXX1XXXXXXX
009C                NUM & IF & PROCLR & IORLD & M1PM1BS & PMCTRINC
009C 0000000000000000 01110XXX1XXXXXXX XXXX1XXXXXXX1XXX XXXX1XXXXXXX
009D                NUM CON1L2 & IF ,,RPCT & PROCLR & PRSHF & OKSHF & LOADREG
009D 0000100110010000 01001XXXXXXXXXXX XXXXXXXXXXXX11X1 0111111XXXXX
009E                NUM & RETURN
009E 0000000000000000 01010XXXXXXXXXXX XXXXXXXXXXXXXXXX XXXXXXXXXXXX
```

Figure 2 A section of "wide word" microcode prepared for a typical parallel processor control unit. The code was assembled with the aid of a "meta-assembler", which allows the designer to define rapidly an "assembly language" for his machine so that instructions can be written in easily remembered alphabetic character groups. The meta-assembler then converts the alphabetic groups into sets of ones, zeros, and X's, according to previously defined relationships between alphabetic groups and sets of ones and zeros. The output listing depicts the rows of alphabetic letter groups prepared by the hardware designer, followed by the equivalent "assembled" rows of ones, zeros, and X's generated by the meta-assembler. The code represented in this figure is the main control program for the uppermost microprogram control unit depicted in Figure 3.

1.3. High Computational Demand Tasks

For a small class of tasks which require processors capable of throughput in the range of 2×10^8 to 5×10^9 operations/second, none of the approaches described earlier is adequate; with present digital device technology, special measures are always required to achieve such high computational rates. These tasks are likely to remain the least frequently encountered, particularly in the biomedical world. However, the demand for such high computational power is already becoming substantial in the aerospace, military, seismic, and earth resources disciplines. As a single example, the millions of high spatial resolution multispectral images generated by the United States Landsat D Earth Resources Satellite, planned to be operational by 1981, will overwhelm the capacity of the fastest available processors. Nonetheless, applications in the biomedical sciences for very high capacity computers do occasionally occur.

In early 1980 several multimillion dollar general-purpose scientific computers are under development which will ultimately be capable of executing hundreds of millions to several billion arithmetic operations per second [13,14]. Although the availability of very large machines is increasing, they will not be widely accessible for several years. Achievement of computational rates above several hundred million arithmetic operations per second, in a sufficiently cost conservative manner to allow more widespread usage than can be expected for the general-purpose giant computers, will require the development of special-purpose machines optimized to execute a very small class of well understood algorithms. Though limited in flexibility, highly specialized processors can be very efficient in comparison to general-purpose computers since all arithmetic elements not required to execute a preselected class of algorithms are carefully eliminated from their design.

A recent biomedical research project requiring computational rates approaching several billion arithmetic operations per second is an advanced generation truly three-dimensional real-time x-ray computed tomography capability, the Dynamic Spatial Reconstructor (DSR). Unlike commercially available x-ray computed tomography machines [1], which collect in 5-20 seconds sufficient projection data to reconstruct only a single cross-sectional image, the DSR will collect within an 11 msec duration sufficient projection data to reconstruct up to 240 adjacent 1 mm thick cross sections encompassing a cylindrical volume of tissue (e.g., the thoracic or abdominal contents) 22 cm in axial extent and 24 cm in diameter [3]. Since the entire data collection procedure can be repeated 60 times each second, a scan lasting only ten seconds produces sufficient projection data to reconstruct up to 150,000 cross sections [15]. Reconstruction and appropriate three-dimensional display of these cross sections results in a time varying, truly three-dimensional x-ray image of the structure under study, with potentially powerful biomedical research and clinical diagnostic possibilities [16]. If such an x-ray scanning capability is to prove useful in biomedical research and clinical diagnostic environments, the duration necessary to completely process and display the volumetric images must be reduced to at most a few minutes for a few seconds of actual data collection. Since the best throughput times achieved to date using large minicomputers combined with presently available programmable array processors is approximately 5-20 seconds per cross section, it was determined that several orders of magnitude speed improvement would be necessary to achieve the required throughput, equivalent to a computational rate of at least several billion arithmetic operations per second. Since such a large throughput did not appear supportable even by next-generation programmable array processors of the type depicted in Figure 1, it was recognized that a special-purpose processor executing a limited subclass of image reconstruction algorithms would have to be developed.

Figure 3 is a schematic diagram of a special-purpose parallel hardware processor designed to execute several closely related reconstruction algorithms [15]. In accord with earlier comments regarding optimum control strategies for a parallel processor system, the design will employ two separate control units to govern the operation of multiple interlinked, cooperating arithmetic sections, each executing a portion of the entire image reconstruction algorithm; Figure 2 is actually the main microcode control program prepared for the uppermost of the two microprogram controllers depicted in Figure 3. The arithmetic unit depicted in the upper portion of the figure executes a linear filtration operation on individual projection data vectors each containing up to 512 elements, and then transfers its intermediate results to the multiple processors in the lower portion of the figure, which complete the remaining portions of the algorithm. In its full embodiment, the processor will consist of 29 separate arithmetic sections, each executing a portion of the procedure in parallel. A small scale engineering prototype model of the parallel processor design of Figure 3 has been developed to verify basic architectural concepts. The system design, which includes a built-in self-testing hardware capability (see below), is intended as a verification vehicle for software subroutines for the microprogram controllers. Although the engineering prototype executes a limited set of parallel operations every 160-200 nsec, the next-generation full scale processor will execute a much larger number of parallel operations every 35-40 nsec, resulting in an eventual capability in the range of 3-4 billion fixed precision arithmetic operations per sec.

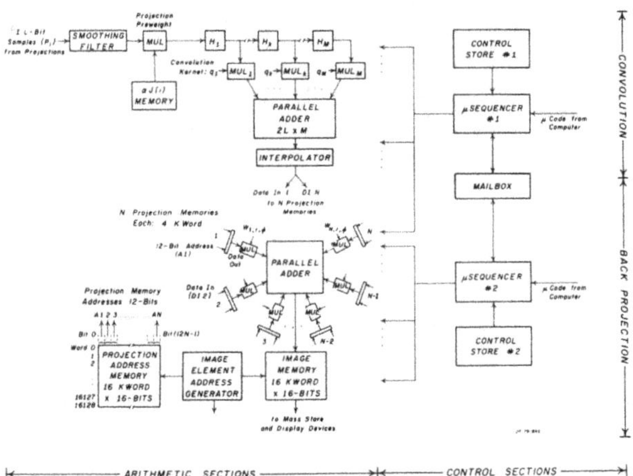

Figure 3 Design for a special-purpose parallel pipeline processor to execute high-speed image reconstructions for x-ray computed tomography. Note pair of interlocked microprogram control units which operate the filter subprocessor and back projection subprocessor, respectively. (Reproduced with permission from [7])

The design and development of a special-purpose processor with very narrowly defined capabilities employing presently available automated design aids (see below) generally requires several years of engineering effort, from the original assessment of the numerical analytic characteristics of the algorithms to be executed [15], through the final operational verification of the full scale processor. Hence, such a special design can only be justified in those instances in which neither microcomputers, programmable array processors, nor large general-purpose mainframe computers will yield sufficient cost-effective computational throughput to satisfy the operational constraints of the complete system. However, as will be described later, improvements in the methods by which digital designers develop the detailed architecture of a new computer promise in the near future to decrease significantly the time required for this procedure.

1.4. Incorporation of Improved Device Technology in Processor Design

1.4.1. Very Large Scale Integrated Circuitry

Incorporation of advanced digital device technologies into new processor architectures can often simultaneously result in a simplification in their design and an increase in processor capability and flexibility. The impact of ever increasing levels of circuit density has already been illustrated in the description of the newest families of single component 16-bit and 32-bit microprocessors, which in effect will allow algorithms previously executable only on large minicomputers to be supported with considerably less hardware and at considerably lower cost. The newest of these single component microprocessors have been made possible because the photolithographic processes by which these integrated circuits are fabricated have become so sophisticated that a single silicon "chip" can contain from 50,000 to 100,000 active logic gates. By comparison, ten years ago a state of the art component contained approximately one hundred such gates.

1.4.2. Ultra High-Speed Integrated Circuitry

An additional advance in the state of the integrated circuit art which will become increasingly important, particularly for the fabrication of ultra high-speed processors, is the development of extremely fast digital devices with both high circuit density and subnanosecond logic gate propagation delays [17]. For purposes of comparison, gate delays in the newest single component microprocessors are in the 2-5 nsec range. The new families of ultra high-speed components will allow the redesign of several traditional architectures to achieve increases in throughput and/or performance/cost ratios by factors of 3-5 while executing the same instruction sets. These new subnanosecond devices, of a type referred to as emitter coupled logic (ECL), are being incorporated into the next generations of giant commercial computers [14] and programmable array processors [8] of the type depicted in Figure 1, into highly specialized processors such as that depicted in Figure 3, and also into the designs of very powerful signal processing computers under development for the military [13].

These new subnanosecond device technologies are under investigation at the Mayo Foundation for possible use in the fabrication of the next generations of ultra high-speed special-purpose image processing and reconstruction computers [15,17]. Using conventional transistor-transistor logic (TTL) device technology with 3-6 nsec gate propagation delays, system clock rates much in excess of 25 MHz have in the past resulted in processors with poor immunity to externally and internally generated electrical noise, resulting in frequent transient, unrepeatable errors. Using an earlier family of emitter coupled logic exhibiting 2 nsec gate delays, it was possible to fabricate large special-purpose processors containing in excess of four thousand integrated circuits and employing a 40 MHz system clock [2]. Several applications now envisioned for special-purpose high-speed computers will routinely require clock rates in the range of 75-150 MHz.

To verify the performance improvement which might be achieved with the newest subnanosecond devices over that available from less advanced technologies, several prototype processors have been designed and rigorously tested in our laboratories. For example, we have recently fabricated an engineering prototype nine element linear filter processor, the architecture of which exploits the even-function symmetry required of all filter kernels employed in computed tomographic reconstruction algorithms [18]. The prototype filter processor, which contains approximately one hundred integrated circuits, was designed to allow operation at very high system clock rates. Figure 4 depicts measurements from selected test points while the processor was operating at a clock rate of 125 MHz. The device is capable of filtering an entire vector containing five hundred elements in five microseconds (this processing rate exceeds that of present generation programmable array processors by a factor of roughly a thousand). The high-speed oscilloscope traces depict the 125 MHz clock waveform, as well as single bit-lines at the final output and at various other locations within the functioning processor. Measurements of individual signal traces indicated that the combined worst-case noise from all sources, including wiring crosstalk, contamination introduced by the terminators, and voltage bus noise, is approximately 160 mV peak-to-peak (low to high signal excursion for this logic family is 800 mV). The high performance and high noise immunity of this circuit is typical of several larger systems designed in our laboratories, further strengthening the belief that very powerful processors can be fabricated with the new families of logic.

Performance improvements due to increases both in speed and integrated circuit packing density will continue for the foreseeable future. Advances in the lithographic, fabrication, and packaging technologies employed in the manufacture of high-speed integrated circuits will result in speed improvements by factors of two every two or three years throughout the 1980s. For example, in late 1979 the intrinsic gate delays of subnanosecond ECL devices, when measured in specialized test circuit configurations representative of a small portion of a computer system, would not permit reliable multi-component circuit operation at system clock rates in excess of 250 MHz [17]. Figure 5 depicts results measured in early 1980 from the same test circuit configuration fabricated with integrated circuits encapsulated in ceramic packages recently redesigned to circumvent several deficiencies encountered earlier [17]. The performance of these new components is significantly improved; system clock rates above 450 MHz were achieved. This approximate doubling of circuit speed implies that the same number of components can perform twice as much computation, or that the same computation rates can be achieved with fewer components and at lower total cost. Additional improvement in the speed of these components resulting from advances in integrated circuit fabrication techniques is likely during the next two or three years.

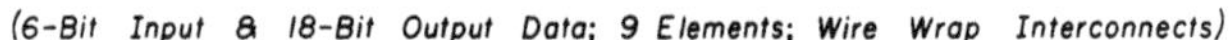

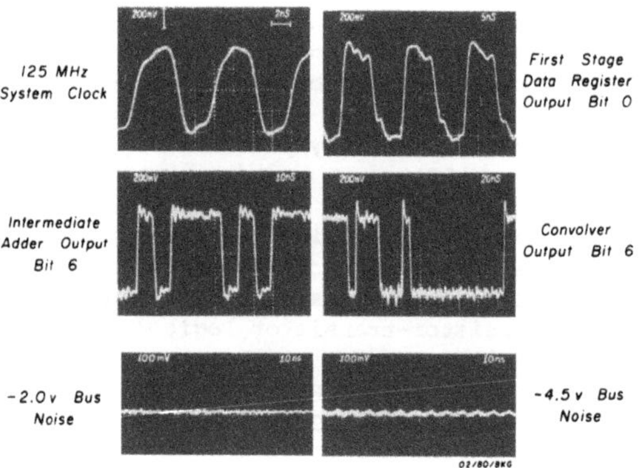

Figure 4 Operation of prototype direct convolution filter processor fabricated with subnanosecond emitter coupled logic. Note particularly the high system clock rate, short rise/fall times, and low system noise levels. (Reproduced with permission from [7])

(454 MHz System Clock via Square Wave Oscillator;
Carriers Bump Soldered to PC Board)

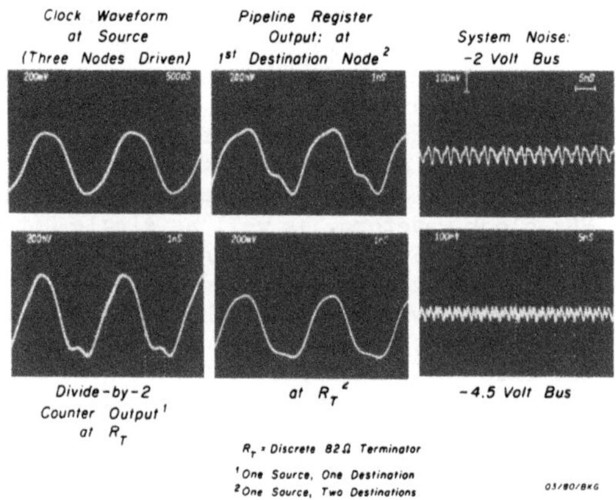

Figure 5 Operation of a prototype digital test circuit fabricated with subnanosecond emitter coupled logic, exploiting a new method for encapsulation of the silicon integrated circuits. The test circuit, which simulates a small portion of the arithmetic unit of a digital computer, operated correctly at the highest system clock rate achieved in our laboratory to date with this family of logic. Improved

speed performance in the test circuit implies that higher throughput than possible heretofore can be similarly attained in larger systems using these fabrication techniques.

1.4.3. Configurable Gate Arrays

Computer designers are well aware that the cost of a processor which is to be replicated many times is proportional to the total number of integrated circuits used in its fabrication; hence, the cost of such a processor can be markedly reduced by employing high density integrated circuits incorporating a large portion of the entire processor. Until very recently, custom designs for large scale integrated circuits were feasible only for those devices, e.g., fixed precision multipliers, which were in such high demand that production runs in the tens of thousands of components could be virtually guaranteed. The extremely high cost of new LSI circuit designs has effectively precluded the use of custom components in the processors of all but one or two very large vendors, even if dozens of machines are to be fabricated.

The custom design of special integrated circuits has been simplified by the recent commercial introduction of powerful "design stations" composed of a large graphics display unit, a minicomputer, and special computer programs to aid the engineer in the development procedure; nonetheless, the full-time effort of a specialist is frequently required for a year or more to complete the design of a custom component of low to medium complexity. However, a compromise approach is becoming available, in which a single large scale integrated circuit structure containing several thousand individual unconnected logic gates is mass produced, with the final interconnection of the individual gate elements carried out with highly automated equipment during the final stage of fabrication at a very low per-design cost. These general purposal LSI components, termed "configurable gate arrays" (CGAs), presently contain more than 1200 unconnected gates; similar designs soon to be available will contain two to four thousand equivalent gates, a capacity which is not even close to the maximum size limit imposed by technological constraints. These devices will also exhibit propagation delays in the range of .5-6 nsec with moderate levels of power dissipation. As an example of the improvements in processor performance to be gained by exploiting CGAs, the prototype convolution filter processor of one hundred integrated circuits which provided the data for Figure 4 could easily be placed on a single 2000 gate CGA. A fully augmented direct convolution filter processor of a similar design would require approximately 800 of the currently available subnanosecond ECL integrated circuits; the same design could be reduced to a parts count of approximately 25-30 CGA components of only three distinct device types, which would execute an entire direct filtration of a 500 element fixed precision vector in less than 2 microseconds [18].

1.5. Fault Isolation, Diagnosis and Self-Test Features Required for Advanced Scientific Processors

The increasing complexity of all types of computer-like devices, including large mainframe general-purpose machines, advanced special-purpose programmable array processors, and single component microcomputers, is creating a severe problem for the ultimate users of these systems. When such a machine suffers a hardware malfunction, the users of the machine are frequently initially unaware of the malfunction; when the problem finally becomes obvious, the owner commonly possesses neither the knowledge nor the specialized equipment to diagnose and correct the fault. The inaccessibility of local support personnel capable of correcting such problems is particularly acute in the biomedical world, where the investigators using the computer are usually untrained in computer hardware technology. The solution to this dilemma is that the devices must be designed to diagnose their own hardware malfunctions, and to specify to the user the steps required to correct the faults. Minicomputer vendors are now incorporating hardware into their processors which permit a computer in the vendor's factory to test a faulty machine remotely via a dial-up telephone link, and indicate precisely that portion of the computer (generally one or a few cards containing integrated circuitry) which must be replaced. An alternate method, now gaining acceptance, provides sufficient dedicated internal hardware for complete self-testing of the machine. However, most computer vendors have been slow to adopt this latter approach; many minicomputers and almost all array processors have no such capability. There is a growing concensus, however, that "testability" should be built into a processor at the individual integrated circuit level, i.e., that portions of the silicon "real estate" of LSI and VLSI microprocessors and of large configurable gate arrays should be dedicated to self-test and diagnosis functions; such a capability for a microprocessor could include a small program stored on-chip in read-only-memory which could be executed by transmitting a "test" command on a reserved pin of the integrated circuit. The stored test program would exercise every capability of the integrated circuit, and signal with a coded message if an internal error was detected. This type of built-in testing is not available on present generation microprocessors, but is likely to become so in the next generation. In the case of the CGA devices, which are likely to be dedicated to the pipelined execution of arithmetic instructions, a small amount of extra logic will be included to permit the complete and rapid testing of every bit pathway in the entire integrated circuit whenever desired, at full operating speed if necessary. At present, built-in test features are incorporated into a processor almost as an afterthought; by including test features on every component, the processor designers will be able to implement exhaustive automatic fault diagnosis into their machines. The inclusion of self-test features is now nearly mandatory; advanced device technology and high density circuitry are both the cause of and the cure for the problem of undiagnosable machine failures.

1.6. Computer-Aided Design Software for Rapid Development of New Machine Architecture

The logical and physical complexity of all types of digital processors has been roughly doubling every two years since the late 1960s; as a result, modern machines containing 75,000 to one-quarter million logic gates are now commonplace. Regardless of whether these gates are physically distributed among thousands of integrated circuits, as is still true for mainframe computers, or are all placed on a single integrated circuit, as is the case for advanced single component microprocessors in the 70,000-100,000 gate complexity range, the designs of these devices are becoming too complex for engineers to develop within a reasonable duration using pencil and paper methods. In an effort to reduce the engineer's design burden, during the past five years there has been an increasing effort to develop special sets of operator-interactive computer programs, called computer-aided design (CAD) packages, which assist the engineers at every stage of the design process. Via interaction with a computer terminal, the engineers can specify the component-by-component logical design of a subsystem. Using appropriate keyboard commands and a light pen or X-Y cursor, the individual logical blocks or components are retrieved from a pre-established file and drawn onto the screen of the computer terminal in the desired topological relationships; interconnecting wires are then specified by the engineer, and are incorporated into the hardware design by the CAD program. As the design process proceeds, the CAD program provides the designer with information required to verify the correctness of his design, including worst case timing limits on all subsections of the processor and inadvertent design conflicts which violate pre-established design rules. With the aid of these same programs, the physical wiring layouts and component locations of the individual circuit boards can be established and verified for accuracy prior to actual fabrication. Although the power and flexibility of CAD software are growing rapidly, the sophistication of the CAD programs frequently limits the complexity of a design which can be attempted, and not the device fabrication technology itself (frequently the same CAD programs can design either an entire processor containing many components, or the detailed layout of a single high density integrated circuit).

Figure 6 is a schematic diagram of the step-by-step design of a logic board, as executed by a computer-aided-design program developed in our laboratory and specifically optimized for the design rules of high-speed ECL. In Step 1, the designer specifies a set of typical physical elements, in this example an off-board signal connector (labelled E1) and a pattern of contact points for a single integrated circuit (labelled E2). Pin positions are then numbered, and the correct physical dimensions between the contact pads, as well as the electrical characteristics of each contact pad (e.g., "pins 1 and 16 committed to the ground plane, pin 8 commited to the -5.2 V power plane") are specified. In Step 2, a "row" of connectors and a "row" of integrated circuit locations are generated by a horizontally moving (row-wise) "step-and-repeat" propagation of the patterns. In Step 3, a column-wise step-and-repeat propagation of the row types established in Step 2 is used to define an entire logic board, which for this example contains two rows of two board connectors each, and one row of two integrated circuit patterns. In the final step (Result) all pin numbers and physical and electrical descriptions established in Step 1 are added to the board layout created in Step 3. By this mechanism the Mayo-developed CAD program allows an engineer to specify the layout details of very large circuit boards containing several hundred integrated circuits; software compilation of the board to produce the physical and electrical specifications employed in its physical fabrication require a few minutes of computer time. A board contining 200 integrated circuits, forty 40-pin connectors, 200 terminator packages, 400 capacitors, and 12500 contact points was recently laid out in a few hours and "compiled" in less than five minutes. In later phases of the CAD program, the electrical characteristics of individual circuit component types are specified; logical hardware designs are then mapped into physically available part types, interconnects are established and tested for design errors, a worst case timing simulation is carried out, and the design is then released for fabrication. Special software aids are also available to assist the designer during the initial checkout of the hardware, and in its maintenance thereafter. These same principles, and in many cases the same software packages, can be applied to the design of the CGA devices discussed previously. It is only by the use of such computer aids that the development time and risk for new processor designs can be reduced to acceptable levels.

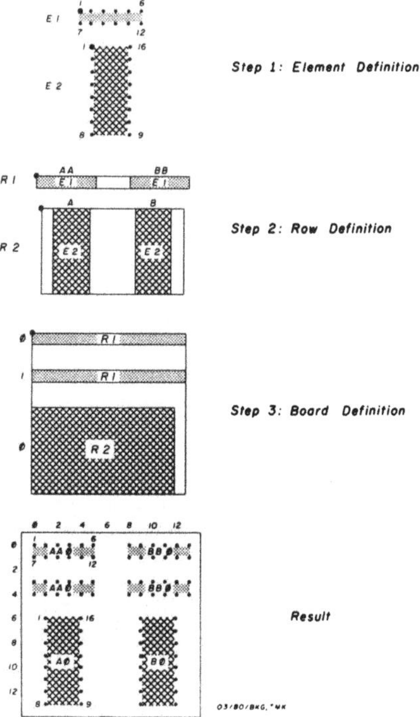

Figure 6 Diagrammatic representation of operator-interactive engineering design of a large logic board for special-purpose processors, using special computer-aided

design (CAD) software programs. Several types of physical elements are first established; the board is then built up by "step-and-repeat" methods (see text).

2. ACKNOWLEDGMENTS

R. D. Beistad, A. Chu, and D. A. Schwab for technical assistance; D. C. Darling, E. C. Quarve, M. C. Fynbo, D. Vander Schaff, M. A. Engesser, I. E. Donovan, and L. O. Johnson for assistance in preparation of text and figures.

2.1. Grant Acknowledgments

This investigation was supported in part by U. S. Public Health Service Grant HL-04664, RR-00007 from the National Institutes of Health; Grant F33615-79-C-1875 from the U. S. Air Force, a grant from the Fannie E. Rippel Foundation, and the contribution of specialized digital components by Fairchild Camera and Instrument Corporation.

3. REFERENCES

1. A. C. Kak, "Computerized tomography with x-ray, emission, and ultrasound sources," Proceedings of the IEEE, 1979, 67(9), pp. 1245-1272.

2. B. K. Gilbert, M. T. Storma, C. E. James, L. W. Hobrock, E. S. Yang, K. C. Ballard, and E. H. Wood, "A real-time hardware system for digital processing of wide-band video images," IEEE Transactions on Computers, 1976, C-25(11), pp. 1089-1100.

3. R. A. Robb, E. L. Ritman, B. K. Gilbert, J. H. Kinsey, L. D. Harris, and E. H. Wood, "The DSR - a high-speed three-dimensional x-ray computed tomography system for dynamic spatial reconstruction of the heart and circulation," IEEE Transactions on Nuclear Science, 1979, NS-26(2), Part 2, pp. 2713-2717.

4. S. P. Morse, W. B. Pohlman, and B. W. Revenel, "The Intel 8086 Microprocessor: A 16-bit evolution of the 8080," IEEE Computer Magazine, 1978, 11(6), pp. 18-27.

5. E. Stritter and T. Gunter, "A microprocessor architecture for a changing world: The Motorola 68000," IEEE Computer Magazine, 1979, 12(2), pp. 43-52.

6. N. A. Alexandridis, "Bit sliced microprocessor architecture," IEEE Computer Magazine, 1978, 11(6), pp. 56-81.

7. B. K. Gilbert and L. D. Harris, "Advances in processor, display, and device technology for biomedical image processing," IEEE Transactions on Nuclear Science NS-27(3) (June) 1980 (In Press).

8. Advanced Flexible Processor Microcode Cross Assembler Reference Manual, Document 77900500. Control Data Corporation, Minneapolis, 1979.

9. L. D. Wittie, "Architectures for large networks of microcomputers," Proceedings of the IEEE Computer Society Workshop on Interconnection Networks for Parallel and Distributed Processing, West Lafayette, Indiana, April 21-22, 1980, IEEE Press, New York (In Press).

10. M. J. B. Duff, "CLIP4: a large scale integrated circuit array parallel processor," Third International Joint Conference on Pattern Recognition, 1976, pp. 728-732.

11. A. P. Reeves, "A systematically designed binary array processor," IEEE Transactions on Computers, 1980, C-29(4), pp. 278-287.

12. S. M. Ornstein, W. R. Crowther, M. F. Kraley, R. O. Bressler, A. Michel, and F. E. Heart, "Pluribus - a reliable multiprocessor," Proceedings of the AFIPS National Computer Conference, Anaheim, 1975, 44, pp. 551-559.

13. T. M. McWilliams, "The SCALD timing verifier: a new approach to timing constraints in large digital systems," Proceedings of the 1980 IEEE International Symposium on Circuits and Systems, 1980, IEEE Publication #80CH1564-4, pp. 415-423.

14. H. Stopper, "The BCML circuit and packaging system," IEEE Transactions on Components, Hybrids, and Manufacturing Technology, 1980, CHMT-3(1), pp. 110-120.

15. B. K. Gilbert, A. Chu, D. E. Atkins, E. E. Swartzlander, Jr., and E. L. Ritman, "Ultra high-speed transaxial image reconstruction of the heart, lungs, and circulation via numerical approximation methods and optimized processor architecture," Computers and Biomedical Research, 1979, 12(1), pp. 17-38.

16. E. L. Ritman, J. H. Kinsey, R. A. Robb, L. D. Harris, and B. K. Gilbert, "Physics and technical considerations in the design of the DSR: A high temporal resolution volume scanner," American Journal of Roentgenology, 1980, 134(2), pp. 369-374.

17. B. K. Gilbert, L. M. Krueger, and R. D. Beistad, "Design of prototype digital processors employing subnanosecond emitter coupled logic and rapid fabrication techniques," IEEE Transactions on Components, Hybrids, and Manufacturing Technology, 1980, CHMT-3(1), pp. 125-134.

18. B. K. Gilbert, S. K. Kenue, R. A. Robb, A. Chu, A. H. Lent, and E. E. Swartzlander, Jr., "Rapid execution of fan beam image reconstruction algorithms using efficient computational techniques and special-purpose processors," IEEE Transactions on Biomedical Engineering, 1980, BME-27 (12) (In Press).

MATHEMATICS OF DIGITIZATION OF BINARY IMAGES

by

Jean SERRA, Ph,D., Mining Eng.
Centre de Morphologie Mathématique
Ecole des Mines de Paris
35 Rue St-Honoré 77305 Fontainebleau (France)

ABSTRACT

Image transformation and measurements are defined either in the plane (R^2) or on regular lattices of points. Each of the two versions is a mathematical model, the former being more adapted to questions such as rotations, similarities, convergence, and relationships with physical properties, the latter being more accessible to numerical treatment. The key idea of the paper is the following: the only notion which has a physical meaning with respect to digitization is the pair: "set model-morphological criterion". This point of view leads to a definition of digitization linking models to criteria. From this standpoint 3 questions have been considered:

- Transformations digitizable for the most extensive set-class in morphology (i.e. the closed sets $F(R^2)$). A theorem is given according to which the increasing and upper semi-continuous mapping are digitizable for the closed sets.

- Transformations preserving honotopy. It is shown that if $x \in F(R^2)$ and its complement X^c are both open as a compact disk B with radius $a > 0$, then and only then, their intersections by an hexagonal lattice with spacing $\leq$ a generate graphs preserve the original homotopy.

- The digitization of some stereological parameters, in the context of the convex ring model, is studied.

1. INTRODUCTION

Between the digitation of an image stored in a computer and the object it represents, there is always a loss of information. For example, if the object is a red blood cell smear, two cells which are separated in reality can be digitized as impinging images if the resolution is faulty.

A fundamental question thus arises: how can image processing best accentuate or eliminate the difference between the real and the digitized image. Suppose, for example, that we wish to count the red blood cells mentioned above; we could, of course, apply a classic particle counting algorithm. But even if the results are correct with respect to the digitized image, they will contain as many errors as there are cells that touch after digitization. Alternatively, we can use an ultimate eroding algorithm (J. Serra 1981) which marks individually the centers of the particles comprising the object, even if they touch. In this case the digitization errors do not influence the validity of the final results.

The question of the physical significance of digital algorithms thus arises. In this presentation we shall address ourselves to the more limited case of the digitization of binary images. The principal results are the following:

1. The most reliable algorithms i.e. the only ones which always minimize the fluctuations due to digitization, are those we call the increasing transofrmations. Thus, the surface is always a reliable estimation, but the perimeter is not.

2. If we require that the digital image have the same particle structure and contain the same holes as the real object (we would say that it has the same homotopy) it is necessary and sufficient that the object be rather regular i.e. that it is morphologically open and closed by a disk of radius r, and that the spacing of the pixels of the digital lattice be inferior to $r/\sqrt{2}$ (square lattice) or to r(hexagonal lattice).

These mathematical results orient the designing of the digital image processors toward algorithms of the increasing type, and towards certain methods of validity testing for digital algorithms.

In addition, these results show that when one designs special purpose digital image processors it is preferable to adopt the hexagonal lattice rather than the square one.

2. THE SPACES R^2 AND Z^2

In image analysis, the zone of the space belonging to the same material (microscopy) or exhibiting the same texture (LANDSAT images) are usually modelled by sets of points in the Euclidean plane R^2. However, these images are most often obtained by scanning which provides digital data, i.e. functions defined over the space Z^2 of the pairs of integers. The purpose of this paper is to study the relationships between these two continuous and discrete approaches (the mathematical structure of Z^2 is that of a module).

Here a few topological comments are necessary. To handle digitization correctly, we must be able to express in R^2 how a sequence $\{X_i\}$ of sets tends toward a limit X. On the other hand, we have to restrict the class $\mathcal{P}(R^2)$ of all the possible parts of R^2. Indeed the Euclidean space is too rich for our purpose. For example, a set such as "all the points with irrational coordinates of the plane" has absolutely no physical meaning. To simplify things, pseudo-distance ρ, from point x to set X, can be defined as follows:

$$\rho(x,X) = \inf_{y \in X} d(x,y) \qquad x \in R^2 \quad , X \in \mathcal{P}(R^2)$$

where d is the Euclidean distance. With respect to ρ, there is no difference between a set X and its topological closure $\bar{X}$ (i.e. X plus its boundary), since $\rho(x,X) = \rho(x,\bar{X})$, $\forall$ x, $\forall$ X. In other words, all the notions derived from ρ will not be related to the parts $\mathcal{P}(R^2)$ of R^2, but to the equivalence classes of sets which have the same closure. For example, the points with irrational coordinates of R^2, and the whole plane itself will be considered as identical. Hence it now suffices to concentrate upon the class $\mathcal{F}(R^2)$ of the closed sets of R^2. The pseudo-distance ρ generates a topology, called intersection topology. G. Matheron (1969) (1975) and D. G. Kendall (1974) exhaustively studied it in a more general frame than R^2 (for a simpler presentation see also J. Serra (1980) Ch. III). By definition, a sequence

$\{X_i\}$, $x_i \in F$ converges towards a limit $X \in F$ if and only if, for any $x \in R^2$, the sequence $\rho\{x, X_i\}$ converges toward $\rho\{x,X\}$ in R_+. From this standpoint, we can derive all the basic topological notions, such as neighborhoods, continuity, semi-continuity etc... We quote only one result for it will be useful below. An increasing mapping Ψ from F into itself (or more generally from $F \times F \to F$) is upper semi-continuous (u.s.c.) if and only if $X_i \downarrow X$ in F implies $\Psi(X_i) \downarrow \Psi(X)$ in F. ($X_i \downarrow X$ means $X_{i+1} \subset X_i$ and $X = \bigcap_i X_i$; Ψ is said to be increasing when $X \subset Y \Rightarrow \Psi(X) \subset \Psi(Y)$).

Another notion, useful in what follows, is that of dilation. The dilate $Y = X + B$ of X by B is the set of points $x - b$, where $x \in X$ and $b \in B$ (Serra 1965-1980). If B is symmetrical with respect to the origin, we have $X + B = \bigcup_{x \in X} \bigcup_{b \in B} (x + y)$. The operation of dilation is defined in R^2 as well as in Z^2.

3. REPRESENTATION

We must accept the unfortunate fact that the two spaces R^2 and Z^2 are not isomorphic since there are several different ways to interpret the same module in Euclidean space. The notion of representation will be the go-between that links the two spaces.

Definition. Let $X \in F(R^2)$ and k a positive integer. With each pair (X,k) we associate the representation $C(X,k)$, where C is a mapping from $F \times N^+$ onto F such that the range of the mapping is isomorphic to $P(Z^2)$; i.e. there exists a one-to-one and onto mapping Y of the range of C in F and $P(Z^2)$. Therefore T^{-1} exists and we have:

$$(1) \qquad \forall \hat{X} \in P(Z^2), \quad X \in F,\ k \in N^+ : T^{-1}(\hat{X}) = C(X,k)$$

A few examples of the most common representations is the best way to procede. To avoid confusion throughout this section we will put a "hat" on sets and transformations that relate to $P(Z^2)$.

a - The lattice representation

Let u and u' be two independent vectors of R^2 starting from the origin O. A lattice L in R^2 is the set of all of the extremities x that satisfy :

$$(2) \qquad Ox = \hat{x}_1\, u + \hat{x}_2\, u' \text{ where } (\hat{x}_1, \hat{x}_2) \in Z^2$$

The two sets of Fig. 1 a and b show the basic ways of constructing lattices, namely the square lattice (u = (o,a) ; u' = (a,o)) and the hexagonal lattice (u = (a,o), u' = $(\frac{a}{2}, \frac{a\sqrt{3}}{2})$), where a is a positive constant called the lattice unit. Replacing a with $a_k = a.2^{-k}$ results in a new lattice L_k that contains the original one, as well as all intermediary lattices of units $a_i (1 \leq i \leq k)$. Associate with lattice L_k a small cell $C_k(o)$ centered at the origin and congruent to $u_k + u'_k$; i.e. a rhomb or a square depending on the type of lattice. Let $L_k(y)$ denote L_k translated by a $y \in C_k(o)$. Over all y in $C_k(o)$, the union of the $L_k(y)$'s covers the plan R^2.

Similarly, we can turn the lattice through an angle $\alpha \in [0,2\pi]$, resulting in $L_k(y,\alpha)$. In what follows, no distinction is made between the hexagonal or the square mode when the property under study is valid in both cases. To construct a representation from L_k is now straightforward. For any $X \in F$ we have :

$$(3) \qquad C(X,k) = X \cap L_k \text{ and } T = (\hat{x}_1, \hat{x}_2) : \hat{x}_1\, u_k + \hat{u}_2\, u'_k \in C(X,k)$$

b - The covering representation

The covering representation is commonly used in image analysis to digitally code the curves in R^2 (H. Freeman, 1971) ; our main interest in it is that it is exactly right for digitization the increasing mappings. Start from the lattice L_k.

With each point $x \in L_k$ associate the elementary cell $\{x\} \oplus C_k(o) = C_k(x)$ which is translated from the origin to the point x. Over all x in L_k, the union of the $C(x)$'s covers R^2. Then the covering representation C)X,k) of $x \in F$ is defined to be the union of <u>the cells</u> $C_k(x)$ <u>which hit X</u> :

$$(4) \qquad C(X,k) = \{ \bigcup C_k(x) \; ; \; x \in L_k, \; C_k(x) \cap x \neq \emptyset \} = [\, (x \oplus C_k) \cap (L_k \oplus C_k)]$$

The covering representation satisfies the two important properties :

i) For any $X \in F$, $\lim_{k\to\infty} C(X,k) = X$ in F. Figure 2 illustrates this point.

ii) With respect to the dilations in R^2 and in Z^2, we have :

$$C(x \oplus B,k) = [(x \oplus C_k) \cap L_k] \oplus [(B + C_k) \cap L_k] \oplus 2\, C_k$$

$$= T^{-1} \{T[C(X,k)] \,\hat{\oplus}\, T\, [C(B,k)]\} \oplus C_k$$

the covering representation of $X \oplus B$ is the inverse image of a digital dilation of the digital images of X and B, modulo a dilation by C_k.

d - <u>The planar graph representation</u>

Strictly speaking, the planar graph representation is just an extension of the lattice representation. Starting from a set $X \in F\ (R^2)$ and its square and hexagonal lattice representations $X \cap L$, it is extremely easy to add sets of edges D to the representations in order to associate planar graphs $(X \cap L, D)$ with them (the various modes of obtaining such graphs, shown in Fig. 3, are clear enough, and we no longer need to define them). All these planar graphs are defined on the Euclidean plane. However it is easy to see (Serra, 1980) that they correspond to strictly digital graphs (one-to-one and onto mappings) which can be treated by digital algorithms. Therefore, they are representations of X. They appear in questions involving the connectivity of X. In particular, one says that a planar graph representation $(X \cap L, D)$ preserves the homotopy of X when X and $(X \cap L, D)$ exhibit the same structure of particles and holes (a more precise definition is given in Serra, 1980).

4. THE DIGITIZATION CONCEPT

a - <u>Two counter examples</u>

The tools are honed; it only remains to bridge the gap from digital to continuous morphologies. The following two examples illustrate where the problems lie.

i) Are the Poisson points

A first approach would be to consider the intersection of a set X of Poisson points with the sequence of lattices L_k, $k \in N^+$. We might hope that as k increases, X becomes better and better known. Unfortunately, this is not the case; the intersection $X \cap L_k$ remains empty, no matter how large k: The lattices only "catch" those points with rational coordinates which have zero probability in the Poisson process. On the other hand, by starting from the covering lattice, we "catch" all the Poisson points by dilating them. How sure are we this "parasite" dilation will not upset any subsequent morphological transformation?

ii) Connectivity number for the Boolean model.

Consider a very simple set X, a 2-D Boolean formulation with convex primary grains, together with a very simple parameter N, the connectivity number of the compact subset X Z, i.e. the number of its particles minus their holes. By probabilistic means we can calculate the mathematical expectation of N, as well as that of the digital connectivity numbers N' and N" of the hexagonal and octogonal graphs associated with $X \cap Z \cap L_k$. It is curious that as the lattice spacing a_k becomes infinitesimally small, the two numbers E(N') and E(N") tend toward different limits that are both distinct from the true value E(N) : Relative errors are enormous, as much as 200% (Serra, 1980).

b- The definition of digitization

The first example in 3-a showed that the various representations are not equivalent in R^2, although they are all isomorphic to $\mathcal{P}(Z^2)$. The lesson learned from the second example is probably deeper: the question is not to know whether a set of R^2 is digitalizable or not - the only thing with a physical meaning is the pair "morphological criterion - set model". The subject of digitization stems from consideration of only this pair. The more demanding the criterion, the less numerous the accessible sets are.
In reality, the structure of the physical space is unknown to us; we can be sure that it is neither R^2(nor R^3) nor Z^2. At ultra-microscopic scales, the rocks and the biological structures appear as molecules, themselves sophisticated organizations of substructures, etc.... In fact, the space itself changes. But that is not our problem; in morphology, we simply want to make chemical, physical or physiolocigal properties of the bodies correspond to their geometry at a given scale, or for a limited range of scales. Some of these properties are relevant to the Euclidean space (partial differential equations for mechanics, hydrodynamics, etc.... optical magnifications; mechanical rotations of a microscopic states) while others are relevant to the digital mathematical structures (in the Texture Analyser for example). A digitization theory should make the two space models coherent with respect to each other, rather than deciding which fits best with the physical world. The following definition of digitization reflects this approach.

Definition. Let $U(\mathcal{F})$ be a sub-class of the closed sets and Ψ a class of morphological transformations mapping U into $\mathcal{F}$. A pair $(X,\psi) \in U \times \Psi$, is said to be digitalizable when there exists a representation. $\mathcal{C}(U,N^+)$ and a digital algorithm $\hat{\psi}$ from $\mathcal{P}(Z^2)$ onto itself, such that:

$$(5) \qquad \forall\ (X,\psi) \in (U \times \Psi),\ k\to\infty \Rightarrow \mathcal{T}^{-1}\ \hat{\psi}\ \mathcal{T}\ (\mathcal{C}(X,k)) \to \psi\ (X) \text{ in } \mathcal{F}$$

Figure 4 illustrates the steps involved in the digitization.

Notes:
1 - Conversely, a class $\hat{\Psi}$ of digital algorithms has a Euclidean interpretation if there exists a class (U, Ψ) and a representation $\mathcal{C}$ such that for each pair $(X,\psi) \in (U, \Psi)$, relation (5) is satisfied.

2 - The preceding definition is immediately extendable to parameters which are mappings $U\to R$ (the real numbers) in the Euclidean case, and mappings $\mathcal{P}(Z^2)\to N$ (the integers) in the digital case.
Equipped with this definition, we now try to answer the following three important questions:
α - If we take U to be the largest possible class, i.e. $\mathcal{F}$ itself, what are the transformations ψ such that the pair (X, ψ), $X \in \mathcal{F}$, is digitalizable ?

β - If the transformations $\psi \in \Psi$ depend only the homotopy of X, what is the class U $(\mathcal{F})$ which is digitizable?

γ - Are the basic stereological parameters digitizable?
(the answers are given by theorems, the proofs of which can be found in Serre (1980)).

5. DIGITIZABLE TRANSFORMATION FOR THE CLASS $\mathcal{F}$

We do not claim that the following theorem generates all possible digitizable transformations on the class $\mathcal{F}$. However the resulting class obtained from dilations, intersections and their finite iterations, is rather broad.

Theorem 1 : Any mapping Ψ from $\mathcal{F}$ into itself that is increasing, translation invariant and upper semi-continuous is digitizable. In particular, erosion, dilation, morphological opening and closing, and the size distributions, are all digitizable

REMARKS :

1 - Physically speaking, theorem 1 means that the increasing mappings do not further "complicate" the initial set X, and even often frees it from small details. As a result, all of the sets, even the most tortuous such as fractal sets, can be investigated by using dilations, erosions, and size distributions.

2 - We might wonder whether a similar theorem can be proved if we replace the increasing condition and the semi-continuity condition with one of continuity. Unfortunately it can not, as is well known by experimenters who have tried to digitalize rotations.

3 - There are independent repercussions of theorem (1) on random closed sets. By Choquet's theorem, a random closed set is characterized by dilations, which is a digitalizable operation. Hence statistical inference for random sets is always possible, but must avoid non increasing transformations such as connectivity number.

6. HOMOTOPY AND DIGITIZATION

Theorem 2 : Let $X \in \mathcal{F}(R^2)$ be a closed set, X^c be its complement, and $(\mathcal{C}(X),D)$ and $(\mathcal{C}(X^c),D)$ their respective planar graph representations induced by a hexagonal lattice with origin y, orientation α and spacing a_k. These representations preserve the homotopy of X if and only if X and X^c are open with respect to the compact disk $B(a_k)$ of radius a_k.

Corollary : The class of compact sets satisfying conditions i) and ii) of theorem 2 is digitalizable for the morphological transformations depending only on the homotopy of X.

Remarks :

1 - Theorem 2 generalizes to 2-D sets, the well-known result due to Shannon that the highest harmonic detectable in a signal has a frequency equal to one half the sampling frequency.

2 - Neither the origin y nor the orientation α of the lattice L_k appeared in the proof, and so theorem 2 remains valid for any displacement of L_k. If α is fixed, then the disk $B(a_k)$ can be repalced by the hexagon of side a_k. If the lattice is square, the theorem can be transposed by taking $a_k\sqrt{2}$ for the radius of B. In other words, for a given sampling frequency a_k, the hexagonal lattice tolerates a weaker hypothesis on the structure of the object than does the square lattice (or equivalently, it tolerates a larger spacing, given equal hypotheses).

3 - Quite apart from giving us a class of sets that are digitizable with respect to homotopy theorem 2 can also be used for digital images, to condense data for example.

7. MINKOWSKI FUNCTIONALS AND DIGITIZATION

The three Minkowski functionals in R^2 are the area, the perimeter and the connectivity number ; they are the basic-measurements for 2-D sets. Since the Lebesgue measure is increasing, translation invariant and upper semi-continuous on $\mathcal{F}(R^2)$, the area of $X \in \mathcal{F}$ is digitizable with respect to the covering representation. As for the connectivity number, it is digitizable only for the set model involved in theorem 2 (although it is defined for a broader class of sets (R^2).

The case of the perimeter U(X) is less straightforward. This notion can be defined for the compact sets satisfying theorem 2, as well as for the finite unions of compact convex sets, or more generally for the class of the normal bodies (Hadwiger (1959)). In any case, we can interpret it via Crofton's formula as the rotation average of the total projection $D(X, \alpha)$ in direction α ; this turns out to be just the right link needed to go from the perimeter to its digitization. We have:

$$(6) \qquad U(X) = \int_0^{\pi} D(X,\alpha)\ dx = \int_0^{\pi} dx \int_{-\infty}^{+\infty} N\ [X \cap \Delta(y,\alpha)]\ dy$$

where Dy is an ordinate axis orthogonal to direction α and where $N\ [X \quad \Delta(y,\alpha)]$ is the number of intercepts of X by the straight line of direction α and ordinate y. More over;

Theorem 3 : Let X be a set of the convex ring, $D(X,\alpha)$ its total porjection in direction α, and let L_k be a lattice having α as a principal direction, and let N_α (01) be the intercept number in direction α of the digital version of X according to the covering representation. Then $D(X,\alpha)$ is digitizable and, as $k\to\infty$,

$$a_k \frac{\sqrt{3}}{2}\ N_\alpha(0,1) \to D(X,\alpha) \qquad \text{(hexagonal lattice)}$$

$$a_k\ N_\alpha\ (0,1) \to D(X,\alpha) \qquad \text{(square lattice)}$$

The quantity $D(X,\alpha)$ being continuous in α, the perimeter $U(X)$ can be approximated by averaging over different lattice directions according to relation (6).

REMARK : Due to Crofton's formula we were able to estimate the perimeter $U(X)$ without having to localize or digitalize the boundary ∂X, which is fortunate. For even if we could build a digital contour tending toward ∂X, it would not necessarily mean that its length tends toward ∂X. In the literature, one sometimes finds studies devoted to perimeter estimations based on contour following. The contour following techniques act on digital graphs through segmentation, component labelling, etc..., i.e. they use notions which deal with connectivity. On the contrary, a sufficient digital tool used to estimate $U(X)$ is the module structure of Z^2, and is independent of all graphs.

CONCLUSIONS

Space limitation did not allow us to present some other interesting results (digitizability of the convex hull for the compact sets, but not for the closed sets ; lack of digitizability of the general notion of a skeleton ; etc...., see Serra (1980)). The above results illustrate a few important lessons. Theoretically speaking, they suggest that we preferably use increasing transformations (when possible), and also that we modify some concepts (the skeleton for example). Practically speaking, the above theorems result in some good workable tests :

a - When possible, change the magnification factor before digitization. If perimeter estimates increase slightly with the magnification, then the conditions of Theorem 3 are fulfilled. If not, then one must restrict oneself to using increasing transformations and to area measurements.

b - For a given magnification, move and turn the object by analogue means, then digitize and compute the connectivity number. If it stays constant for any bounded portion of the object that is completely contained in the digitizing mask, then one can assume that the conditions of Theorem 2 are fulfilled and hence perform homotopic analyses. If not, then abandon connectivity or try to see if the connectivity number stays invariant under analogue displacements followed by a small digital opening.

c - If the image is closed and open with respect to a small digital convex set, then it is oversampled and one would do better to reduce the magnification rate.

REFERENCES

G. BERNROIDER (1977) The foundation of computational geometry : theory and application of the point-lattice concept within modern structure analysis (in Lecture Notes in Biomathematics n° 23, Springer-Verlag, 1978).

H. HADWIGER (1957) Vorlesungen über Inhalt, Oberfläche and Isoperimetrie (Springer, Berlin).

G. MATHERON (1975) Random Sets and Integral Geometry (Wiley and Sons, New York).

A. ROSENFELD, A.C. KAK (1976) Digital Picture Processing (Academic Press, London).

J. SERRA (1981) Image Analysis and Mathematical Morphology (Academic Press, London).

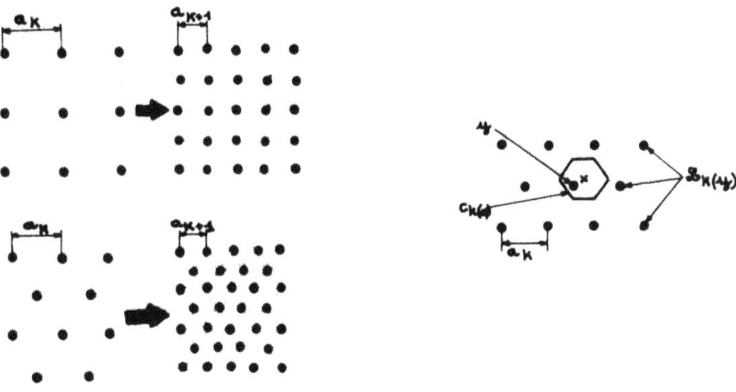

Figure 1 : a, b - Hexagonal and square lattices of size a_k

c - Translation of lattice over the basic cell $C_k(o)$

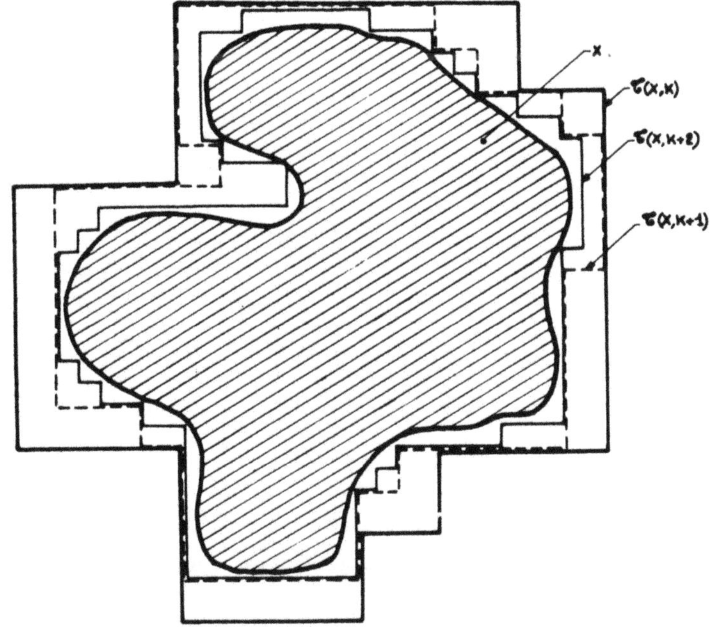

Figure 2 : Decreasing sequence of covering representations of X.

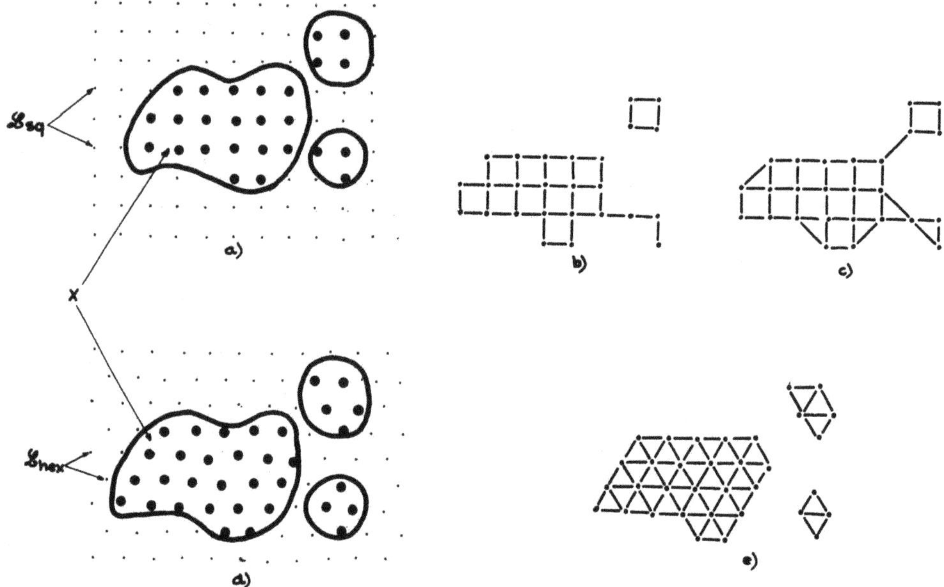

Figure 3 : a) and d) - Set X and its square and hexagonal lattice representation ($X \cap \mathcal{L}_{sq}$ and $X \cap \mathcal{L}_{hex}$ resp.)

b) and c) - planar graphs on $X \cap \mathcal{L}_{sq}$ (square and octogonal graphs resp.)

e) - planar graph on $X \cap \mathcal{L}_{hex}$

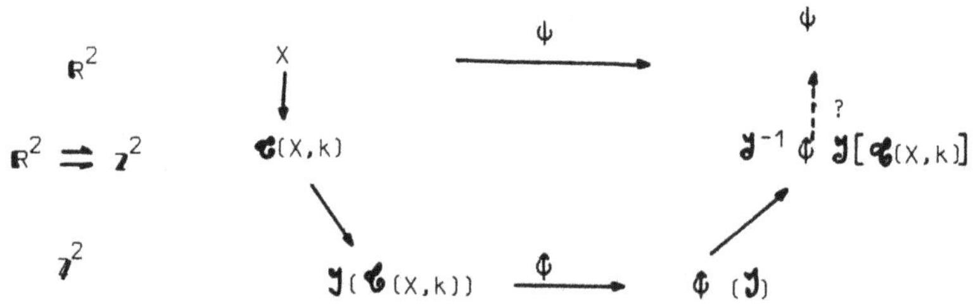

Figure 4 : The **digitization** approach

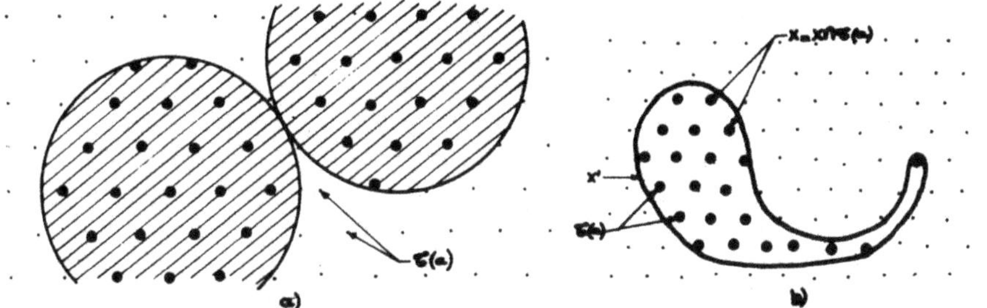

Figure 5 : a - X is connected and opened by $B(a_k)$, but the graph ($\mathscr{C}(X)$,D) id disconnected.

b - X^c is opened by $B(a_k)$; X, X $\ominus$ $B(a_k)$ and X $\oplus$ $B(a_k)$ exhibit the same connectivity. Nevertheless, ($\mathscr{C}(X)$,D) may be disconnected).

CELLULAR COMPUTERS AND BIOMEDICAL IMAGE PROCESSING

by
Stanley R. Sternberg

Environmental Research Institute of Michigan
and
University of Michigan
Ann Arbor, Michigan 48107
U.S.A.

ABSTRACT

Image processing operations are defined which permit image processing algorithms to be written as algebraic expressions whose variables are whole images. Highly parallel cellular computer architectures for evaluating these expressions are presented. Examples of processing algorithms and processed images from radioventriculography, microscopy and two-dimensional gel electrophoresis are presented.

INTRODUCTION

Rapid technological advances in biomedical instrumentation and computer hardware and software technologies for image processing are now drawing together two historically disparate areas, life science and computer science-engineering. Effective combination of these disciplines now promises to yield major advances in clinical medicine and life science research. New instrumentation for digital radiography and ultrasound, computed tomography and nuclear medicine, for quantitative autoradiography and light and electron microscopy, and for two-dimensional gel electrophoresis have already greatly advanced our understanding of normal and abnormal biological processes. Concurrent new developments in computer based image processing, such as practical implementation of the principles of cellular automata have produced new classes of special purpose computer hardware and software capable of processing images at least two orders of magnitude faster than the fastest conventional sequential computers.

CELLULAR COMPUTERS

The serial nature of conventional computers seems to restrict, or at least obscure, their usefulness as image or picture processors. Since each computer instruction typically affects only one or two pieces of data, manipulations of an entire image must be accomplished through explicit iteration which costs heavily in both time and conceptual distraction. The picture processing approach we are investigating avoids these problems by defining a set of operations which act on images as a whole. This provides an efficient conceptual framework for picture processing tasks. In addition, the cellular nature of these operations allows them to be implemented in computer hardware architectures employing a high degree of parallelism, thus eliminating the costs of iteration. We have coined the term cytocomputer after the Greek "cyto" meaning cell to describe the resulting picture processing computer. First and second generation cytocomputers have been developed at the Environmental Research Institute of Michigan (ERIM).

Cytocomputer image processing operations are based on the concepts of cellular automata. Each cell or picture element of an image is subjected to a sequence of time discrete transformations, the transformed value of a cell being determined by the initial values of a finite group of cells composing its neighborhood. Each image transformation is performed in an individual cytocomputer processing element referred to as a processing stage. A cytocomputer consists of a serial pipeline of programmable processing stages, where each stage in the pipeline performs a single transformation on an entire image. Pictures are entered into a cytocomputer in a line-scanned format and progress through the pipeline of processing stages at a real-time rate. Following an initial delay to fill the pipeline, images can be processed at the same rate they are scanned.

A cellular system constitutes a "space" in which automaton events can take place. Governing the events are simple rules which precisely formulate what kind of action can occur in the system. The cellular space consists of an infinite n-dimensional Euclidean space together with a neighborhood relation which gives, for each cell in the space, a list of cells which are its neighbors. A cellular system is specified by assigning to each cell a "cell state" and a rule which gives the state of a cell at discrete time t + 1 as a function of its own state and the state of its neighbors at time t, called the "transition function."

Cellular spaces and digital images share a common conceptual framework. Each picture element of a digital image can be thought of as a cell in a given state. If we define a neighborhood relationship and a cell transition function on a digital image, then application of the transition function will cause the configuration of cell states forming the image to be modified or transformed into new configurations. Of particular interest is the question of whether there exist neighborhood relationships and transition functions which will cause images to be transformed in predictable and useful manners.

The image processing approach we are investigating differs from conventional methods in that the basic manipulative informational unit is pictorial and deals with images as a whole. Image processing is treated as a computation involving images as variables in algebraic expressions. These expressions may combine several images through both logical and geometric relationships. Finally, highly efficient cellular computer architectures are realizable for implementing the computation automatically.

IMAGE ALGEBRA

Image processor architecture and language for image processing are opposite sides of the same coin and are inseparable. Image processor design and image processing language development cannot proceed independently of one another. Theories of computer design and formal language complement each other and fuse traditionally disjoint hardware and software areas into image processing systems.

Formal theories of cellular automata have demonstrated the computational universality of the cellular machine. The conceptual similarity of cellular components and digital images is strongly suggestive of a cellular automata approach to image processor architecture. By contrast, a strong link between digital image processing and formal language has yet to be convincingly established. This is because image processing languages have invariably dealt with pixels (picture elements) as their atomic (primitive) variables. But a pixel is not a picture just as an individual cell of a cellular computer is not a computer. Rather, a formal language of image processing should deal with pictures as the primitives of the language, and the operators embodied in a picture processing language should be specified between whole images and not iteratively on picture fragments.

The language development we put forward here is formal in the sense that what we describe is an algebra of image processing. The variables of the image algebra are pictures, or, more precisely, images, of any size, color, time sequence or dimension. The notion that any image can be formulated as a binary image in an augmented space forms the basis of our approach.

Let E^n denote the set of all points in Euclidean n-space and let $p = (x_1, x_2, \ldots, x_n)$ represent a point of E^n. With each set A belonging to E^n is associated a <u>binary image</u>, an n-dimensional composition in black and white, where the point p is black in the binary image if and only if $p \in A$; otherwise p is white. A binary image in E^2 is a silhouette, a composition in black and white which partitions the plane into regions of foreground (black) and background (white). A binary image in E^3 is a partitioning of a volume into points belonging to the surface and interior of objects (black) and points belonging to the space surrounding those objects (white). The notion of a binary image augments the usual notion of a black and white picture by specifying a coordinate system for the picture.

The intersection of any two binary images A and B in E^n, written $A \cap B$, is the binary image which is black at all points p which are black in both A and B. Symbolically,

$$A \cap B = \{p \mid p \in A \text{ and } p \in B\}.$$

The union of A and B, written $A \cup B$, is the binary image which is black at all points p which are black in A or black in B (or black in both). Symbolically,

$$A \cup B = \{p \mid p \in A \text{ or } p \in B\}.$$

Let Ω be a universal binary image (all black) and A a binary image. The complement of A is the binary image which interchanges the colors black and white in A. Symbolically,

$$\bar{A} = \{p \mid p \in \Omega \text{ and } p \notin A\}.$$

Denote two points $(x_1, x_2, \ldots, x_n)$ and $(y_1, y_2, \ldots, y_n)$ of E^n by p and q, respectively. The vector sum p + q is the point

$$p + q = (x_1 + y_1, x_2 + y_2, \ldots, x_n + y_n),$$

while the vector difference p - q is the point

$$p - q = (x_1 - y_1, x_2 - y_2, \ldots, x_n - y_n),$$

both in E^n.

Scaling a binary image A in E^n by a real-valued constant s multiplies the coordinates of the points p belonging to A by s,

$$sA = \{sp \mid p \in A\}$$

where

$$sp = (sx_1, sx_2, \ldots, sx_n).$$

Similarly, we can define vector scaling of a binary image A in E^n by the n-dimensional vector $\vec{s}$ whose elements are scalars $s_1, s_2, \ldots, s_n$ as

$$\vec{s}A = \{\vec{s}p \mid p \in A\}$$

where

$$\vec{s}p = (s_1x_1, s_2x_2, \ldots, s_nx_n).$$

If A is a binary image of E^n and p a point in E^n, then the translation of A by p is the binary image of E^n given in terms of vector sums as

$$A_p = \{a + p \mid a \in A\}.$$

Translation of a binary image A by a point p shifts the origin of A to p. If A_{b_1}, A_{b_2}, ..., A_{b_n} are translations of the binary image A by the black points of the binary image $B = \{b_1, b_2, \ldots, b_n\}$, then the union of the translations of A by the black points of B is called the dilation of A by B and is symbolized

$$A \oplus B = \bigcup_{b_i \in B} A_{b_i}$$

Figure 1 illustrates the dilation operation.

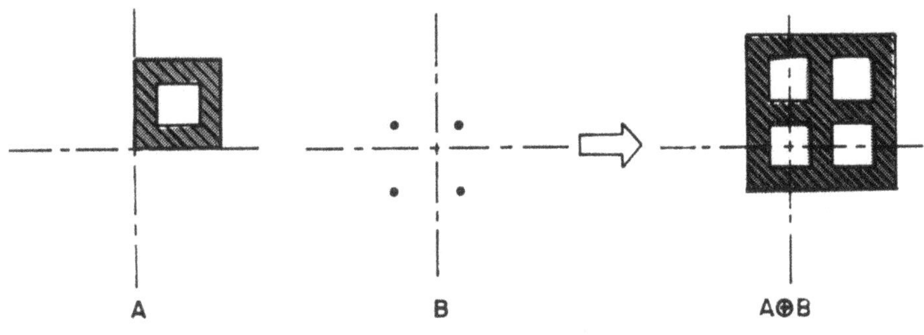

FIGURE 1. DILATION

The operational dual of dilation is erosion. The erosion of a binary image A by a binary image B is black at a point p if and only if every black point in the translation of B to p is also black in A. Symbolically,

$$A \ominus B = \{p \mid B_p \subseteq A\}.$$

Figure 2 illustrates the erosion operation.

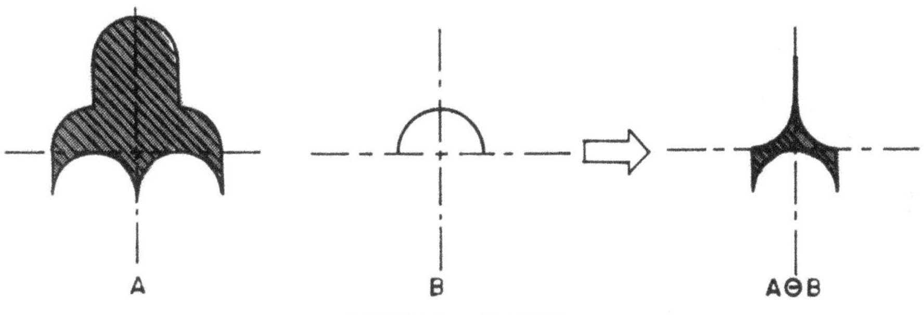

FIGURE 2. EROSION

Dilation as a set addition operator was employed by Minkowski [1], although Mandelbrodt [2] suggests that G. Cantor first employed dilation by "balls" as a set smoothing operation. Lyusternik [3] refers to the dilation of polyhedra as mixing. Matheron [4] and Serra [5] defined the dual operation erosion as a set inclusion operator although the definitions given here, independently derived by Sternberg [6] and further developed by Holsztynski [7], differ slightly in form from that set forth by Matheron and Serra.

The dual nature of dilation and erosion is geometric rather than logical and involves a geometric complement as well as a logical complement. The geometric complement of a binary image is called its <u>reflection</u>. The reflection of a binary image B is that binary image B´ which is symmetric with B about the origin, that is

$$B' = \{-p \mid p \in B\}.$$

The geometric duality of dilation and erosion is expressed by the relationships

$$\overline{A \oplus B} = \overline{A} \ominus B'$$

and

$$\overline{A \ominus B} = \overline{A} \oplus B'.$$

Geometric duality contrasts with logical duality (DeMorgan's Law)

$$\overline{A \cup B} = \overline{A} \cap \overline{B}$$

and

$$\overline{A \cap B} = \overline{A} \cup \overline{B}.$$

Figure 3 illustrates the geometric duality principle of dilation and erosion.

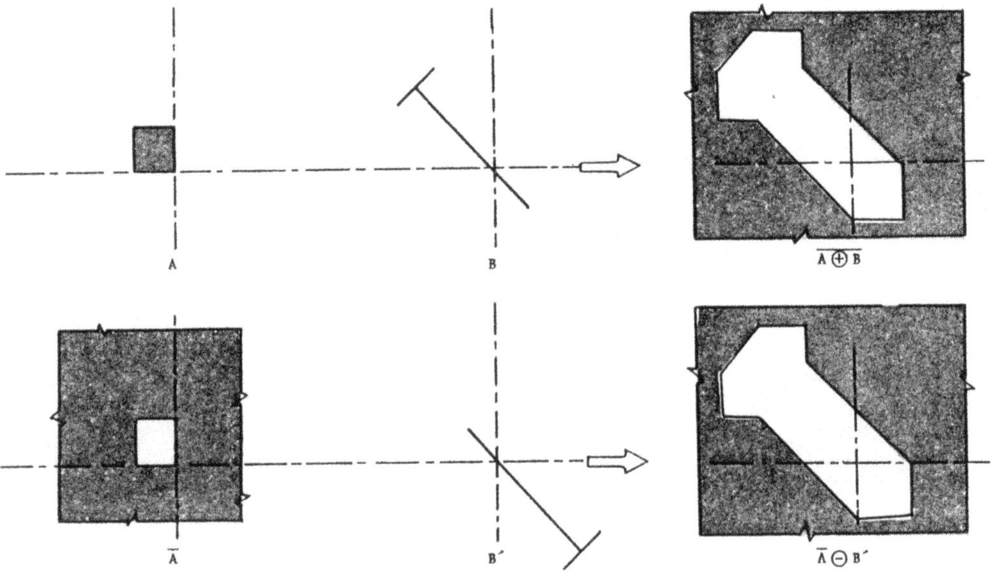

FIGURE 3. DILATION AND EROSION AS DUAL OPERATIONS.

GREYVALUED IMAGES

A binary image in n-dimensional space is a function which assigns the color black or white represented by the integers 1 and 0 respectively to points in that space. A <u>greyvalued image</u> is a function which assigns a real number $y \in \mathcal{R}$ to each point in n-space. The range of y corresponds to the range of tonal variation ascribed to a point. If y denotes the greyvalue of a given point $p = (x_1, x_2, \ldots, x_n)$ in n-space, then the given point can be represented in an augmented binary space E^{n+1}, the given point written as an (n + 1)-tuple $p^* = (x_1, x_2, \ldots, x_n, x_{n+1})$ where $x_{n+1} = y$. If A is a set of points in n-space and if G is a function which assigns a greyvalue y to each point of A, then G(A) is a greyvalued image having a binary image representation in (n+1)-space, that is, the greyvalued image G(A) in n-space corresponds to a binary image A* in (n+1)-space, where $p^* = (x_1, x_2, \ldots, x_n, x_{n+1})$ is an element of A^* if and only if $p = (x_1, x_2, \ldots, x_n)$ is an element of A and the greyvalue of p is x_{n+1}. We say that p^* has the value of 1 if $p^* \in A^*$ and zero otherwise in keeping with our binary image convention.

Thus a greyvalued image in 2-space such as a continuous-tone photograph can be denoted by a binary image in 3-space. The binary image in 3-space consists of black sheets, not necessarily connected, representing the single-valued greyvalue function. In this form, the binary image in augmented space is referred to as a _greyvalue surface_.

We could apply the functions of the image algebra directly to greyvalue surfaces, but to do so would be analogous to restricting ourselves to line drawings in 2-space. Since we prefer to deal with foreground-background representations in 2-space where the foreground, or black region, has solid form, we also prefer to deal with the binary image representation of a greyvalued image in solid form. For this reason, we introduce the concept of an _umbra_.

Umbra means shadow, or more particularly, the volume of space that falls in shadow. If A is a greyvalued image in n-space and A^* is its greyvalue surface in (n+1)-space, then the umbra of A, denoted U(A), is a binary image in (n+1)-space where

$$U(A) = A^* \oplus X'_{n+1}$$

where the binary image X'_{n+1} consists of points belonging to the reflection of the non-negative X_{n+1} axis. Thus, a point $p^* = (x_1, \ldots, x_{n+1})$ is black in the umbra representation of a greyvalued image if and only if the greyvalue of the point $p = (x_1, \ldots, x_n)$ in the greyvalued image is greater than or equal to x_{n+1}. A one-dimensional greyvalued image and its two-dimensional greyvalue surface and umbra are illustrated in Figure 4.

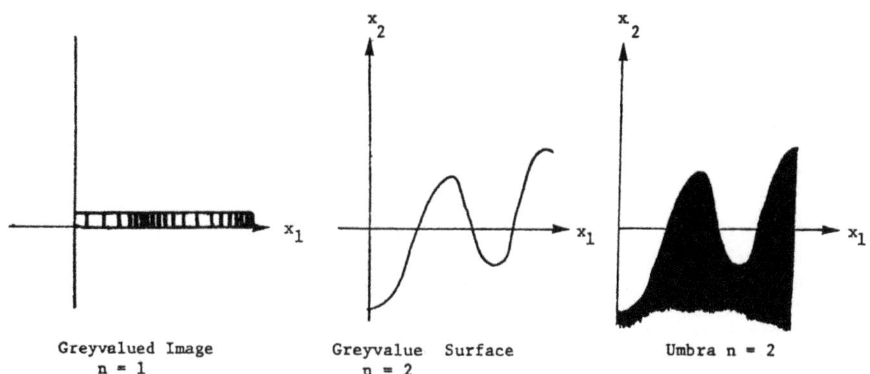

FIGURE 4. UMBRA REPRESENTATION OF A ONE-DIMENSIONAL GREYVALUED IMAGE

The concept of the umbra representation of a greyvalued image permits the extension of the image algebra from binary images to greyvalued images. Unions and intersections of binary umbras are binary umbras. Dilations and erosions of binary umbras are binary umbras.

IMAGE PROCESSOR ARCHITECTURE

Image processing algorithms are constructed as well-formed strings of primitives which are either variables representing binary images or binary image operations. The image being processed by an algorithm is referred to as the active image. Other images referred to in an image-algebraic expression are called reference images. An image processing algorithm consists of modifying the active image by logically or geometrically combining it with reference images or with previously modified active images.

The operations desired for image processing, described above in algebraic notation, are easily implemented in a parallel processor designed for cellular transformations. Each picture element (pixel) of a digitized image can be thought of as a cell in a given state. If we define a neighborhood relationship and a pixel transition function on a digital image, application of the transition function in parallel across the cellular space will cause the configuration of pixel states forming the image to be modified, or transformed, into new configurations as shown in Figure 5.

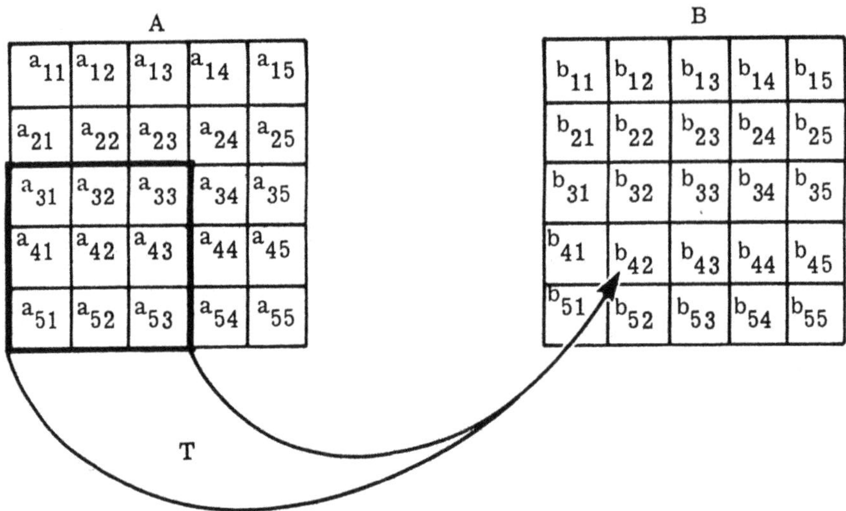

FIGURE 5. NEIGHBORHOOD TRANSFORM OF PIXEL $A_{4,2}$, 3 x 3 WINDOW

The neighborhood relationship on a cellular array determines the set of reference images which may be employed in a single neighborhood transformation. The neighborhood relationship is more generally called the reference image <u>window</u>. All reference images employed in a dilation or erosion transformation must be subimages of the reference image window. Figure 6 illustrates a commonly used reference image window. The example of Figure 7 is a subimage of that window; hence it is an <u>elementary reference image</u>.

Now consider a lattice of cells, where each cell of the lattice has connections with a finite collection of other cells. These other cells comprise its input, and the geometric pattern of the cells used as input to a given cell is exactly that of the points in the reference image window. Figure 8 illustrates the connection pattern for the window configuration shown in Figure 6. As shown in Figure 9, each cell of the cellular array consists of a single bit register for storing the state of the cell and a logic module which computes the new value of the cell state register as

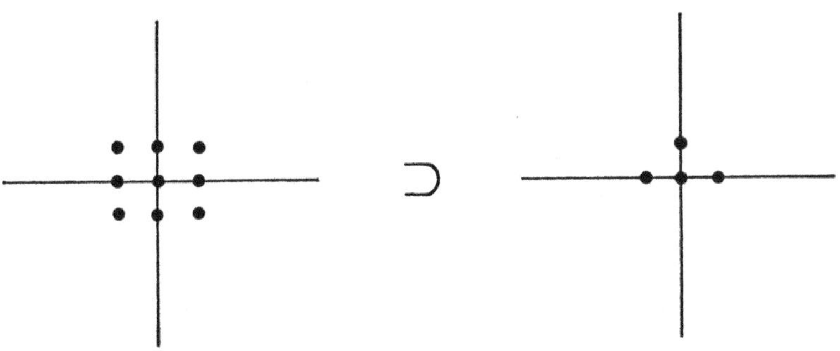

FIGURE 6. EXAMPLE OF A REFERENCE IMAGE WINDOW (IMAGE W)

FIGURE 7. SUBIMAGE B OF W

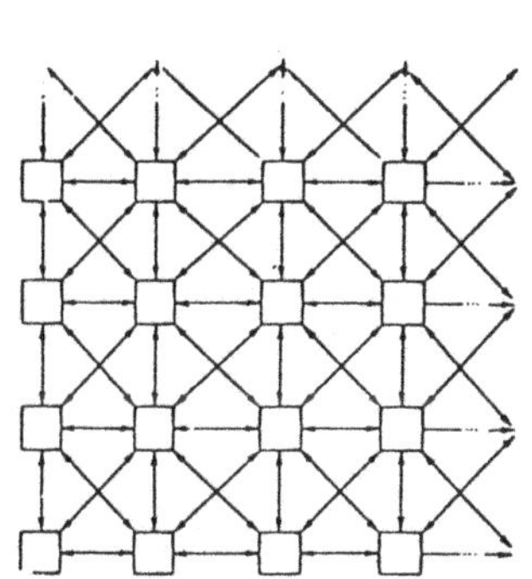

FIGURE 8. CELLULAR ARRAY WITH 3 x 3 WINDOW

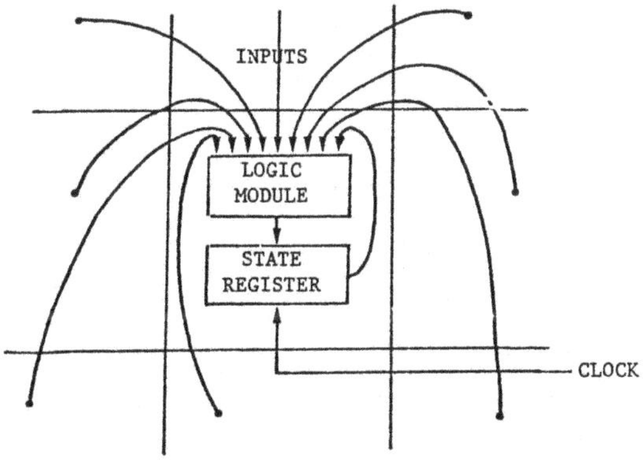

FIGURE 9. DETAIL OF CELLULAR ARRAY SHOWING CELL COMPONENTS

a function of the cell input. For example, in the illustrated case above, each cell logic module receives input from nine state registers, the eight surrounding cells and the state register of the given cell. Upon application of a common clock pulse to each cell in the array, all cell state registers are transitioned from their previous state to a new state as given by the output of the logic module.

Suppose that a digital binary image A is stored in such a cellular array and we wish to compute $A \ominus B$ where B is the subimage of W given in Figure 7. Then the logic module of each cell should implement a boolean function of its inputs such that its output is a 1 only if the inputs from the four cells denoted by B are all 1, the states of the other cells in the window being immaterial or "don't cares", i.e., the state of cell p is determined by an "AND"ing of the cells designated by B.

Upon receipt of a clock pulse, all cells in the logical array simultaneously change state, the resulting binary image being identically $A \ominus B$ through the definition of erosion,

$$A \ominus B = \{p \mid B_p \subseteq A\}.$$

Dilation in the logical cellular array follows from the definition of dilation as

$$A \oplus B = \{p \mid B'_p \nsubseteq \overline{A}\}.$$

Here the center cell p takes state 1 only when the inputs from the cells in the window designated by the reflected reference image B' are not all 0; in other words, cell p of the binary image $A \oplus B$ is black when the "OR"ing of the cell states designated by B' is 1. In either case, dilation or erosion, the new state of each cell in the array is computed by application of a programmable boolean function of a finite group of cells comprising a window of inputs to the given cell. Geometric operations of dilating or eroding by subimages of the window are implemented in a single clock cycle.

Most image processing algorithms require operations with reference images which are larger than neighborhood windows practical to implement in hardware. In these cases, the reference image is decomposed into subimages which fit the window. The binary reference image B in an image-algebraic expression may be replaced by either the union or dilation of binary subimages. If $B = B_1 \cup B_2$, then

$$A \oplus B = (A \oplus B_1) \cup (A \oplus B_2) \qquad A \cup B = (A \cup B_1) \cup B_2$$

$$A \ominus B = (A \ominus B_1) \cap (A \ominus B_2) \qquad A \cap B = (A \cap B_1) \cup (A \cap B_2)$$

$$B' = B_1' \cup B_2' \qquad \bar{B} = \bar{B}_1 \cap \bar{B}_2$$

and if $B = B_1 \oplus B_2$, then

$$A \oplus B = (A \oplus B_1) \oplus B_2 \qquad B' = B_1' \oplus B_2'$$

$$A \ominus B = (A \ominus B_1) \ominus B_2 \qquad \bar{B} = \bar{B}_1 \ominus B_2'$$

The most obvious architecture for implementing iterative neighborhood transformations is the cellular array. In a cellular array, one processor exists for each pixel in the image. These processors communicate with their window neighbors to perform neighborhood operations. Although such an architecture can be very fast, it has drawbacks; for instance, N^2 processors are needed to process an N x N image.

The practical shortcomings of cellular array image processors led ERIM to develop an alternative parallel structure, the cytocomputer. Lougheed and McCubbrey [8] compare cytocomputer and cellular array processor architectures and show that the cytocomputer architecture can have several advantages over the array architecture, such as low complexity, high bandwidth, and considerable architectural flexibility. First proposed by Sternberg [9] in 1976, a cytocomputer (Figure 10) consists of a serial pipeline of neighborhood processing stages, with a common clock, in which each stage in the pipeline performs a single neighborhood transformation of an entire image. Pictures are entered into the pipeline as a stream of pixels in sequential line-scanned format and progress through the pipeline of processing stages at a constant rate. Following the initial latency to fill the pipeline, processed images are produced at the same rate they are entered. Shift registers within each stage store two contiguous scan lines while window registers hold the 9 neighborhood pixels which constitute the 3 x 3 window input of a neighborhood logic module. This module performs a preprogrammed transformation of the center pixel based on the values of the center and its eight neighbors. Neighborhood logic transformations are computed

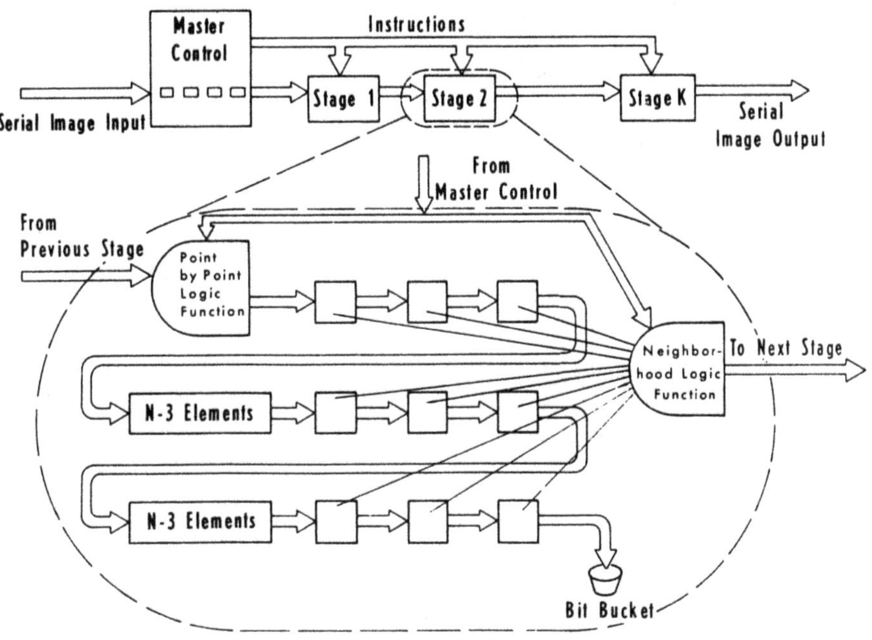

FIGURE 10. PIPELINE IMAGE PROCESSOR
(N = linelength)

within the data transfer clock period, allowing the output of a stage to appear at the same rate as its input. At each discrete time interval, a new pixel is clocked into the stage. Simultaneously, the contents of all delay units are shifted one element. In addition, operations which do not involve the states of a pixel's neighbors, such as greyvalue scaling, bit setting, etc., are performed in a separate point-by-point logic section to simplify the neighborhood logic circuit.

To visualize the transformation process, imagine a 3 x 3 window moving across an image array as shown in Figure 11. The processing stage storage section shows the contents of the latches after pixel $A_{6,6}$ has been read. The contents of the neighborhood latches allow the stage to compute the transformed value of the pixel in the

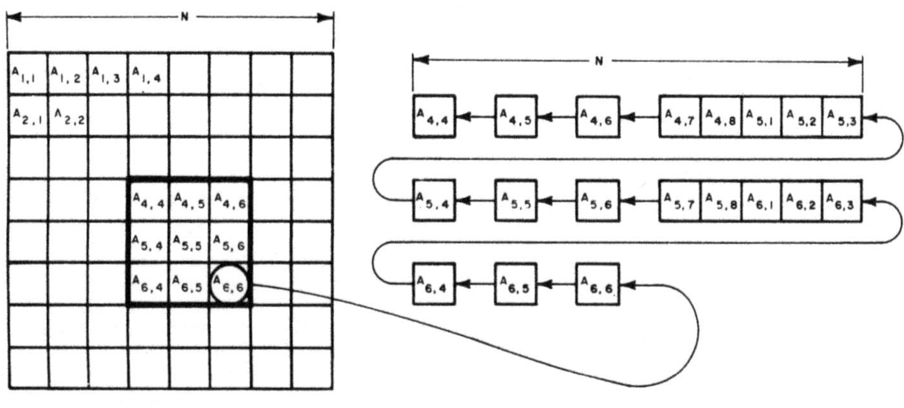

FIGURE 11. MOVING WINDOW IMPLEMENTED WITH SHIFT REGISTER STORAGE

center latch, $A_{5,5}$. This transformed pixel becomes an element of the serial input to the next stage. From this example, one can see that the latency of a stage is equal to N + 2 time steps, N being the linelength. One can now visualize a series of 3 x 3 windows following each other across the image, each one processing the previous stage's output as shown in Figure 12. (There are a number of schemes for handling the boundaries of the image. Our first generation hardware surrounded the image with a border of "frame" pixels which were not modified in the transformations.)

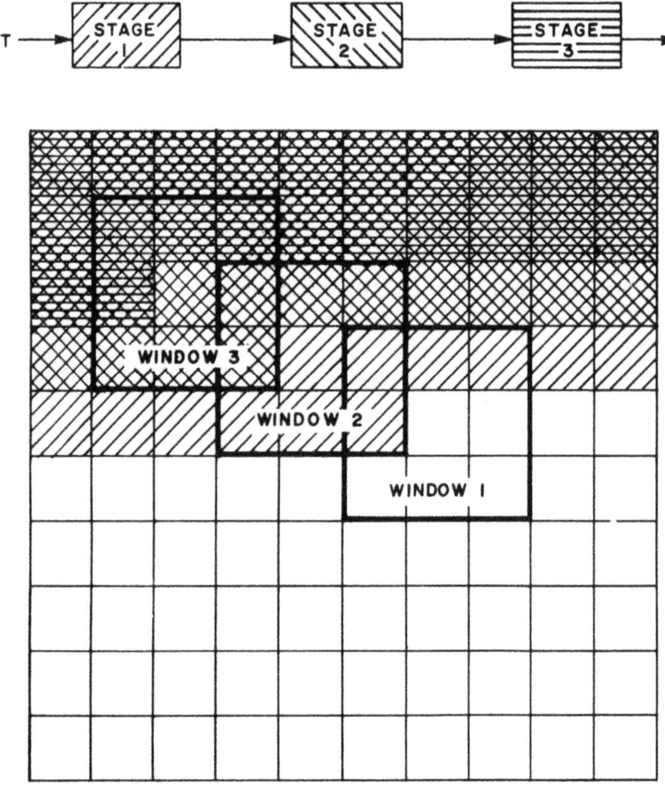

FIGURE 12. THREE-STEP IMAGE TRANSFORMATION SHOWING WINDOW RELATIONSHIPS DURING EXECUTION

Transformations implemented in a cytocomputer stage fall into two main categories. One class, referred to as silhouette (2-D) transforms, apply the image algebra operations to planar binary images. The other class, called umbra (3-D) transforms, performs the same set of operations on greyvalued images, where the greyvalue represents the brightness of a picture point or its height above an arbitrary reference plane. In the case of the umbra transforms, the reference images are umbras of subimages of a 3 x 3 x 3 cubic window.

IMAGE PROCESSING

The result of an image transformation is invariant of the orientation of the image only if the reference images employed in the transformation process are rotationally invariant. Images of disks and balls (disks and balls are solid, circles and spheres are shells) are most frequently employed as reference images in cytocomputer image processing. Figure 13 illustrates a greyvalued image of a ball having a 104 pixel

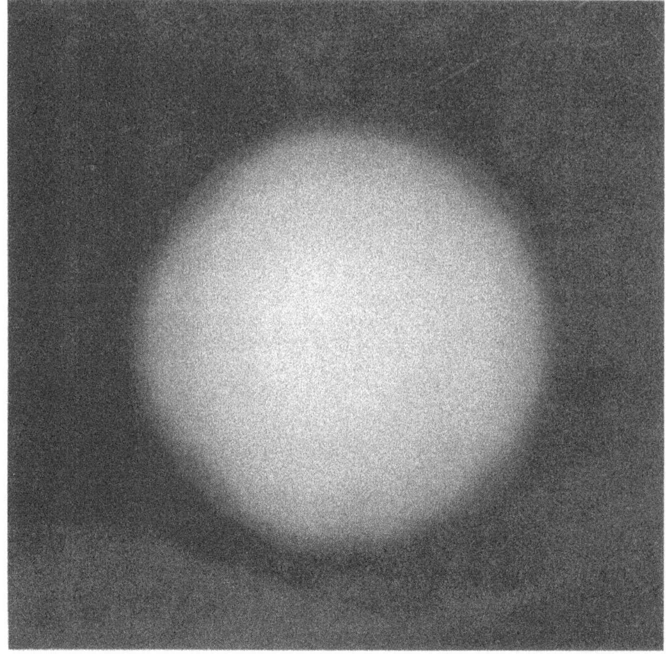

FIGURE 13. GREYVALUED IMAGE OF BALL — RADIUS 104 PIXELS

radius. The image was generated by starting with an active image of a single non-zero pixel and iteratively dilating by 104 elemental reference images selected from a 3 x 3 x 3 window. The algorithm was written by Peter F. Lambeck of ERIM. It generates balls of any radius.

It is difficult to visualize the three-dimensional structure of a reference image when the third dimension is presented as a brightness level. The procedure SHADE transforms an image whose height is encoded as brightness into a greyvalued image which is easily visualized as a three-dimensional structure. The greylevels resulting from the SHADE transformation appear visually to arise from a light source illuminating the structure, when in actuality the transform employs only dilation and <u>image sums</u> and <u>image differences</u>. An image sum or difference, denoted by the symbols "+" and "-" respectively, denotes a pixel-by-pixel addition or subtraction of brightness level. (Vector sum and difference operations which employ the same symbolic notation are distinguishable from context.)

Denote the greyvalued active image undergoing shading as A and let P_1 and P_2 be binary images each consisting of a single black point

$$P_1 = \{p | x_1 = 1, x_2 = 0, x_3 = 0\}$$

and

$$P_2 = \{p | x_1 = 0, x_2 = 1, x_3 = 0\}.$$

Now form intermediate greyvalued images I_1, I_2 and I_3 from A, P_1 and P_2 as

$$I_1 = (A \oplus P_1) - (A \oplus P_1')$$

$$I_2 = (A \oplus P_2) - (A \oplus P_2')$$

$$I_3 = (A \oplus P_1 \oplus P_2) - (A \oplus P_1' \oplus P_2').$$

Then the shaded active image may be obtained from the intermediate images as

$$\mathrm{SHADE}(A) = \frac{1}{3}(I_1 + I_2 + I_3) + \text{greyconstant}$$

where the variable greyconstant is determined such that SHADE(A) has no negative valued pixels. The SHADE procedure as applied to the greyvalued image of the ball in Figure 1 is illustrated in Figure 14.

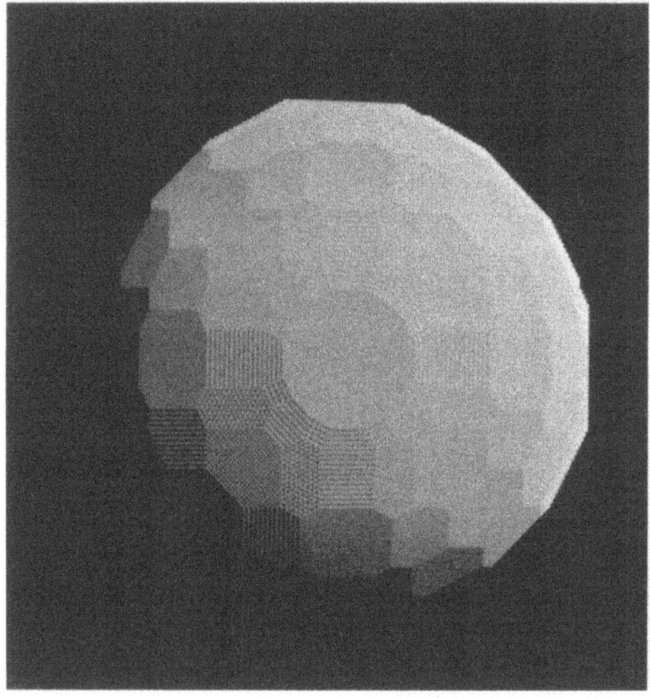

FIGURE 14. SHADED BALL — RADIUS 104 PIXELS

From the geometric interpretations of erosion and dilation, we most naturally draw definitions for two new transformation procedures on binary images which are expressable in terms of erosion and dilation. First, the opening of a binary image A by a binary image B is the union of all translations of B which are included in A. Symbolically denoting the opening of A by B as OPEN(A,B), we can write

$$\mathrm{OPEN}(A,B) = \bigcup_{p \in (A \ominus B)} B_p$$

since $p \in (A \ominus B)$ if and only if $B_p \subseteq A$. Now the union of all translations of a binary image B by the black points of a binary image $(A \ominus B)$ is by definition the dilation of B by $(A \ominus B)$. Since dilation is commutative, we can then write

$$\text{OPEN}(A,B) = (A \ominus B) \oplus B.$$

Closing is the dual of opening and is most easily defined in terms of the complement of A and the reflection of B. The complement of the closing of A by B is the union of all translations of B' which are included in $\bar{A}$. Denoting the closing of A by B symbolically as CLOSE(A,B), we can write

$$\overline{\text{CLOSE}(A,B)} = \bigcup_{p \in (\bar{A} \ominus B')} B'_p$$

since $p \in (\bar{A} \ominus B')$ if and only if $B'_p \subseteq \bar{A}$. Now the union of all translations of a binary image B' by the black points of a binary image $(\bar{A} \ominus B')$ is the dilation of B' by $(\bar{A} \ominus B')$. Since dilation is commutative, we can then rewrite the complement of the closing of A by B as

$$\overline{\text{CLOSE}(A,B)} = (\bar{A} \ominus B') \oplus B'$$

from which we can apply duality and obtain an expression for the closing of A by B as simply

$$\text{CLOSE}(A,B) = (A \oplus B) \ominus B.$$

Application of opening and closing by three-dimensional reference images is illustrated by the segmentation of high-resolution digital images of human urinary bladder epithelium (Figure 15). Several images for cytocomputer analysis were provided by Judith M. S. Prewitt of the National Institute of Health, Bethesda, Maryland, who is developing a theoretical foundation for computer-based automation of histology by application of graph-theoretic and syntactic models to tissues [10]. The hematoxylin-stained sections show nuclei which are well defined but with coarse chromatin patterns. Closing of the greyvalued image A of Figure 15 by a ball of radius 5, denoted B_5, produces an intermediate image I illustrated in Figure 16,

$$I = \text{CLOSE}(A,\ B_5).$$

The closing operation fills in the small dark chromatin patterns in the cell nuclei so that application of the process of opening image I by a ball of radius 5 will discriminate bright regions of the nuclei from bright regions in the surrounding cytoplasm,

$$J = \text{OPEN}(I,\ B_5).$$

Image J is illustrated in Figure 17. Following closing and opening procedures, a simple thresholding operation described in an image algebra sense as the intersection of the plane W,

$$W = \{p \mid x_3 = \text{thresholdvalue}\},$$

with the umbra of image J gives the segmented image S of Figure 18,

$$S = \text{THRESH}\ (J,\ \text{thresholdvalue})$$

where

$$\text{THRESH}\ (J,\ \text{thresholdvalue}) = J \cap W.$$

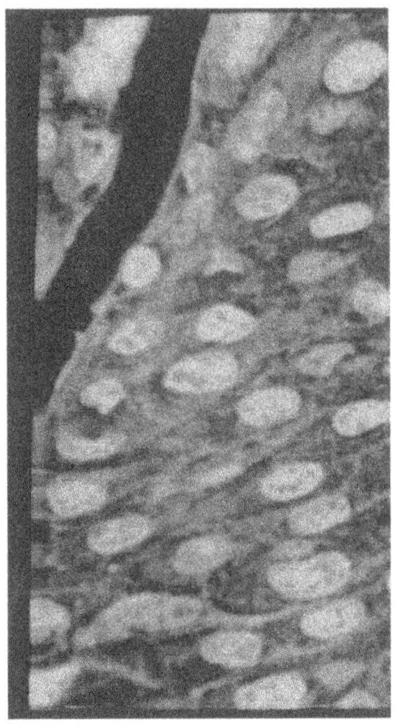

FIGURE 15. STAINED BLADDER EPITHELIUM (IMAGE A)

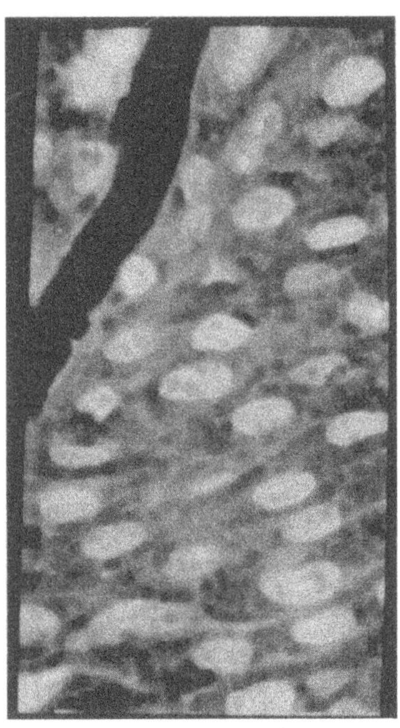

FIGURE 16. CLOSING OF IMAGE A (IMAGE I)

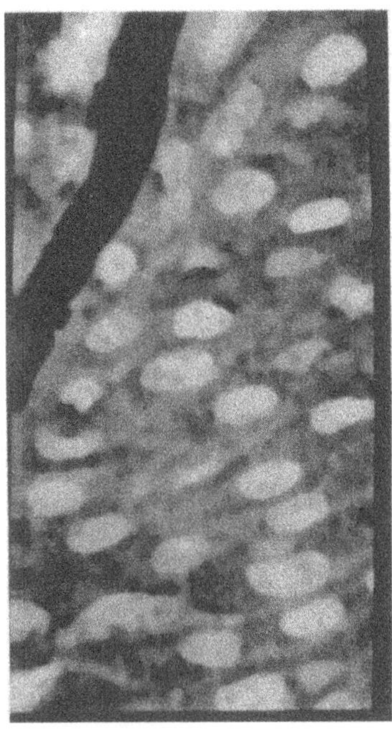

FIGURE 17. OPENING OF IMAGE I (IMAGE J)

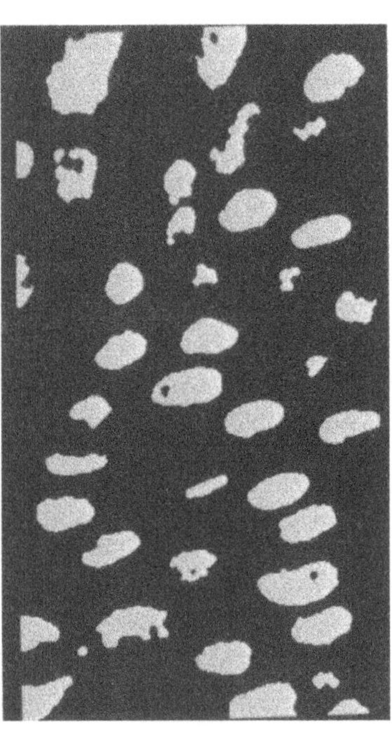

FIGURE 18. SEGMENTED NUCLEI (IMAGE S)

Alternating application of opening and closing by balls of increasing radii is termed isotropic filtering because the transformed image is smoothed independent of the orientation of its surfaces. The procedure ISOFIL is

$$O_1 = OPEN(A, B_1)$$

$$C_1 = CLOSE(O_1, B_1)$$

$$O_2 = OPEN(C_1, B_2)$$

$$C_2 = CLOSE(O_2, B_2)$$

$$\vdots$$

$$O_n = OPEN(C_{n-1}, B_n)$$

$$ISOFIL(A, B_n) = CLOSE(O_n, B_n)$$

where B_n denotes a ball of radius n. Isotropic filtering is illustrated by application to nuclear ventriculograms provided for cytocomputer processing by James H. Thrall and Bertram Pitt of the University of Michigan School of Medicine.

Imaging of the cardiovascular system has become an essential part in establishing the diagnosis of many cardiovascular diseases, especially coronary artery disease and in assessing the degree of functional impairment. Quantification of image parameters has been a well recognized goal in cardiac diagnosis for over two decades. Based on results of tedious hand calculations and more recently, semi-automated analyses, there is now an overwhelming consensus that quantification not only increases diagnostic accuracy but provides significant data not obtainable from qualitative image analysis alone.

The first step in quantitative image processing is contour mapping to define the limits of cardiac structures, most importantly the left ventricle. This step has remained a major stumbling block in meeting the requirements for an ideal quantitative analysis system. A time-gated nuclear bloodpool study is illustrated in Figure 19. The resolution of the individual cardiac images is 32 x 32 pixels with 6 bits of intensity information which limits the accuracy of left ventricle contour mapping. Therefore, the first step of the cytocomputer contour mapping procedure is a rescaling of the original image, A, by 4, meaning that greyvalued image $4 * A$ is 128 x 128 pixels by 8 bits intensity.

The scaled greyvalued image is next isotropic-filtered by opening and closing with balls B_r up to a radius of 4. The result, expressed as

$$I = ISOFIL(4 * A, B_4)$$

is shown in Figure 20. The data of greyvalued image I may be more naturally visualized as the anatomical structure which it represents if we apply the procedure SHADE to I. Greyvalued image SHADE(I) is shown in Figure 21.

The most frequently encountered difficulty in automatically processing nuclear ventriculograms is finding the interventricular septum, the valley between the hump in the center, the left ventricle, and the adjacent hump, the right ventricle. The method employed here is to "roll a ball" whose diameter is wider than the valley over the umbra I, the theory being that the ball will touch the umbra almost everywhere except at points in the valley, and hence differentiate it. The method of rolling the ball over the umbra is closing, a translating ball being indistinguishable from a rolling one.

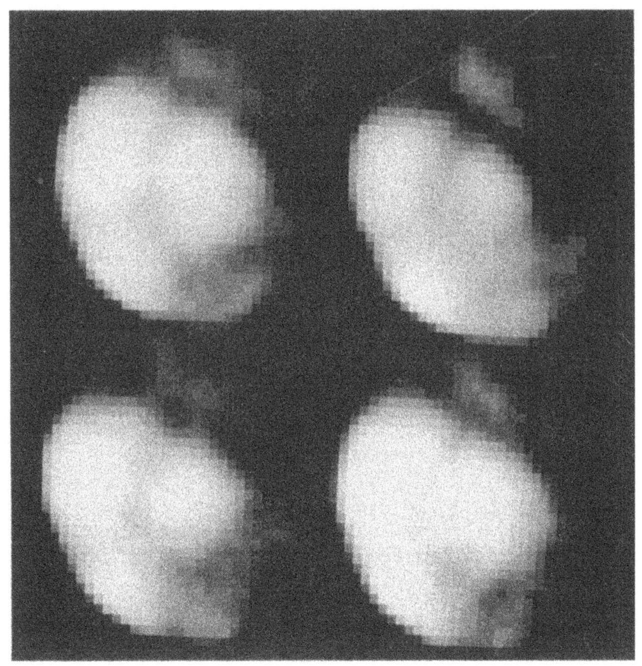

FIGURE 19. NUCLEAR VENTRICULOGRAMS (IMAGE A)

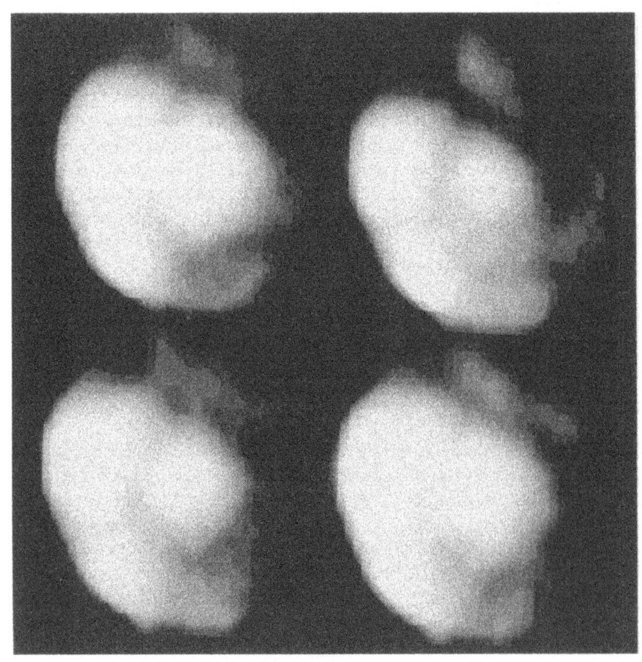

FIGURE 20. SCALED AND ISOTROPIC-FILTERED VENTRICULOGRAMS (IMAGE I)

Hence,

$$J = \mathrm{OVERBALL}(I,\ B_{49})$$

where

$$\mathrm{OVERBALL}(I,\ B_{49}) = \mathrm{CLOSE}(I,\ B_{49}) - I$$

and B_{49} is a ball of radius 49. Greyvalued image J is shown in Figure 22.

Rolling the same ball under the grayvalue surface of I is the method employed here to differentiate the remaining left ventricle boundaries, hence

$$K = \mathrm{UNDERBALL}(I,\ B_{49})$$

where

$$\mathrm{UNDERBALL}(I,\ B_{49}) = I - \mathrm{OPEN}(I,\ B_{49}).$$

Greyvalued image K is shown in Figure 23.

To combine edge information from greyvalued images J and K, we take their image difference. First, however, we vector scale the intensity of J by 2 to increase contrast in the septum region,

$$L = K - (1,\ 1,\ 2) * J.$$

Greyvalued image L is shown in Figure 24.

Thresholding greyvalued image L produces the silhouettes M shown in Figure 25,

$$M = \mathrm{THRESH}(L,\ \mathrm{thresholdvalue}).$$

In a step of the procedure not illustrated nor explained, the connected region covering the point at the center of each frame of image M is isolated from the remaining nonzero portion of the image. Call this procedure ISOLATE,

$$N = \mathrm{ISOLATE}(M).$$

Next, image N is isotropic-filtered by disks D_r,

$$D_r = \left\{ p \,|\, x_1^2 + x_2^2 \le r^2,\ x_3 = 0 \right\},$$

up to a disk radius of 4, which smooths the jagged edges of the thresholded left ventricles

$$O = \mathrm{ISOFIL}(N,\ D_4).$$

The edges of image O uniformly underestimate the perceived ventricular boundaries. Therefore, we dilate O by a disk of radius 6,

$$P = O \oplus D_6.$$

Figure 26 shows the union of image O and the dilated edge of image P, namely,

$$Q = (P \oplus D_2) \cap \overline{P}.$$

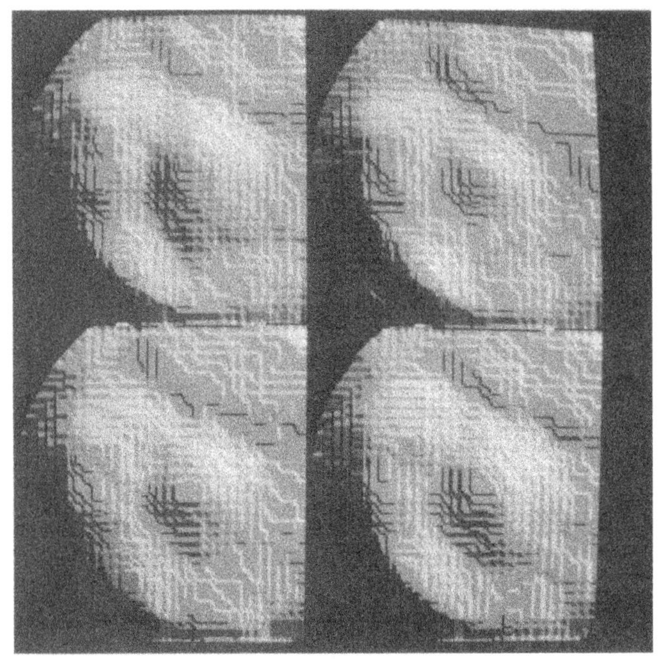

FIGURE 21. SHADED VENTRICULOGRAMS

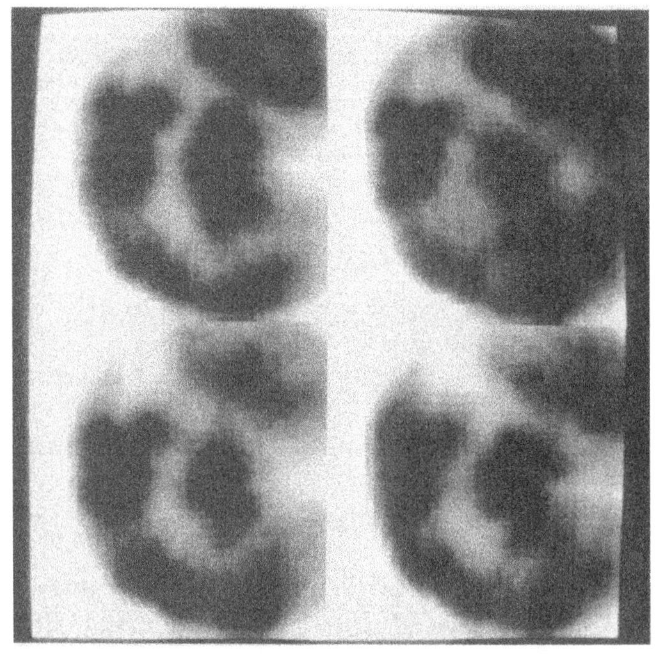

FIGURE 22. NUCLEAR VENTRICULOGRAMS PROCESSED
FOR ENHANCED SEPTUM (IMAGE J)

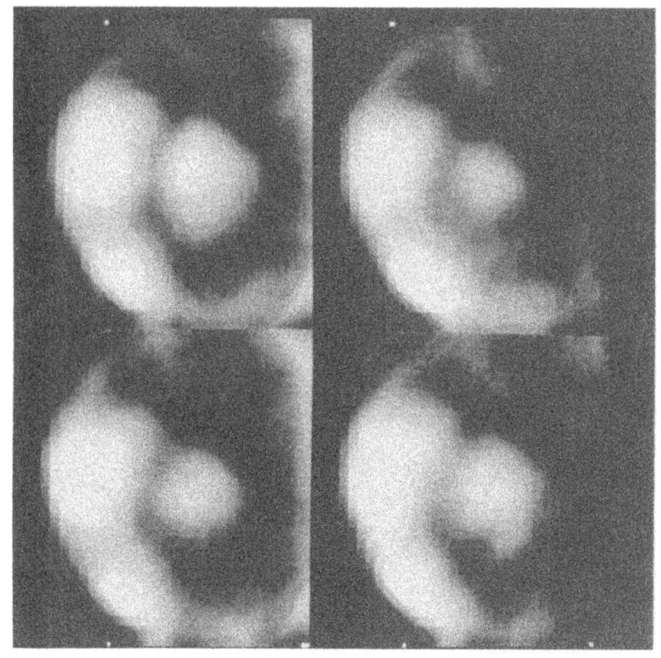

FIGURE 23. BACKGROUND-NORMALIZED NUCLEAR VENTRICULOGRAM (IMAGE K)

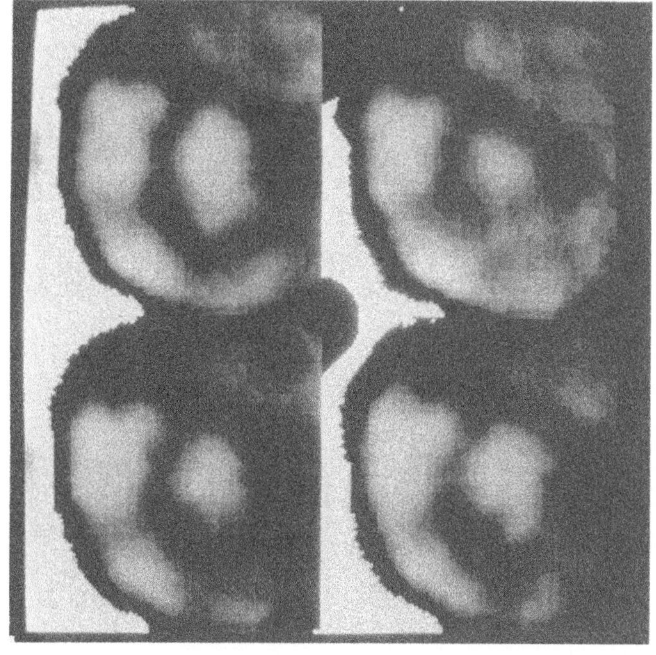

FIGURE 24. EDGE ENHANCED NUCLEAR VENTRICULOGRAM (IMAGE L)

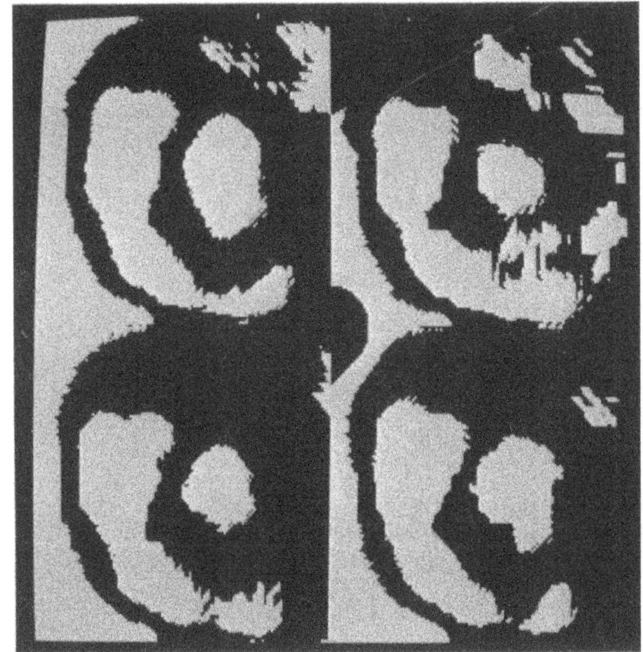

FIGURE 25. THRESHOLDED NUCLEAR VENTRICULOGRAM (IMAGE M)

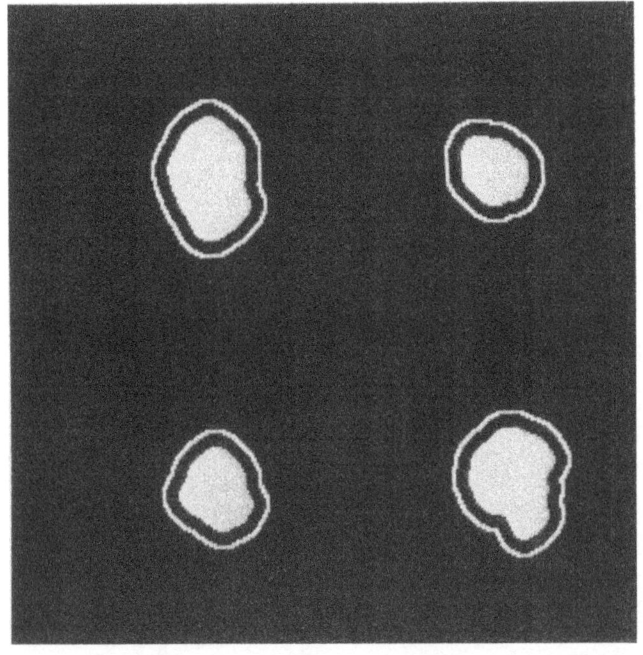

FIGURE 26. EDGE CUES OF LEFT VENTRICLES (IMAGES O and Q)

Image Q, as is symbolically implied, is the image which cues the determined ventricular boundaries onto the shaded greyvalued images, shown in Figure 27. The procedure CUE is not explained.

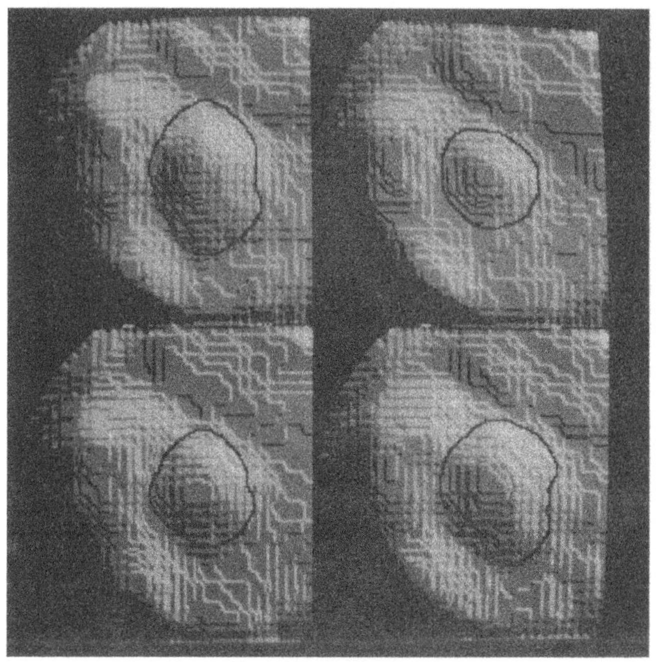

FIGURE 27. LEFT VENTRICLE EDGES ON SHADED VENTRICULOGRAMS

There is a significant concern today about man's exposure to environmental elements, especially those agents which may be carcinogens or mutagens. As a step in quantifying the impact of mutagenic agents on human populations, techniques are being developed for the detection of mutations and for estimating the mutation rate in sample populations. James V. Neel of the University of Michigan School of Medicine has employed electrophoretic methods to detect protein structural alterations which reflect changes in genetic material. Recently, two-dimensional electrophoresis systems in which proteins are separated according to charge in one direction and on the bases of subunit molecular weight in the second direction have been developed. The significant practical advantage of the 2-D gel system is that many proteins are identified on a single gel.

Digitized images of 2-D electrophoretic gels of hair follicles and blood lymphocytes were obtained from Drs. Norman and Leigh Anderson at Argonne National Laboratories and subjected to cytocomputer processing by Michael Skolnick of ERIM. The gel images obtained from the Andersons were digitized to 256 grey levels at a resolution of approximately 1500 scan lines at 1500 picture elements per line. Figure 28 displays one of the lymphocyte images at 512 x 512 x 8 bits resolution. Figure 29 is a 256 x 256 detail of that image with negated greyvalues.

Differences in various portions of the gel image are mainly attributable to variations in the background levels in the immediate vicinity of each spot, a situation which would make background removal by conventional histogram methods impractical. Background removal, performed in the context of a cytocomputer procedure as background normalization, is accomplished by conceptually rolling a ball whose diameter

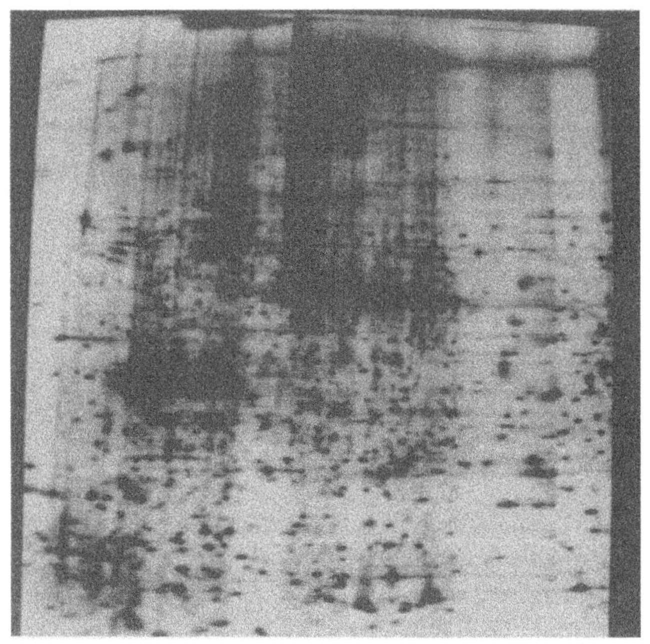

FIGURE 28. 2-D ELECTROPHORETIC GEL
OF BLOOD LYMPHOCYTES

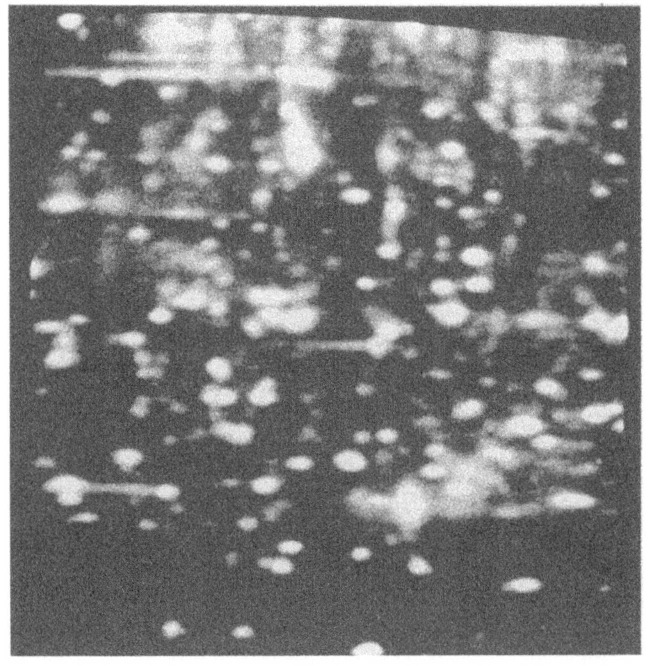

FIGURE 29. DETAIL OF THE IMAGE OF FIGURE 28

is larger than the expected spot widths along the underside of the greyvalue surface of the gel image umbra. The locus of all points in threespace overlapped by the rolling ball is the background estimate, since the ball cannot penetrate the narrow confines of the spot peaks. The background normalized image of Figure 29 is shown in Figure 30.

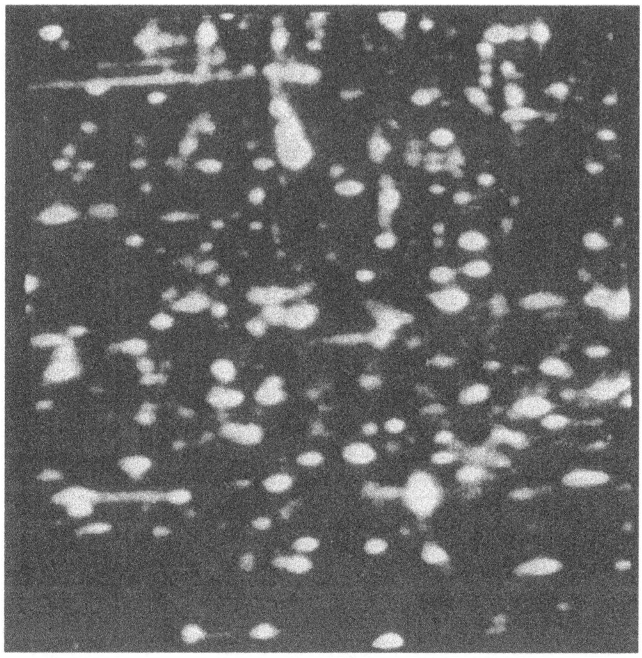

FIGURE 30. BACKGROUND-NORMALIZED DETAIL

Individual spot peaks are local maxima on the greyvalue surface of the gel image. Local maxima are detected by a cytocomputer procedure of iterative neighborhood transformations. Detected local maxima having a greyvalue greater than a preselected minimum are shown in Figure 31 superimposed on the shaded and shadowed image of Figure 30. Shadowing is a cytocomputer procedure.

The digitized electrophoretic gels exhibit strong local linearity. Therefore, it is not unreasonable to expect that uniquely identical local constellations of spots will occur in different gels of the same cell type. This has been experimentally validated.

Figure 32 shows a composite of details from four gel images of lymphocytes taken from four different individuals of the same family. Those spots marked by a + sign have been found by a cytocomputer procedure to be common to all four gels. The establishment of invariant protein spots and the detection of variations not previously observed forms the basis for mutation estimates by 2-D electrophoretic and image processing methods.

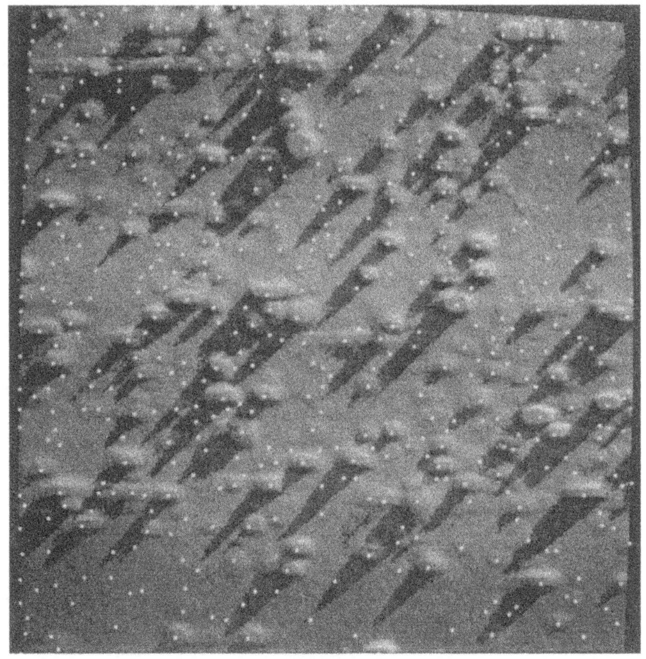

FIGURE 31. DETECTED SPOTS SHOWN ON SHADED AND SHADOWED GEL IMAGE

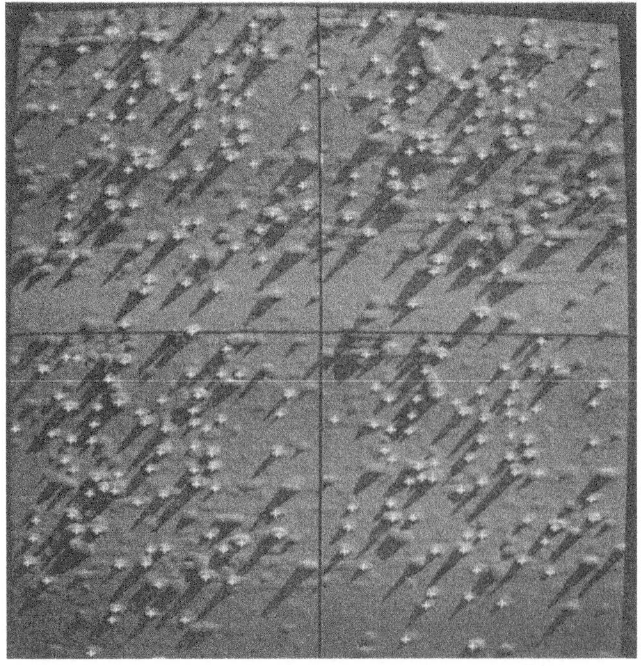

FIGURE 32. DETECTED CONSTELLATIONS OF SPOTS

CONCLUSION

This paper has attempted to present a unified approach to the subjects of a formal language for image processing, a computer architecture for image processing, and biomedical image processing. It is this writer's personal conviction that language, machine and application should not be segmented for study and that parallel learning processes link progress in language, machine and application understanding. For after all, parallel processing is the paradigm of this presentation.

ACKNOWLEDGEMENTS

The content of this paper is the product of the efforts of far too many people to personally acknowledge here. Let it suffice to extend my gratitude to Mary St. John for typing and coordinating production of the finished draft and to Richard Legault for his long and continued support of cytocomputer research.

REFERENCES

[1] Hancock, Harris, Development of the Minkowski Geometry of Numbers, Volumes 1 and 2, Dover, 1961.

[2] Mandelbrot, B., Fractals - Form, Chance, and Dimension, W. H. Freeman and Co., San Francisco, 1977, p. 287.

[3] Lyusternik, L. A., Convex Figures and Polyhedra, D. C. Heath and Co., Boston, 1966.

[4] Matheron, G., Random Sets and Integral Geometry, Wiley and Sons, New York, 1976.

[5] Serra, J., Lectures on Image Analysis by Mathematical Morphology, Fontainebleau, N-475, Juillet, 1976.

[6] Sternberg, S. R., "Parallel Architectures for Image Processing," Proceedings of the IEEE Computer Society's 3rd International Computer Software and Applications Conference, 1979.

[7] Holsztynski, W., "An Introduction to the Theory of Translation Invariant Transformations and Cytocomputers," ERIM Internal Report, December, 1977.

[8] Lougheed, R. M., McCubbrey, D. L., "The Cytocomputer: A Practical Pipelined Image Processor," Proceedings of the 7th International Symposium on Computer Architecture, 1980.

[9] Sternberg, S. R., "Automatic Image Processor," U.S. Patent 4,167,728, September 11, 1979.

[10] Prewitt, J. M. S.,"Canonical Representations for Tissues and Textures," Proceedings of the IEEE Computer Society's 3rd International Computer Software and Applications Conference, 1979.

BIOMEDICAL PARALLEL IMAGE PROCESSING ON PROPAL 2

by
P. Roux, J. Richalet
ADERSA-GERBIOS
2, avenue du 1er Mai
91120 PALAISEAU
(France)

ABSTRACT

PROPAL 2 is a mini parallel associative computer with an SIMD architecture. Each Processing Element (PE) works in a serial bit mode, with words of variable length from 1 to 256 bits. The most sophisticated feature of this computer is a special bus called "ascenseur" which allows an easy loading of data from the host computer and performs shifting of information from one PE to others. The assembly language is an overset of the MITRA SEMS assembler. Thus programming is done in FORTRAN through assembly language subroutines in order to improve the already existing software. The ability to work on variable length words gives PROPAL 2 a great efficiency in picture processing. On large picture processing problems (scaling - filtering - convolution - feature extraction ...), the computation time T_p of PROPAL 2 is given by :

$$T_p \simeq 1{,}4 \; T_M/NPE$$

where T_M is the computation time of a standard mini-computer (with floating point arithmetic unit) and NPE the number of elementary processors.

Compared to a SEMS MITRA 15-35, PROPAL 2 with "128 PE" being a standard configuration, the average gain to be expected is close to 90, but it depends on the problem. Real interactivity, which is a key problem in picture processing is then achieved.

A practical application will be shown.

1. INTRODUCTION

Most minicomputers lack processing power especially when large amounts of data are to be handled as in picture processing. PROPAL 2 is designed to fill the gap between mini and large computers using a lowcost parallel repetitive structure.

2. COMPUTER ARCHITECTURE

As we know there are 4 main computer architectures types (see figure 1).

2.1 Single Input, Single Data stream type (SISD)

A single processing unit works with a single set of instructions in sequential way on unique stream of data.

2.2 Pipe line type

Some algorithms may be cut down into intermediate steps. Each step will be relegated to a specialized processing unit. Input data will be processed in n intermediate steps from the data acquisition to the final result. Thus, for each computer cycle, n data are processed simultaneously. Therefore each data unit seems to be computed in $1/n$ cycle time.

2.3 Multiple Instruction - Multiple Data stream type (MIMD)

This is a multiprocessor type of organization : a large number of processing units work independantly on specific data with interactions.

But there are many communication problems between the processors and the synchronization task is so difficult that the parallelisation level cannot exceed ten.

2.4 Single Instruction - Multiple Data stream type (SIMD)

In this type of computer a great number of processing elements work simultaneously under the same instruction stream on different data streams. This structure is well suited for high performance computers ; the most famous being Illiac 4 of the Illinois University [1].

3. PROPAL 2 ARCHITECTURE

PROPAL 2 belongs to the SIMD type [2] ; it is divided into two main parts, a sequential unit and a parallel processor.

3.1 The sequential unit of PROPAL 2 is used as a 16 bit-microprogrammed minicomputer and controls the parallel processor.

The basic structure of the sequential unit of PROPAL 2 includes :

- an arithmetic and logic unit
- 32 general purpose registers
- two accumulators
- one input buffer.

This unit can handle a system of interrupts, a suspension at the micro-level and one-level submicroroutines.

The sequential unit is microprogrammed and microprogrammable and has a cycle from 100 ns to 250 ns.

3.2 The parallel processor is made of processing elements (PE) whose number may be chosen between 128 and 2048 (see figure 2).

A PE (figure 3) is a bit serial processor, i.e. it works sequentially bit by bit ; is composed of a memory, an ALU, and a slice of the "lift register" ("ascenseur" ®).

The memory has a two level hierarchy :

M1 : a working memory of 256 bits of high access speed (35 ns) ;

M2 : a storage memory of 16K bits of low access speed (450 ns).

The ALU is a serial unit which can do boolean operations, fast addition with automatic carry, fast multiplication on two variables and conditional shift. It is made of fast boolean operator, a fast serial parallel multiplier and a fast adder. Associated with that ALU, there is a special Tag (D-Tag) which can be considered either as a true accumulator or as an activity flag.

The "lift register" is a system made of 16 bits/PE. It can be used :

- as a two address register (read and write)
- as a highway of interconnection between PEs (see figure 4).

It can be seen as a vertical bidirectional shift register of 1 or 16 bits of width, able to shift data of 1 or 16 bits from one PE to the next one in 50 ns or in 150 ns, depending on the clock used for this purpose (external or internal clock). The "lift register" can be recirculated or loaded with input data, coming from the microprocessor or from a peripheral.

The solution of the "lift register" is the best economical choice for PE interconnections (mainly due to the fact that it takes only one micro-instruction to transfer 16 bits from one PE to its neighbour).

4. MICROPROGRAMMING PROPAL 2

The microprogramming of PROPAL 2 has only one level, thus enabling it to work at great speed. The time required for each micro-instruction depends on its nature : 100 ns to load the accumulator, 200 ns for a test or for a conditional branch, 250 ns in case of tests and conditional branching when associated with the loading of a register .

All the micro-instructions associated with the parallel processor require at least 150 ns.

The micro-instruction of PROPAL 2 has two different fields of 48 bits :

- . the control unit field ;
- . the parallel processor field.

The whole system sequence is generated by the control unit field ; thus that field is always necessary. The mapping of the microprogram control memory is of 2K words of 48 bits for the control unit and 2K words of 96 bits for the control unit and the parallel processor. These fields are divided into 9 subfields for the Control Unit and 12 for the parallel processor.

To make microprogramming easier, different software aids are available a micro assembler, a micro implantor and a micro simulator.

5. INSTRUCTION SET

The user may use a programming language which is an overset of the MITRA SEMS assembler

The control unit emulates the MITRA 15 code for the sequential functions. The special parallel functions are defined by a user code in this assembler.

Thus, PROPAL 2 is directly imbedded in the MITRA system by way of its assembly language, but it is also interfaced with available high-level languages such as FORTRAN callable subroutines.

Parallel function may be divided into four main categories :

- . function between values contained in two zones
- . function between a common value and a zone
- . shift functions
- . I/O functions.

The first two types of macro-instructions can perform :

- . boolean operations
- . arithmetic operations
- . semantic operations (max, min, greater than ...).

The other types are :

- . shift and recirculation of a zone, upward and downward of one or many positions ;
- . input/output by a shift function with the reading and the writing of data in the memory of the sequential unit, etc.

We define a "zone" as a block of data containing a number of NB bits (with NB $\in$ [1, 256]) for each PE. The address of the Lowest Bit is the same for each PE.

We define "common values" as data of NB bits which can be applied to every PE. Those data are contained in the sequential unit program memory.

6. PACKAGING OF PROPAL 2

The basic configuration (128 PEs) consists of only one rack with a maximum of 33 printed boards :

- 1 for the control unit
- 1 for the micro-control memory
- 2 for the communication with the host computer
- 2 for the interface cards necessary for PROPAL itself (between the CU and the PEs)
- 16 for the PE boards.

Each PE board is composed of 8 complete PEs, with their memories (256 bits of fast bipolar memory, and 4K or 16K bits of MOS memory), with their "lift register" and input output circuits. The technology used is Skottky and Low Power Skottky TTL. The size of the board is 280 – 400 mm.

7. AN IMAGE PARALLEL PROCESSING TECHNIQUE : CHROMOSOME "SKELETONIZATION" [3 à 8]

We shall see now an application of PROPAL 2 that exemplifies the power of this computer :

The average human nucleated cell contains 23 pairs of chromosomes. Chromosome skeletonization is used in analyzing deviations from the normal structure.

A chromosome consists of two identical chromatids, which are usually parallel, formed at a visible structure known as the centromere.

Through staining during the metaphase of mitosis, we can measure the discriminant features of the chromosomes which are the length of the chromatids and the position of the centromere.

From a 50 line X 50 column binarized photo using PROPAL 2 we can operate simultaneously on the whole image.

Let us consider the algorithm :

We use a two step-iterative method, one step for the horizontal direction and the second one for the vertical direction.

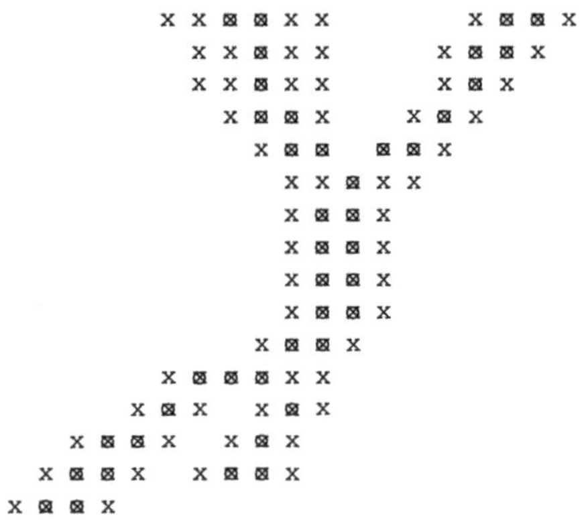

```
          x x ⊠ ⊠ x x         x ⊠ ⊠ x
            x x ⊠ x x       x ⊠ ⊠ x
            x x ⊠ x x       x ⊠ x
              x ⊠ ⊠ x     x ⊠ x
                x ⊠ ⊠   ⊠ ⊠ x
                  x x ⊠ x x
                  x ⊠ ⊠ x
                  x ⊠ ⊠ x
                  x ⊠ ⊠ x
                  x ⊠ ⊠ x
                x ⊠ ⊠ x
          x ⊠ ⊠ ⊠ x x
        x ⊠ x   x ⊠ x
    x ⊠ ⊠ x   x ⊠ x
  x ⊠ ⊠ x   x ⊠ ⊠ x
x ⊠ ⊠ x
```

Figure 10 - Chromosome skeletonization

x : raw chromosome
⊠ : skeleton

Let us describe the horizontal step procedure :

1 - Save horizontal bands which only have one pixel thickness (*) ;

2 - Save vertical bands which have one pixel width (*) ;

3 - Outline erasing, i.e. erase pixels whose left and right neighbours are different ;

4 - Continuity problems, i.e. do not erase outline pixels which are the neighbour of another outline pixel from another subset ;

5 - Restore the saved pixels in the residual picture ;

6 - Stop computing if the new picture duplicates the previous one.

In the figure 10, we see both the original chromosome picture and the skeleton.

Each step of this process is computed on this picture in 4 ms by PROPAL 2.

Results

For a 50 x 50 image we have a performance ratio equal to 125 between the parallel algorithm on a 64 PE-PROPAL 2 and the sequential algorithm on a SEMS MITRA 15-35.

The reason for this difference in execution time comes from the fact that in a sequential algorithm the image is processed point by point. On the contrary in PROPAL 2 each line is computed simultaneously on a variable length bit field ("Zone").

8. SUMMARY

Picture processing needs :

- very fast processing
- storage of a great amount of data
- true interactivity
- versatility
- programmability.

One answer is to use SIMD type of parallel processors because SIMD is a convenient trade-off between power and cost. PROPAL 2 works on serial elementary processors with words of variable length which is especially suited to picture processing. Computing power now permits a true interactivity. A better share of the work to be done is then possible : tedious computing is done by the computer, intelligent decisions and evaluations are done by man.

Programmable computers in this fast developping domain of picture processing, where specifications vary rapidly, compete very well with dedicated hardware.

(*) Necessary because the skeleton is an outline set.

REFERENCES

1. G.H. Barnes & Al., "The Illiac IV Computer", IEEE T. Computer, Vol. C-17 August 1968, 746-757.

2. C. Timsit, "The PROPAL II Computer", Proceedings of the 1978 International Conference on Parallel Processing, IEEE Catalog n° 78CH1321.9C.

3. A. Rosenfeld, Joan S. Weszka, "Picture Recognition and Scene Analysis", Computer, May 1976, V9N5.

4. R.P. Bishop, I.T. Young, "The Automated Classification of Mitotic Phase for Human Chromosome Spreads", The Journal of Histochemistry and Cytochemistry, Vol. 25, n° 7, 1977, 730-740.

5. P. Marthon, A. Bruel, G. Biguet, "Squelettisation par calcul d'une fonction discriminante sur un voisinage de 8 points", 2è Congrès AFCET-INRIA Reconnaissance des formes et intelligence artificielle, Toulouse, 1979, 107-114.

6. J. Piper, E. Granum, D. Rutovitz, H. Ruttledge, "Automation of Chromosome Analysis", 2è Congrès AFCET-IRIA, Reconnaissance des formes et intelligences artificielle, Toulouse, 1979.

7. R.J.P. Le Gô, "Image-processing automation for chromosome analysis", In : Mutagen induced chromosome damage in man, Edinburg, July 1977, (Evans, H.J., Lloyd, D.C.) Edinburg, University Press 1978, 322-325.

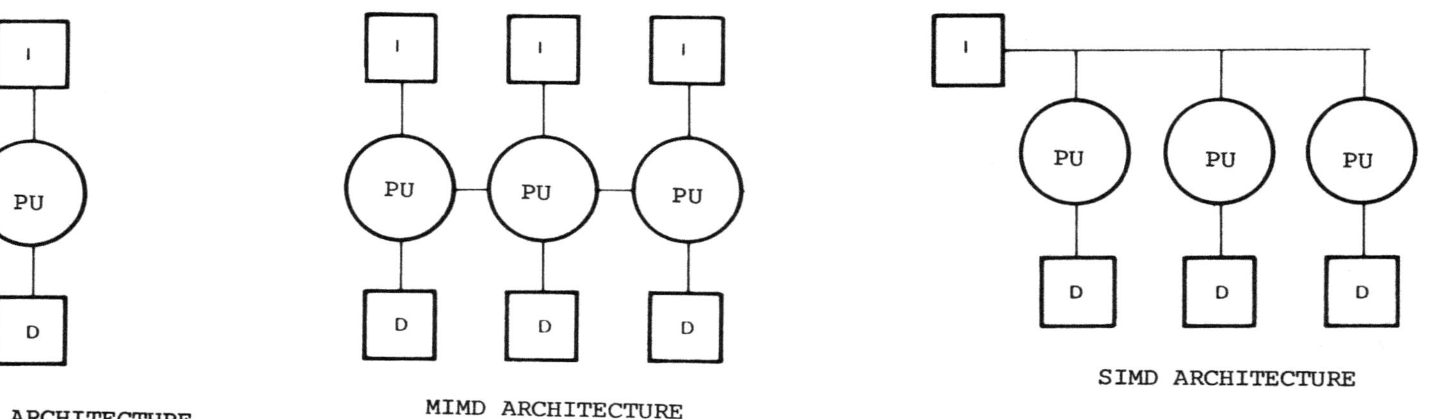

Figure 1 - Main computer architectures

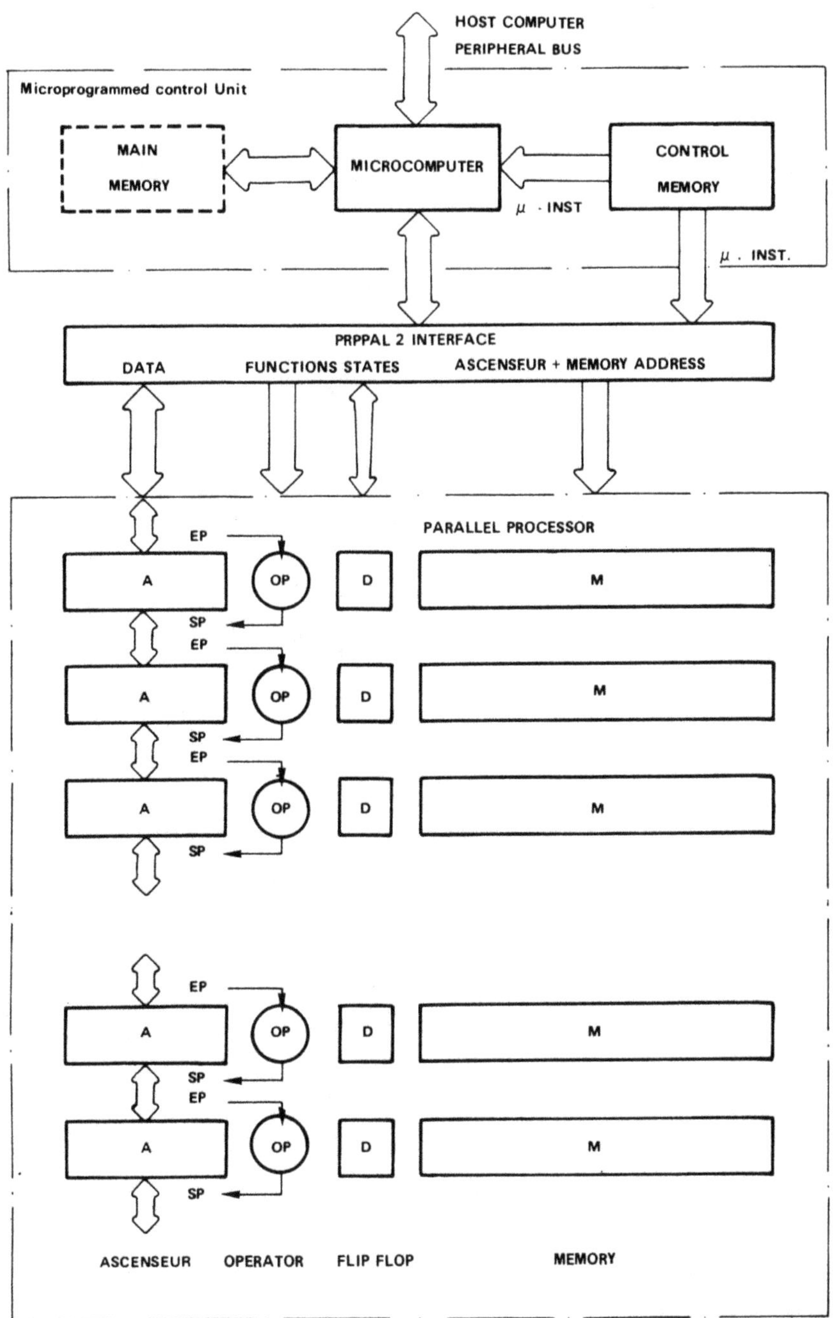

Figure 2 - Basic PROPAL 2 structure

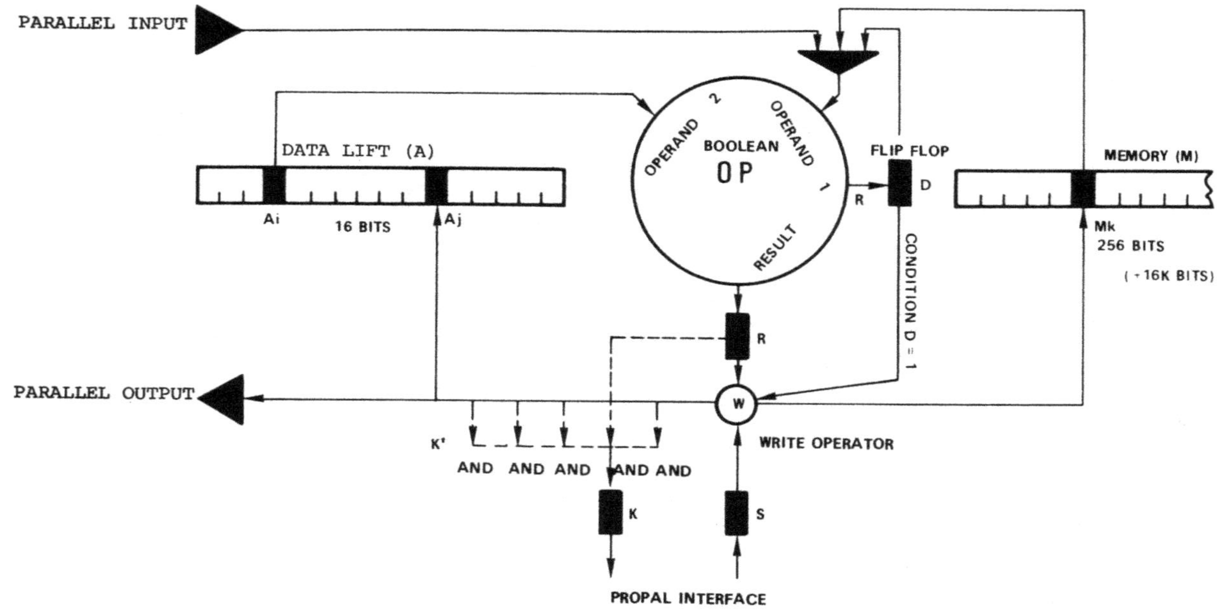

Figure 3 - Elementary functions

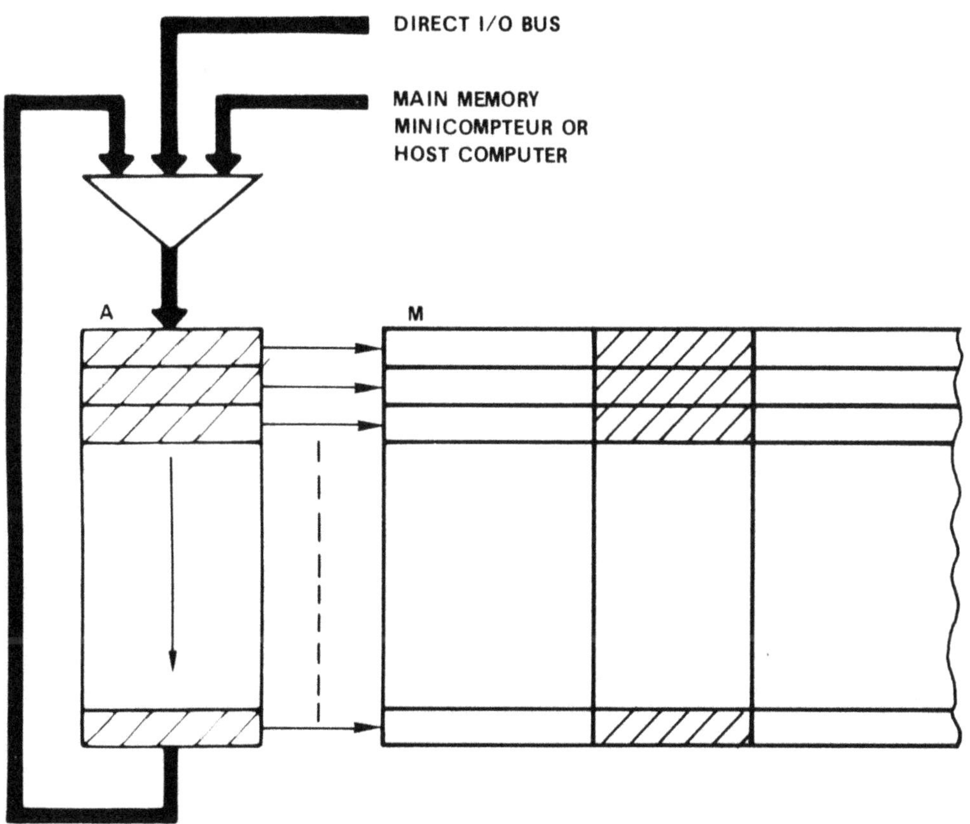

Figure 4 - Use of "Ascenseur" for data lift and loop input/output

LIST OF PARTICIPANTS

United States

Dr. Ruzena Bajcsy
The Moore School of Electrical Engineering
University of Pennsylvania
200 South 33rd Street
Philadelphia, Pennsylvania 19104

Dr. B. Greg Brown
Cardiology Section
Wadsworth Veterans Hospital
Wilshire and Sawtelle Boulevards
Los Angeles, California 90073

* Norman Caplan, Director
Division of Electrical, Computer, and Systems Engineering
National Science Foundation
1800 G. Street
Washington, D. C. 20550

Dr. K. R. Castleman
Jet Propulsion Laboratory
California Institute of Technology
Pasadena, California 91103

Dr. R. C. Eggleton
School of Medicine Indiana University
1219 West Michigan
Indianapolis, Indiana 46202

Dr. Barry K. Gilbert
Biodynamics Research Unit
Department of Physiology and Biophysics
Mayo Foundation
Rochester, Minnesota 55901

Dr. Steven Johnson
Department of Bioengineering
University of Utah
Salt Lake City, Utah 84112

Dr. Leopold G. Koss
Montefiore Hospital and Medical Center, 111, East 210th Street
Bronx, New York 10467

Dr. Charles A. Mistretta
Clinical Sciences Center
Department of Radiology E 3/316
University of Wisconsin
Madison, Wisconsin 53711

Dr. Orhan Nalcioglu
Department of Radiological Scienc
University of California
Irvine, California 92717

Dr. Judith Prewitt
Division of Computer Research and Technology N.I.H. Building 12
Room 2053
Bethesda, Maryland 20205

Dr. Jack Sklansky
School of Engineering
University of California
Irvine, California 92717

Dr. Stanley Sternberg
Environment Research Inst. of Michigan, P.O. Box 8618
Ann Arbor, Michigan 48107

Dr. M. M. Ter Pogossian
School of Medicine
Washington University
St. Louis, Missouri 63110

Dr. Robert C. Waag
Box 648, Diagnostic Radiology
University of Rochester Medical Center
Rochester, New York 14627

** Dr. H. S. Stiehl
Technische Universitat Berlin
Fachbereich 20
Informatik Forschungsgruppe
1 Berlin 10 Einsteinufer 35-37

* Observer from United States
** Observer from Germany

LIST OF PARTICIPANTS (continued)

M. Alain Lansiart
2, rue de la Source Perdue
91190 GIF SUR YVETTE

Dr. RJP Le Go
Dept. de Protection
SRPE But 05
92260 Fontenay Aux Roses

M. Fernand Meyer
Centre de Morphologie Maths
35, rue St. Honore
77305 Fontainebleau

M. Fernand Meyer
Centre de Morphologie Moths
35, rue St. Honore
77305 Fontainebleau

** Dr. Ploem
Silvius Laboratories
P.O. Box 722
Leiden 2405 PAYS BAS THE NETHERLANDS

Dr. Leandre Pourcelot
Faculte de Medecine
Labo de Biophysique
37032 Tours Cedex

M. Jacques Richalet
ADERSA/GERBIOS
2, Av. du 1er Mai
91120 Palaiseau

M. Patrice Roux
Adersa/Gerbios
2, Av. du 1er Moi
91120 Palaiseau

M. Jean Serra
Centre de Morphologie Math
35, rue St. Honore
77305 Fontainebleau

M. E. Tournier
Leti-ceng
85 X
38041 Grenoble Cedex

Mme F. Veillon
IMAG
53 X
38041 Grenoble Cedex

** Observer from The Netherlands

Dr. Jean Pierre Marc Vergnes
Inserm Fr 40
Service Neurologie Chu Purpan
31052 Toulouse Cedex

Mme V. Von Hagen
Labo de Microscopie quantitative
74, rue Marcel Cachin
93000 Bobigny

M. Wendel
Institut de Physique
3, rue de L'Universite
67084 Strasbourg Cedex

www.ingramcontent.com/pod-product-compliance
Ingram Content Group UK Ltd.
Pitfield, Milton Keynes, MK11 3LW, UK
UKHW061656190726
13853UKWH00008B/2232

* 9 7 8 3 6 4 2 9 3 2 1 9 9 *